Traumatic Brain Injury: Associated Speech, Language and Swallowing Disorders

Neurogenic Communication Disorders Series

SERIES EDITOR
Leonard L. LaPointe, Ph. D.

Developmental Motor Speech Disorders
Michael A. Crary

Cognitive-Communicative Abilities Following Brain Injury: A Functional Approach
Leila L. Hartley

Pediatric Traumatic Brain Injury: Proactive Intervention
Jean L. Blosser and Roberta DePompei

Mild Traumatic Brain Injury: A Therapy and Resource Manual
Betsy S. Green, Kristin M. Stevens, and Tracey D. W. Wolde

Linguistic Levels in Aphasia
Evy Visch-Brink and Roelien Bastiaanse

Traumatic Brain Injury: Associated Speech, Language and Swallowing Disorders
Bruce E. Murdoch and Deborah G. Theodoros

Traumatic Brain Injury: Associated Speech, Language and Swallowing Disorders

Bruce E. Murdoch, Ph.D.
Professor and Head
Department of Speech Pathology and Audiology
The University of Queensland
Australia

Deborah G. Theodoros, Ph.D.
Senior Lecturer in Speech Pathology
Department of Speech Pathology and Audiology
The University of Queensland
Australia

SINGULAR
™
THOMSON LEARNING

SINGULAR

™

THOMSON LEARNING

NOTICE TO THE READER

Singular Staff:

Business Unit Director:
William Brottmiller

Acquisitions Editor:
Marie Linvill

Developmental Editor:
Kristin Banach

Editorial Assistant:
Cara Jenkins

Executive Marketing Manager:
Dawn Gerrain

Channel Manager:
Kathryn A. Bamberger

Project Editor:
Mary Ellen Cox

Production Coordinator:
John Mickelbank

Art/Design Coordinator:
Sandy Doyle

Library of Congress Cataloging-in-Publication Data

Murdoch, B.E., 1950-
Traumatic brain injury: associated speech, language, swallowing disorders/ by Bruce E. Murdoch and Deborah G. Theodoros.
p. cm.
Includes bibliographical references.
ISBN 0-7693-0017-0 (alk. paper)
1. Brain damage— Complications.
2. Deglutition disorders.
3. Speech disorders.
4. Language disorders.
I. Theodoros, Deborah G.
II. Title.

RC387.5 .M87 2001
616.8'047—dc21
00-052371

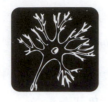

Contents

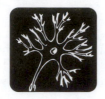

Foreword

The brain is a marvelous thing. It has been called the only human organ capable of studying itself. While the metaphoric heart has been rhapsodized in song and sonnet much more frequently, the brain and its peculiar music have met increasing attention, not only popularly, but notably from researchers, scholars, educators, and clinicians who must deal with attempts to understand it. Advances in neural imaging, digital technology, and virtual environments are increasingly helping us probe the depths of neural mystery. In this new century, we will see neuroscience become much less tainted by superstition than in previous times. Advances in understanding ourselves, particularly our neural inner selves, will require the evolution of our language as well, and prefixed terms such as neurophilosophy, neurosociology, neuroesthetics, neurodeterminism, and even neuropantheism may well work their way into our academic and clinical lexicons. Another concept, and perhaps new term that may gain favor, is neuropragmatism. The clinical science of understanding the pragmatic impact of neuropathology will continue to be bumped along by evolving knowledge of the brain and the needs of the people who suffer brain damage. Appreciation of the consequences and impact of neural impairment, and its inevitable effect on life participation and activity, is slowly creating a presence on the horizon that may well be of equal importance as the fascinating theoretic justifications of neuroscience. And there is plenty of impact, particularly when humans are visited with traumatic, diffusing, debilitating brain injury with all its life affecting consequences.

When the human nervous system goes awry, the cost is enormous. Direct and indirect economic impact of brain disorders in the United States has been estimated to be over 400 billion dollars. It is impossible to measure the toll that brain disorders extract in terms of human agony from victims and their families. Each disruption of delicate neural balance can cause problems in moving, sensing, eating, thinking, and a rich array of human behaviors. Certainly not the least of these are those unique human attributes involved in communication. To speak, to understand, to write, to read, to remember, to create, to calculate, to plan, to reason . . . and myriad other cognitive and communicative acts, are the sparks and essence of human interaction. When they are lost or impaired, isolation can result, or at the very least, quality of life can be compromised.

Traumatic brain injury (TBI) has painful penalties of its own. A majority of traumatic brain injury survivors are under the age of 30. The costs of severe brain injury often exceed 4 million dollars. A survivor of severe brain injury faces 5 to 10 years of intensive services and rehabilitation. Every five minutes, someone dies from a head injury. Every five minutes, someone becomes permanently disabled due to a head injury. Even so-called mild traumatic brain injury can cause cognitive impairments serious enough to alter a person's ability to enjoy life or be able to work and earn a living.

This book is about those many sequelae and consequences that arise from TBI that affect human cognitive and communication functions. The authors and contributors of this book are both rising stars and internationally recognized experts on human communication and cognition and its disorders. I have had first hand knowledge of these Australian professionals since experiencing a study sabbatical with them, and subsequently, two three-year terms as a visiting professor doing collaborative research and clinical teaching with them. I have watched them at work and at play. They engage in each with delight, dedication, and heartiness. The corpus of their work is evidence of the seriousness of their scholarly pursuits. This book is another prime bit of confirmation of their values of thoroughness, scholarly acumen, and impressive clinical expertise. The work represented in this book is carefully grounded in sound theory, research, and a series of objective and carefully designed studies. The meticulousness of the laboratory is never far away from the conclusions drawn in the clinic. In addition to the strong science evident in this work, the authors point to a humane side as well. The positivism expressed in the concepts and activities of rehabilitation, relearning, intervention, recovery, adjustment, acceptance, and reintegration are rewards that can be extracted from the colossal challenge of traumatic brain injury. Tragedy can be followed by recovery of improved life quality. All of this can be hastened by sound clinical science and shrewd clinical insight. Both of those qualities are amply demonstrated in this book.

Leonard L. LaPointe, Ph.D.
Francis Eppes Professor of Communication Disorders
Florida State University
Tallahassee, FL
and
Editor-in-Chief, *Journal of Medical Speech-Language Pathology*

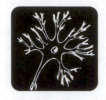

Preface

John, a 20-year-old male, sustained a severe traumatic brain injury (TBI) in a motor vehicle accident. As a result of the diffuse brain damage sustained in the accident, John now exhibits a range of long-term neurological deficits which include physical impairments as well as cognitive, communicative and swallowing disabilities. Collectively, these impairments have reduced John's quality-of-life and have prevented his return to work and study, leading to financial difficulty. In addition, the presence of communicative impairments in the form of motor speech and language disorders have impaired his ability to interact with other people, including his family and friends, leading to John's social isolation. The presence of a swallowing disorder has also necessitated John being placed on a swallowing program by his speech-language pathologist.

The range of disabilities exhibited by John is typical of those seen in people who experience brain damage as a result of severe head trauma. Unfortunately, it is only in recent years that the importance of communication and swallowing abilities, to the long-term quality-of-life survivors of TBI, has begun to be recognized. In past years the perceived importance of speech, language and swallowing disorders, following TBI, to various health professionals, has been diminished by a range of factors including: A lack of appropriate terminology to adequately describe the disorders; a lack of quantifiable research data regarding the nature of speech, language and swallowing disorders post-TBI; and the perception that communication disorders were of secondary importance to the medical management of people with TBI. Given the increasing prevalence of TBI world-wide, and the serious economic and social consequences of associated communication and swallowing disorders, it is time that the neglect of these sequelae seen in past years be swept aside, and attention focused on the development of effective and long-lasting programs for the treatment of these disorders. As an initial step to the development of these programs, there has been a need for research to properly define the basis and nature of these communication problems as a platform for the development of appropriate treatment goals. To this end, this book provides the reader with a synthesis of our current understanding of the neuropathophysiology and nature of communication and swallowing disorders exhibited by persons with TBI. Chapters dedicated to description and discussion of the various treatments available for each of these disorders are also included.

Finally, the editors wish to thank John and the numerous other individuals with TBI who, despite their disabilities, made themselves available to participate in the various research projects described in this book. If survivors of TBI like John are to enjoy a high quality of life then they need and deserve functional communication and swallowing skills. It is our sincere hope that the publication of this book will be one step towards achieving this goal.

Bruce E. Murdoch
Deborah G. Theodoros

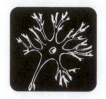

Contributors

Justine Goozée
Department of Speech Pathology and Audiology
The University of Queensland
Queensland, Australia

Fiona Hinchliffe
Department of Speech Pathology and Audiology
The University of Queensland
Queensland, Australia

Angela C. Morgan
Department of Speech Pathology and Audiology
The University of Queensland
Queensland, Australia

Bruce E. Murdoch
Department of Speech Pathology and Audiology
The University of Queensland
Queensland, Australia

Deborah Theodoros
Department of Speech Pathology and Audiology
The University of Queensland
Queensland, Australia

Elizabeth T. Ward
Department of Speech Pathology and Audiology
The University of Queensland
Queensland, Australia

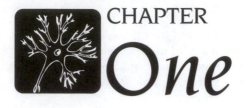

CHAPTER
One

Introduction: Epidemiology, Neuropathophysiology, and Medical Aspects of Traumatic Brain Injury

Bruce E. Murdoch and Deborah G. Theodoros

Introduction

Traumatic brain injury (TBI) has been defined as "an insult to the brain, not of the degenerative or congenital nature, but caused by an external force, that may produce a diminished or altered state of consciousness" (National Head Injury Foundation, 1985). According to this definition, TBI occurs only in those cases where the brain damage is caused by an external force and thereby excludes brain insult resulting from other neurological conditions such as cerebrovascular accidents, tumors, degenerative brain diseases (e.g., Parkinson disease), demyelinating conditions (e.g., multiple sclerosis) and infectious disorders (e.g., encephalitis). TBI, therefore, is the consequence of a head injury in which the severity has been of sufficient magnitude to cause damage to the brain. Head injuries incurred in road traffic accidents, falls, sporting and industrial accidents, or assaults are the most frequent causes of TBI in peacetime.

Communication impairments in the form of speech and/or language disorders are commonly reported sequelae of TBI. When present, these impairments have important negative implications for the long-term quality of life of survivors of TBI. Some authors have suggested that communication abilities may play the pivotal role in determining the quality of survival after head trauma (Najenson, Sazbon, Fiselzon, Becker, & Schechter, 1978). Certainly the presence of a communication disorder reduces the individual's ability to function in situations that require normal receptive and expressive language abilities as well as understandable, efficient, and natural sounding speech (e.g., vocational positions that require independent interaction with the public, etc.). Put simply, the presence of a communication disorder in an adult following TBI may impede the successful return of the individual to study, work, or general social activities, leading to academic failure, loss of vocational standing and social isolation. In the case of a child, following TBI, a communication disorder may affect the developmental process of the individual, leading to impairment of the further acquisition of speech, language, and social skills. The increasing recognition of the potentially devastating effects of communication disorders on the quality of life of TBI survivors has, in recent years, alerted clinicians to the need for the development of new and more effective treatments for these disorders. Likewise, this increased awareness has, over the past two decades, given impetus to increased levels of research aimed at increasing our understanding of speech and language disorders occurring subsequent to TBI. Following the heightened awareness of the potentially devastating effects of communication disorders on individuals with TBI, speech-language pathologists have also, in recent times, become increasingly aware of the high incidence of swallowing impairment (dysphagia) in the TBI population and the subsequent need to develop swallowing programs in their clinical settings. The aim of this book is to provide a synthesis of current knowledge relating to communication and swallowing disorders associated with TBI in children and adults and a rationale and strategies for the assessment and treatment of these disorders.

The communication and swallowing impairments that occur in association with TBI are both complex and heterogeneous in nature. In order to understand the diversity of the communication disorders observed in survivors of TBI and to fully comprehend the various assessment and treatment procedures described later in this book, an understanding of the basic mechanisms of head injury is required. This chapter reviews the epidemiology, etiology, neuropathophysiology, and medical aspects of TBI and provides a basic introduction to the associated communication and swallowing disorders. Subsequent chapters of the current book are devoted to detailed analyses of the various speech, language, and swallowing impairments seen in TBI, together with a description of appropriate assessment and treatment strategies.

Classification of TBI

Brain injuries arising from head trauma are generally classified into two broad types: nonpenetrating (closed) injuries and penetrating (open) brain injuries. In nonpenetrating injuries, the membranes (meninges) covering the brain remain intact, even though the skull may be fractured. Penetrating, or open, brain injuries, on the other hand, occur when the coverings of the brain are ruptured as a result of tearing of the dura mater by skull fragments, as may occur in depressed fractures of the skull, or when the brain is penetrated by some missile such as a bullet or is lacerated by a depressed bone fragment(s).

Nonpenetrating brain injuries tend to be associated with diffuse brain pathology and represent by far the majority of traumatic head injuries incurred in civilian life. In contrast, penetrating head trauma tends to be associated with more focal brain pathology, although diffuse effects also can be observed, and is more common in wartime. Historically, much of what we know about the effects of TBI on speech and language function has come from studies of patients who have sustained penetrating missile wounds in wartime (Luria, 1970; Russell & Espir, 1961). In more recent years, however, emphasis has shifted to research into communication disorders exhibited by patients with TBI injuries of the nonpenetrating, or closed, type. Given that clients with this latter type of TBI constitute the majority of communication-impaired TBI individuals referred to speech-language clinics, speech and language disorders associated with closed head injuries will be the primary focus of the chapters appearing later in the current book. Consistent with this focus, the term "TBI," when used throughout the subsequent chapters, will refer to traumatic brain injury caused by closed head injuries. It should also be noted that because of its widespread use in the TBI literature, the term "head injury" is on occasion used interchangeably with TBI in subsequent chapters.

TBI is also classified according to the level of severity, based on the level of altered consciousness experienced by the patient following the trauma. Altered consciousness levels posttrauma may vary from transient disorientation at one extreme to a deep coma at the other. A patient can be classified as having a mild, moderate, or severe TBI, according to where their level of consciousness fits on this continuum. To date, however, medical professionals have not been able to agree on the measure of altered consciousness to be used in assigning severity levels to TBI. The most commonly used scale, the Glasgow Coma Scale (GCS), (see Table 1-1) was developed by Teasdale and Jennett (1974, 1976) and involves estimation of the depth of coma as a measure of severity within the first 24 hours of the trauma. The patient is assigned a score of between 3 and 15 on the GCS, with points being assigned in the categories of eye opening (ranging from 4 points for spontaneous eye opening to 1 point for no response), best motor response (from 6 points for obeying commands to 1 point for no response), and best verbal response (from 5 points for oriented to 1 point for no response). The greater the score on the GCS, the more conscious the patient, with a total score of 13–15 representing mild TBI, a score of 9–12 indicating a moderate TBI, and a score of 8 or less indicating a severe TBI. As an alternative to the GCS, the severity of TBI is estimated by some medical personnel on the basis of the duration of posttraumatic amnesia

Table 1-1. Glasgow Coma Scale

Eye Openings	Best Verbal Response	Best Motor Response
4. Spontaneous	5. Orientated	6. Responds to verbal commands
3. Nonspecific reaction to speech	4. Confusion, disorientation	5. Localized movement to terminate painful stimulus
2. Response to painful stimulus	3. No sustained or coherent conversation	4. Withdrawal from painful stimulus
1. No response	2. No recognizable words	3. Decorticate posture
	1. No response	2. Decerebrate posture
		1. No response

(Adapted from Teasdale & Jennett, 1974).

(PTA) (Russell, 1932). PTA represents the period from the time the patient regains consciousness but is still in a disoriented and confused state and until the time the patient's memory for ongoing events becomes reliable and accurate. According to the PTA classification system devised by Russell (1932), a mild TBI is one in which the period of coma plus subsequent PTA is less than 1 hour, a moderate TBI involves a period of coma and PTA of 1–24 hours duration, a severe TBI involves a period of coma and PTA of 1–7 days, and a very severe TBI involves a period of coma and PTA extending greater than 7 days.

Epidemiology of TBI

The majority of reports in the literature indicate that the annual incidence of head injury in Western countries is around 200/100,000 population, with the highest incidence occurring in the 15–24-year-old age group (Kraus et al., 1984; Kraus, 1995; Naugle, 1990). Males by far outnumber females, at a ratio of approximately 2–2.5:1. A high male/female ratio of 3–4:1 has been noted during mid-adolescence to early adulthood (Klauber, Barrett-Connor, Marshall, & Bowers, 1981). Fortunately, it has been estimated that in the majority (82%) of head injury cases, the associated brain damage is either mild or nonexistent (Kraus et al., 1984), with the annual incidence of moderate or severe TBI being between 12-14/100,000 and 15-20/100,000 population respectively (Kraus et al., 1984; Tate, McDonald, & Lulham, 1998).

Overall, motor vehicle accidents are by far the most common cause of TBI, accounting for approximately 50% of all head injuries (Naugle, 1990). This is particularly true for the peak incidence age group (i.e., young males 15–24 years of age). Evidence is available, however, to indicate that the predominant cause of TBI varies with the age of the victims. At one extreme of the age span, child abuse and falls are the most common cause of TBI in preschool children (Gjerris, 1986) while at the other extreme, falls are a common cause of TBI in the elderly (aged 75 years and over). Home accidents, including falls, have been reported to be the most common cause of TBI in children aged less than 5 years; motor vehicle accidents in children

5–9 years; and sporting accidents, road traffic accidents, and falls in children 10–14 years of age. It is noteworthy that the type of road traffic accidents experienced by children differ from those of adolescents and adults. Whereas this latter group are primarily involved in high-velocity motor vehicle accidents as drivers, children less than 2 years of age are almost exclusively injured as occupants of motor vehicles, while older children are primarily injured as pedestrians or cyclists. Despite the fact that motor vehicle accidents may not be the most common cause of head injuries in children, reports are available to suggest that traffic accidents may be the cause of most of the long-term morbidity and nearly all of the mortality in the pediatric population. In fact, it appears that, in all age groups—including both adults and children, the most common cause of head injury associated with acute neurologic injury is a motor vehicle accident (Vernon-Levett, 1991).

Biomechanics of Head Injury

The often-devastating neurological deficits, including communication disorders, frequently associated with TBI are the result of complex biomechanical processes associated with a head injury. In order to understand the neuropathophysiological basis of these deficits, it is necessary to understand the basic mechanical forces involved in causing brain damage subsequent to closed head trauma. Briefly, the biomechanical forces involved in closed head injury include compression, acceleration-deceleration, and rotational acceleration, which result in brain tissue being compressed, torn apart by the effects of tension and sheared by rotational forces (Murdoch, 1990).

According to Gennarelli (1993), the application of force to the head results in mechanical loading, which sets off a cascade of physiological events. Mechanical loading can be initiated by either static or dynamic forces. Static loading results from slow or rapid forces applied to a stationary head so that it is crushed (e.g., compression of the head). The more common type of head injury, however, occurs following dynamic loading. This results from a very brief insult, which has either been applied directly to the moveable head (impact) or by impact elsewhere on the body causing a sudden movement of the head (impulsive; e.g., whiplash injury sustained in rear-end motor vehicle collisions). Thus a significant TBI can occur without the victim sustaining a direct blow to the head (Jennett, 1986).

Dynamic loading produces two main mechanical phenomena responsible for pathological changes in closed head injury—contact and inertial loading (acceleration) (Gennarelli, 1993; Katz, 1992; Ommaya & Gennarelli, 1974). Contact loading is a direct result of an impact to the head and leads to local skull distortions or fractures, and contusions or laceration of the brain at the point of contact (i.e., coup contusions). The propagation of shock waves throughout the skull and brain can also occur and may result in small intracerebral hemorrhages in certain vulnerable areas.

Inertial loading, or acceleration, results from head motion generated by either impact or impulsive forces. This event results in translational or rotational acceleration (Gennarelli, 1993; Pang, 1985). *Translational acceleration* occurs when all parts of the body are similarly accelerated, and there is no resultant relative movement taking place among the constituent parts of the brain (Pang, 1985). There is, however, differential movement between the brain and the skull, during which the cortex may repeatedly impact against the sharp internal structures of the skull. The predominant injuries resulting from this mechanism are brain contusions, which occur directly opposite the point of impact (i.e., contrecoup contusions).

Rotational acceleration occurs when the head receives a force that does not pass through its center of gravity. This results in the head assuming an angular acceleration and rotating around its own center of gravity. Such acceleration of the head results in a twisting motion between the brain and the skull and causes shear-strain or distortion of the brain tissue (Bigler, 1990; Pang, 1985). Such distortion of the brain tissue results in the permanent stretching or rupturing of neuronal fibers that interconnect different brain regions. The resultant damage is referred to as diffuse axonal injury (DAI) and is widely distributed, with most lesions occurring in deep white matter areas of the cerebral hemispheres and in the brainstem (Bigler, 1990).

The biomechanics of closed head injury are largely determined by the physical and structural properties of the skull and contents (Holbourn, 1943). The brain is a relatively mobile mass of material within a rigid container (Gurdjian & Gurdjian, 1975; Holbourn, 1943). Holbourn (1943) considered the most important physical properties of the brain to be its comparatively uniform density, its extreme incompressibility, its small resistance to change in shape, and its high susceptibility to shear-strain damage. During rotational acceleration of the head, the brain does not compress but readily changes shape, or distorts, in an attempt to follow the motion of the skull as it rotates about the brain, resulting in shear-strain damage to the brain tissue. Holbourn (1943) described shear-strain distortion as the "type of deformation which occurs in a pack of cards when it is deformed from a neat rectangular pile into an oblique-angled pile" (p. 438). He expounded the view that, following impacts that cause rotational acceleration of the head, shearing distortion takes place in all parts of the brain as it tries to follow the motion of the skull.

At the time of impact, as a result of external forces, the brain moves within the skull, making contact with its rigid walls, with the greatest degree of contact occurring between the soft frontal and temporal lobes and the bony prominences of the skull (e.g., sphenoidal ridge). Consequently, the skull-brain interface also has an important influence on the mechanics of head injury, particularly in relation to sites of lesion (Bigler, 1990). Anatomically, the skull is a spherical vault, with its anterior and middle cranial fossae having rough and irregular bases. The sharp, lesser wing of the sphenoid bone intervenes between these two fossae. The anterior ventral aspect of both frontal lobes of the brain is separated by a bony protuberance of the ethmoid bone, called the crista galli. In adults, the surfaces of the skull in the regions of both the lesser wing of the sphenoid bone and the ethmoid bone are jagged and rough. Many authors view these structures as being directly responsible for the "bruising" of surrounding brain tissues following a closed head injury (Adams, 1975; Bigler, 1990; Ommaya & Gennarelli, 1974). Holbourn (1943) suggested that the anatomical structures in these areas allow the skull to get a good "grip" on the brain, during rotational acceleration.

Differences in the physical and structural properties of children's heads and adult heads have been implicated as at least part of the explanation for the better prognosis for recovery from TBI reported to occur in children as compared to adults

(Levin, Ewing-Cobbs, & Benton, 1983). These latter authors attributed the greater capacity of young children to survive severe closed head injury, as compared with adults, to anatomical and physical features of head injury that differ between the two populations. Jellinger (1983) also suggested that the morphology of cranial injuries in infancy and childhood is different from that in adults. As indicated earlier, according to Holbourn (1943), the type of brain damage that results from a severe head injury depends on the physical properties of the individual's brain and skull. These physical properties are known to differ in a number of ways between children and adults, thereby contributing to different patterns of brain injury following head trauma in each group (Lindenberg & Freytag, 1969). First, an infant's brain weight at birth is 15% of body weight, progressing to only 3% of body weight in adults (Friede, 1973). By the end of the second year of life, brain weight is 75% of the adult brain weight and reaches 90% of adult brain weight by the end of the sixth year (Jellinger, 1983). Second, the existence of unfused sutures and open fontanelles makes the skull of an infant and young child more pliable. Some authors have suggested that, because of its elasticity and greater degree of deformation, the skull of an infant absorbs the energy of the physical impact and thereby protects the brain better than the skull of an adult (Craft, 1972; Menkes & Till, 1995). Other authors, however, believe that the greater pliability of the heads of infants makes them more susceptible to external forces than older children and adults. According to Menkes and Till (1995), although deformation of the head absorbs much of the energy of the impact, thereby reducing the effects of acceleration/deceleration, it adds to the risk of tearing blood vessels. A third anatomical difference in the skulls of children versus adults that may aid a better prognosis in the former group is that unlike adults, the floors of the middle cranial fossa and the orbital roofs in children are relatively smooth and offer little resistance to the shifting brain.

Alternately, the differences reported in the prognosis for recovery following TBI between children and adults may also be related to the different nature of the impacts causing head injury in these two groups (Hendrick, Hardwood-Nash & Hudson, 1964). As described earlier in this chapter, most childhood accidents result from child abuse, falls, or low-speed (20–40 mph) pedestrian or bicycle accidents that involve a motor vehicle. Consequently, many pediatric head injuries are associated with a lesser degree of rotational acceleration and, therefore, presumably a lesser amount of brain damage (Levin, Benton, & Grossman, 1982). Adults, on the other hand, as well as persons in their late teenage years, are more likely to sustain TBI as a result of high-speed motor vehicle accidents, which by their nature are likely to yield greater diffuse brain injury.

Neuropathophysiology of TBI

A knowledge of the neuropathophysiology of closed head injury provides a framework for predicting and understanding the resultant clinical behaviors and contributes insight into brain-behavior relationships. The principal pathologies associated with closed head injury have been categorized in various ways. Typically the divisions involve differentiating focal or diffuse lesions, as well as those that are

Table 1-2. Primary and Secondary Brain Injury After Closed Head Injury

Primary Diffuse Lesions
Diffuse axonal injury
Primary Focal Lesions
Contusions Laceration Basal ganglia hemorrhage Cranial nerve lesions
Secondary Diffuse Lesions and Effects
Cerebral edema Raised intracranial pressure Ischemia Brain shift and herniation Cerebral atrophy and ventricular enlargement
Secondary Focal lesions

Hematoma - extradural
             subdural
             intracranial

primary (immediate on impact) injuries and those that are secondary phenomena not attributable to the impact itself. There is evidence, however, that primary and secondary pathologies combine to form marked heterogeneity of injury (Levin et al., 1982; Pang, 1985). The frequent neuropathophysiological sequelae of closed head injury are summarized in Table 1-2 and discussed further below.

Primary Neuropathophysiological Effects of TBI

Primary brain damage occurs at the moment of impact and is the result of the instantaneous events caused by the blow. This damage frequently constitutes the limiting factor for ideal neurological recovery (Pang, 1985) and includes DAI, contusions, laceration, basal ganglia hemorrhage, and cranial nerve lesions.

Primary Diffuse Lesions

Diffuse cerebral injury, in the form of widespread damage to the axons in the white matter of the brain, produced at the moment of impact is widely considered to be the primary mechanism of brain damage in individuals with closed head injury, and a more important factor in determining outcome than the presence of focal lesions (Adams, Mitchell, Graham, & Doyle, 1977; Gennarelli et al., 1982; Ommaya & Gennarelli, 1974; Strich, 1956, 1961, 1969). This pathological state, also referred to as diffuse axonal injury (DAI) was first described by Strich (1956), who determined the presence of diffuse degeneration of the cerebral white matter in the absence of focal pathology in the brains of four survivors of TBI who were quadriplegic and in a profoundly demented or vegetative state. Strich (1956, 1961) concluded that the severe neurologic deficit manifest in these cases was the result of axonal damage produced by mechanical forces shearing the fibers at the moment of impact.

A number of different areas of the brain have been reported to be commonly affected by DAI subsequent to traumatic head injury, including the subcortical white matter of the cerebral hemispheres, the upper brainstem, the superior cerebellar peduncles, and the basal ganglia (Adams, Graham, Murray, & Scott, 1982; Strich, 1969). The interface between the gray and white matter is also commonly involved, due to shearing between the different tissue types. Magnetic resonance imaging (MRI) has also identified DAI in the brainstem, hippocampus, and corpus callosum, and at interfaces between the brain and dura mater (Guthrie, Mast, Richards, McQuaid, & Pavlakis, 1999).

The concept proposed by Strich (1956, 1961) that DAI is an immediate effect of a closed head injury has often been challenged. Jellinger and Seitelberger (1970), although agreeing that one etiological factor of DAI was mechanical damage to the nerve fibers suggested that vascular, edematous, and anoxic damage to the cerebral cortex and basal ganglia played a significant role in the pathogenesis of white matter changes. Adams et al. (1982), in a study involving a comparison of fatal head trauma cases with and without DAI, failed to find any significant differences between the two groups with respect to the incidence of cerebral edema or hypoxic brain damage. They concluded that DAI occurs immediately, at the time of impact, and is not secondary to any other form of brain damage. Adams et al. (1982) described DAI in terms of a triad of distinctive features: a focal lesion in the corpus callosum; a focal lesion in the dorsolateral quadrants of the rostral brainstem; and microscopic evidence of diffuse damage to axons, such as axonal retraction balls, microglial stars, and degeneration of specific fiber tracts in the white matter.

The findings of Adams et al. (1982) were supported by those of Gennarelli et al. (1982), who induced DAI in the brains of nonhuman primates by means of imparting angular acceleration. DAI identical to that known to occur in humans subsequent to traumatic head injury was produced, and three grades of severity were identified. In the most severe grade, DAI was characterized by a focal lesion in the dorsolateral quadrant of the rostral brainstem in addition to a lesion in the corpus callosum and axonal damage in the cerebral white matter. Gennarelli et al. (1982) concluded that the degree of DAI was directly related to the duration and severity of coma and the clinical outcome. These findings suggest that there exists a continuum of axonal injury, and they were later supported by Blumbergs, Jones, and North (1989) who described similar grades of DAI in humans. According to Adams, Graham, Gennarelli, and Maxwell (1991) even people who have sustained a mild head injury and are rendered unconscious for as little as five minutes after injury, have some degree of DAI.

Although DAI is still largely classed as a primary injury, that classification has been further challenged in recent years by Letarte (1999). He argues that although immediate traumatic axotomy occurs, most of the axonal disruption occurs later. According to Letarte (1999) the majority of axons that will eventually suffer damage remain in continuity immediately after injury, and that it is not until around 6 hours postinjury that the neurofilaments are destroyed and axotomy occurs (Teasdale & Graham, 1998). The model of axonal injury proposed by Letarte (1999) is different from the immediate, irreversible mechanism described by earlier researchers and implies that the deterioration in patients postinjury may be due to this progressive secondary injury, raising the possibility of developing medical strategies to intervene in this progressive degeneration of axons.

Primary Focal Lesions

A brain contusion (bruise) consists of an area of brain tissue characterized by multi-focal capillary hemorrhages, vascular engorgement, and edema. A linear impact on the skull may result in transient distortion and inbending of the bone near the point of impact, causing compression of adjacent brain tissue and bruising of the brain in an area directly below the area of impact. Such contusions, which occur at the point of impact, are termed "coup" contusions. In addition to causing lesions at this site, the impact may cause the brain to strike the skull at a point opposite to the point of trauma, thereby resulting in additional vascular disruption and bruising at this latter site. Contusions of the latter type are termed "contra-coup" contusions. Both coup and contracoup lesions may cause specific and localizable behavioral alterations that accompany closed head injury (Lezak, 1983). The symptoms produced by a brain contusion depend on the size and location of the contusion, and may include speech, language, and swallowing disorders. In that intracellular swelling of adjacent structures is frequently associated with contusions, secondary brain damage may develop, leading some authors to suggest that the clinical significance of contusions lies more in the risk of the secondary injuries caused by the mass effects than the focal damage itself (Gennarelli, 1993).

Irrespective of the point of impact, brain contusions are most often found in the orbital and lateral surfaces of the frontal and temporal lobes, which occupy the anterior and middle cranial fossae (Auerbach, 1986). The frequent presence of contusions in these sites is due to the brain abrading against the irregular and jagged skull surfaces with which it interfaces (Bigler, 1990). Similarly, the frequent occurrence of contusions on the medial surface of the hemispheres and in the corpus callosum are thought to result from the movement of the brain against the falx cerebri and the tentorium (Gurdijian & Gurdijian, 1976). Previously, contusions were considered to occur in cortical regions only; however, computerized tomographic scans have identified contusions within deep areas of the brain.

When a brain contusion is sufficiently severe to cause a visible breach in the continuity of the brain, it is referred to as a laceration. Lacerations are more typically associated with penetrating head injuries than with closed head injuries and tend to be associated with more severe and prolonged neurological sequelae than contusions.

Although intracerebral hematoma associated with closed head injury is usually considered a secondary insult or a primary complication rather than the result of immediate impact injury (Levin et al., 1982), traumatic basal ganglia hematoma has been reported to be indicative of severe primary brain damage (Coloquhoun & Rawlinson, 1989; MacPherson, Teasdale, Dhaker, Allerdyce, & Gailbraith, 1986). A distinct and relatively rare traumatic entity, traumatic basal ganglia hematoma occurs in approximately 3% of severe closed head injuries. Although it can occur in isolation or in association with other intracerebral hematomas and contusions, it is mostly found in patients who have suffered severe diffuse white matter injury (Coloquhoun & Rawlinson, 1989).

A severe closed head injury can cause the dysfunction of a variety of cranial nerves, either by damaging the cranial nerve nuclei in the brainstem or by disrupting the nerves themselves in either their intracranial or extracranial course (Murdoch, 1990). Contusions of the brainstem can damage the cranial nerve nuclei, leading to flaccid paralysis of the muscles innervated by the affected nerves.

In particular, should these affected muscles include the muscles supplied by cranial nerves V, VII, X, or XII, speech disorders may result. The most common cause of damage to the cranial nerves in their intracranial course is fracture of the base of the skull. The facial nerve (VII) is most commonly affected by this condition, leading to flaccid paralysis of the muscles of facial expression. Branches of the facial (VII) and trigeminal (V) nerves may be damaged extracranially by trauma to the face. In general, traumatic cranial nerve palsies are permanent, the exceptions being those resulting from contusions of extracranial branches of the nerves (Murdoch, 1990).

Secondary Neuropathophysiological Effects of TBI

Primary brain injury can generate a variety of secondary insults to the brain, which in turn trigger a pathophysiologic cascade of events. Secondary injury has the potential to be limited with appropriate therapeutic interventions (Gjerris, 1986) and includes cerebral edema, intracranial hemorrhage, ischemic brain damage, pathologic changes associated with increased intracranial pressure (ICP), cerebral atrophy, and ventricular enlargement.

Secondary Diffuse Lesions

According to Bigler (1990) cerebral edema, which involves an increase in brain volume due to an accumulation of excess water in the brain tissue, is "the most common secondary effect of brain injury" (p. 32). Adams, Graham, Scott, Parker, and Doyle (1980) described three types of brain swelling: localized brain swelling, which occurs around a contusion; unilateral brain swelling, which involves diffuse swelling of one cerebral hemisphere; and brain swelling, which involves diffuse swelling of both cerebral hemispheres. Edema resulting from TBI is most commonly vasogenic and results from an increase in the permeability of brain capillaries, which allows water and other solutes to exude out into the extracellular spaces within the brain tissue (Levin et al., 1982; Pang, 1985). Various neuropathological changes may occur as a result of sustained cerebral edema, including stretching and tearing of axonal fibers, compression of brain tissue resulting in cell loss, compression of blood vessels with subsequent infarction of brain tissue, and herniation of the brain (Bigler, 1990).

Elevated ICP occurs when there is an increase in one of the intracranial constituents—blood, brain, cerebrospinal fluid, or extracellular fluid—within the noncompliant skull (Pang, 1985). A sudden increase in ICP is a common finding after closed head injury, most frequently due to the development of extradural, subdural, or intracerebral hematomas or generalized cerebral swelling. Uncontrolled increases in ICP may cause herniation (a shift of part of the brain to another cranial compartment) and can also impede cerebral blood flow, resulting in ischemic brain damage (Levin et al., 1982; Murdoch, 1990; Pang, 1985). Murdoch (1990) described three types of cerebral herniation due to raised ICP following traumatic head injury: transtentorial herniation, in which the medial portions of the temporal lobes are herniated through the tentorial hiatus, due to an increase in the ICP above the level of the tentorium cerebelli; tonsillar herniation, whereby the cerebellar tonsils are displaced down through the foramen magnum; and axial herniation, which occurs when there is a downward displacement of the entire brainstem due to increased ICP.

Transtentorial herniation causes compression of the brainstem and interferes with the functioning of the reticular formation, thereby leading to a deterioration in the level of consciousness. At the same time the third cranial nerve is also compressed, causing pupillary dilation, first on the side of the herniation and later on the other side as well. Eventually, if untreated, compression of the brainstem will lead to death. The level of consciousness and the state of the pupils of the eyes are, therefore, critical factors that require monitoring following closed head injury. The only structure compressed by tonsiller herniation is the medulla, and the first sign of its presence is often respiratory insufficiency or apnea. Although no structures are actually compressed by axial herniation, distortion of the brainstem caused by its downward displacement may cause altered levels of consciousness and changes in respiration.

Ischemic brain damage is also widely recognized as a common sequelae of closed head injury (Adams et al., 1980; Graham, Adams & Doyle, 1978) and ranges from focal necrosis to wide areas of infarction. Although areas of infarction are generally related to the presence of contusions, hematomas, distortion, and herniation of the brain and raised ICP, Adams (1975) also defined a specific category of ischemic brain damage characterized by different patterns of neuronal necrosis and infarction of the brain, which was not directly associated with these factors. Graham and Adams (1971) analyzed 100 cases of closed head injury and discovered an unusually high incidence of diffuse neocortical necrosis even after known causes (e.g., cardiac arrest, status epilepticus, contusions, raised ICP, etc.) were eliminated. In a further study of 151 cases, Graham et al. (1978) confirmed a high incidence (91%) of ischemic brain damage following closed head injury. They also reported that ischemic brain damage following traumatic head injury was more frequently found in the hippocampus (81%) and basal ganglia (79%) than in the cerebral cortex (46%).

The development of cerebral atrophy and ventricular enlargement in the brain following a severe closed head injury has been frequently documented (Bigler, Kurth, Blatter, & Abildskov, 1993; Cullum & Bigler, 1986; Levin, Meyers, Grossman, & Sawer, 1981; Van Dongen & Braakman, 1980). Cullum and Bigler (1986) were able to demonstrate that the average ventricular enlargement in patients with TBI was twice that of the normal person. They also reported the associated presence of marked cortical atrophy following brain injury, which tended to occur more frequently in the frontal and temporal areas of the brain, as well as in a diffuse pattern throughout the cerebral tissue. Traumatically induced cerebral atrophy and ventricular enlargement have been found to be related to subsequent neuropsychological deficits in complex reasoning and problem solving, memory, language, intellect, and social-emotional functioning (Cullum & Bigler, 1986; Levin et al., 1982).

Secondary Focal Lesions

Intracranial hemorrhages are common complications of a closed head injury and may involve bleeding into the extradural, subdural, and subarachnoid spaces; into the ventricles; or directly into the brain tissues (Adams, 1975). Although these hemorrhages may occur immediately following impact, their effects are usually not evident until they are of sufficient volume to act as intracranial space-occupying lesions.

Extradural hematomas usually result from laceration of the middle meningeal artery by fractured bone and involve bleeding between the skull bones and the dura mater (see Figure 1-1). Hematomas of this type usually collect and enlarge fairly rapidly, and signs of ICP become evident within a short period postinjury. Typically, although the

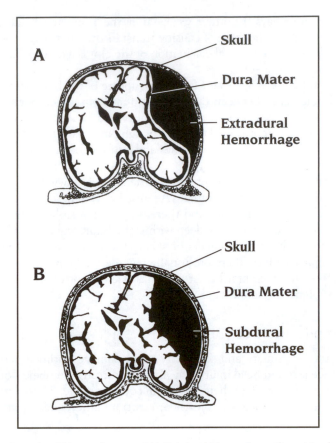

***Figure* 1-1.** a) Extradural Hemorrhage and b) Subdural Hemorrhage (from Murdoch, 1990)

patient may have been knocked unconscious at the time of head injury, consciousness is quickly recovered and then within 1–2 hours the patient becomes increasingly drowsy and develops paralysis down one side of the body as a result of compression of the ipsilateral cerbral hemisphere by the expanding hematoma. Eventually the patient demonstrates pupillary dilation and loses consciousness from compression of the third cranial nerve and brainstem, respectively, as a consequence of herniation of the temporal lobe through the tentorial hiatus. Treatment of an extradural hematoma requires an emergency operation, which involves the drilling of a burr-hole over the bruise site and the evacuation of the clot. If left untreated the patient will die as a result of compression of vital centers (e.g., respiratory centers) in the brainstem. Extradural hemorrhage has been reported to occur in approximately 10% of closed-head-injured persons (Adams et al., 1980).

Subdural hemorrhage is more common than extradural hemorrhage and is attributed to rupture of small blood vessels within the subdural space, leading to bleeding between the dura mater and arachnoid (see Figure 1-1). Adams et al. (1980) recorded an incidence of 45% of subdural hematomas in their series of head-injured subjects. Subdural hematomas develop much more slowly than extradural hematomas and, consequently, although the neurological signs and symptoms resulting from associated increased ICP are the same, they appear at a much later time, in some cases days, in others weeks after the traumatic head injury. If the hematoma develops to the stage of causing transtentorial herniation, as in the case of extradural hematoma, surgical evacuation of the clot is again required to prevent compression of the brainstem.

Subarachnoid hemorrhage occurs following rupture of the blood vessels that cross the subarachnoid space between the arachnoid and pia mater. Such hemorrhages are common occurrences after closed head injury and can be detected by the presence of blood in the cerebrospinal fluid. Although patients with subarachnoid hemorrhages may experience severe headaches and stiffness of the neck for many days, they normally recover spontaneously.

Intracerebral hemorrhages may present in the brain following closed head injury either singularly or in a multiple format (Adams, 1975). These hematomas are usually directly related to contusions and therefore occur mainly in the subfrontal or temporal regions. Those occurring deep within the brain (e.g., in the basal ganglia) are thought to be due to the effects of shear strains on the small vessels at the moment of impact and are therefore usually regarded as primary injuries. An incidence of 42% of intracerebral hematomas has been reported in a study of closed head injury subjects by Adams et al. (1980).

Other Complications of TBI

In addition to the primary and secondary brain damage outlined above, patients who experience a closed head injury may also suffer from a number of other medical complications that may affect their posttrauma quality of life. These further complications include: rhinorrhea and otorrhea; posttraumatic epilepsy; and post traumatic vertigo.

Rhinorrhea and otorrhea

These terms refer to the leakage of cerebrospinal fluid from the nose (rhinorrhea) and ear (otorrhea) subsequent to traumatic head injury. Rhinorrhea occurs following fracture of the frontal bone with associated tearing of the dura mater and arachnoid. Otorrhea, on the other hand, is caused by injuries to the base of the skull. As injuries in this latter region often damage the brainstem as well, otorrhea is of more serious prognostic importance than rhinorrhea. Infections and meningitis are potential hazards of both conditions.

Posttraumatic epilepsy and posttraumatic vertigo

Although not incapacitating, these two complications of closed head injury may have a profound effect on the lifestyle of the head-injured patient. Posttraumatic epilepsy occurs most commonly after penetrating head injuries, the epilepsy being triggered by the formation of scar tissue as a result of brain laceration. The scar may act as an irritating focus to trigger epileptic fits. In some cases, convulsions may occur very shortly after impact (within 24 hours), especially in children. When it occurs in adult head injury cases, however, the epilepsy usually develops within the first 2 years postinjury. Although more common in cases of penetrating head injuries, posttraumatic epilepsy can also occur subsequent to closed head injuries, and may be triggered by the development of subdural hematomas.

Some degree of vertigo accompanied by vomiting and unsteadiness is common after head injury. Posttraumatic vertigo may last for days or weeks or may persist in some cases for many months.

Medical Management of TBI

There are two major components to contemporary treatment of patients with TBI. These include: 1) Rapid evacuation of hematomas and control of increasing ICP; 2) prevention of hypotension and hypoxia and maintenance of cerebral perfusion pressure (CPP) (Letarte, 1999). This current approach, however, has only been implemented since the mid-1980s. It evolved as a consequence of a greater understanding of the mechanisms of cerebral edema and ischemic brain injury brought about by research at the level of cellular physiology.

Until the mid-1980s, the paradigm for treatment of patients with TBI was very much focussed on prevention of increasing ICP. There is evidence that, even from the earliest of times, an awareness existed of the special importance of brain swelling on the outcome from head injury. Archeological findings indicate that in multiple and widespread locations throughout human evolution, trephination was practiced. From the early 1900s to the mid-1950s, rapid evacuation of space-occupying lesions, and particularly hematomas, was the principal treatment for head-injured patients, with surgery being the only available treatment method. This treatment, however, was only made available to patients deemed to have space-occupying lesions and, therefore, eligible for surgery. Consequently many patients who presented as lucid initially went on to deteriorate and often die as the result of untreated space-occupying lesions. Reilly and Adams (1975) reported that many patients with lucid intervals who later died, so-called "talk-and-die" patients, had space-occupying lesions that were potentially treatable. Fortunately, a means of rapidly identifying patients with space-occupying lesions was provided by the introduction of the computerized tomographic (CT) scanner in the mid-1970s. The introduction of this technology also had the effect of intensifying the surgical focus of the treatment of patients with head injury.

Although still focused on the treatment of elevated ICP, nonsurgical therapies for treatment of TBI were introduced in the mid-1950s. The first effective nonoperative treatment for elevated ICP became available with the introduction of urea by Javid and Settlage (1956). Urea was followed by mannitol and in rapid sequence by a series of steroids. Parallel and complimentary to these developments was the description of a technique by Lundberg (1960) that allowed continuous monitoring of ICP. Consequently, by the early 1960s a means of quantifying cerebral edema, as well as methods for treating elevated ICP, was available.

The catalyst to changing the paradigm for treatment of patients with head injury from one that was ICP-centerd to one that also recognized the need to maintain cerebral perfusion was a publication by Miller and Sweet (1978) that highlighted ischemia as a significant threat to patients with head injury. This work culminated in Rosner and coworkers (Rosner, 1995; Rosner & Coley, 1986; Rosner & Daughton, 1990) defining a clinical approach to head injury that recognizes ischemia as of equal importance to edema and mass effect in terms of need for treatment.

Letarte (1999) predicted that in addition to these essential components, a third component in the form of pharmacotherapy will be added to the treatment of patients with TBI early in the new millennium. In particular, pharmacotherapy will aim to combat the neurochemical mediations of secondary injury and will be augmented by new techniques for monitoring brain function such as cerebral blood flow (e.g., Xenon CT), brain metabolism (e.g., positron emission tomography [PET]), and global cerebral oxygenation (e.g., jugular bulb monitoring), among others. Using these new techniques, clinicians will not only be able to view the structure of the injured brain but will also be able to map its blood flow and in so doing monitor the adequacy of attempts to maintain CPP. By being able to monitor the metabolism of the brain, clinicians will be able to track markers of neurologic injury and thereby better estimate the severity of the patient's injuries.

Introduction to Speech, Language, and Swallowing Disorders Subsequent to TBI

Communication impairments in the form of speech and/or language disorders are commonly reported sequelae of traumatic head injury. Archeological evidence suggests that the relationship between traumatic head injury and the occurrence of communication disorders was known to a number of ancient civilizations. Papyrus records indicate that the Egyptians were aware of the relationship as early as 3000–2500 BC (Breasted, 1930). A Roman, Valerius Maximus (30 AD) described a learned man of Athens who lost his memory for words after being struck on the head with a stone. Despite the centuries that this relationship has been known, it is only in recent times that detailed descriptions of the speech and language disorders occurring subsequent to head trauma have started to appear in the literature. Many of the early studies only noted the presence of speech and language disorders in patients who had suffered traumatic head injury without providing detailed descriptions of the disorder (e.g., Lichtheim, 1885; Russell, 1932). It was only following the Second World War that detailed descriptions of posttraumatic language disorders subsequent to penetrating (open) head injuries were published (Goldstein, 1948; Schiller, 1947). Similar analyses of language disorders caused by nonpenetrating (closed) head injuries have only appeared in the literature in any number since the early 1970s. Even as we enter the new millennium, our knowledge of the nature and basis of linguistic impairments following closed head injury remains incomplete, and even the terminology applied to these conditions is somewhat confused and inconsistent. Chapters 9 to 11 of this book provide a detailed description of the language disorders noted to occur in both adults (Chapters 9 and 10) and children (Chapter 11) with TBI. A review of contemporary treatments applicable to persons with TBI presenting with language disorders appears in Chapter 12.

Motor speech disorders occurring subsequent to TBI can take the form of an apraxia of speech and/or a dysarthria. Apraxia of speech is usually thought to result from a disorder in speech motor programming (Canter, Trost, & Burns, 1985; Kent & McNeil, 1987; Kent & Rosenbek, 1983; Pierce, 1991) with some researchers having identified the condition more specifically as a deficit in motor planning, sequencing, control, and/or timing (Kelso & Tuller, 1981; Lebrun, 1989).

In apraxia of speech, the speech disorder is not caused by either paralysis or weakness of the speech production musculature. Rather, the individual has difficulty speaking because of a cerebral lesion that prevents executing voluntary and on command the complex sequence of muscle contractions involved in speaking. Symptoms of apraxia of speech include, but are not limited to: disordered articulation, reduced speech rate, scanning speech, speech initiation difficulties, prosodic disturbance, audible groping, oral posturing, and labored articulatory productions (Lebrun, 1989; Odell, McNeil, Rosenbek, & Hunter, 1990; Wertz, LaPointe, & Rosenbek, 1991). By far the majority of reports in the literature describing the behavioral symptomatology in apraxia of speech, however, are based on examinations of subjects with left hemisphere cerebrovascular disorders. Indeed apraxia of speech has rarely been reported in published studies dealing specifically with patients with TBI, and where it has, the studies have been based on single case reports. Ewing-Cobbs, Fletcher, and Levin (1986) described the features of an apraxia of speech in a 2 year 6 month-old boy subsequent to TBI. The case of a young male in his late twenties who exhibited a moderate apraxia of speech following a motor vehicle accident was presented by Yorkston and Beukelman (1991). Dworkin and Abkarian (1997) described the case of a young man who exhibited an apraxia of speech and a unilateral upper motor neuron dysarthria subsequent to closed head injury and diffuse encephalopathy.

Clinically, TBI patients with an associated apraxia of speech are encountered by speech-language pathologists in their clinics (Yorkston & Beukelman, 1991). In the majority of cases, however, the apraxic patient also exhibits a concomitant language disorder and sometimes a concomitant dysarthria. Particularly in severe TBI cases, it may be difficult for the clinician to isolate the differential effects of the concomitant dysarthria and the apraxia of speech on the patient's speech production, with the affected individual exhibiting dysarthric symptoms (attributed to weakness, slowness, and incoordination of the muscles of the speech mechanism) as well as those caused by a deficit in motor programming. Given the rarity of published reports of apraxia of speech in association with TBI, apraxia of speech will not be dealt with in any further detail in the subsequent chapters of the present book.

Darley, Aronson, and Brown (1969a, b; 1975) have defined dysarthria as "a collective name for a group of speech disorders resulting from disturbances in muscular control over the speech mechanism due to damage of the central or peripheral nervous system. It designates problems in oral communication due to paralysis, weakness or incoordination of the speech musculature" (1969a, p.246). According to this definition, the term "dysarthria" is restricted to those speech disorders associated with pathology of the central and/or peripheral nervous system. It is widely recognized that dysarthria constitutes one of the most persistent sequelae of severe TBI, often persisting beyond the resolution of any concomitant language disorder (Sarno & Levin, 1985). Despite this recognition, the literature relating to the prevalence and natural course of post-TBI dysarthria is unclear. Depending on factors such as the measures used, the stage postinjury when the measures were taken, the population studied, etc., estimates of the prevalence of dysarthria following TBI vary from 8 to 100 percent (Dresser et al., 1973; Groher, 1977, 1983; Sarno, Buonaguro, & Levita, 1986; Rusk, Block, & Lowmann, 1969).

One frequently observed feature of the dysarthria associated with TBI is the persistent nature of the disorder, suggesting that the prognosis for complete resolution of the dysarthric speech disturbance in individuals with severe TBI is poor

(Hartley & Levin, 1990). Despite the persistent nature of dysarthria in TBI, it is only in recent years that some understanding of the effects of nonpenetrating head injuries on the physiological functioning of the major components of the speech production apparatus has been gained. Most reports in the literature have included only clinical descriptions of the speech disturbances, single case studies, or physiological investigations of small groups of TBI cases. Kent, Netsell, and Bauer (1975) in a cinefluorographic study and Lehiste (1965) in an acoustic analysis provided case studies of dysarthria following TBI that detailed deficits in lingual movement, and the slow rate of and incoordination in articulatory activity. However, it was only in the mid-1990s that the first series of studies to comprehensively examine the physiology of the various subsystems of the speech production mechanisms of patients with severe closed head injuries were published (Murdoch, Theodoros, Stokes, & Chenery, 1993; Theodoros & Murdoch, 1994; Theodoros, Murdoch, & Chenery, 1994; Theodoros, Murdoch, & Stokes, 1995; Theodoros, Murdoch, Stokes, & Chenery, 1993). Chapters 2–7 of this book provide a detailed description and discussion of the perceptual, acoustic, and physiological characteristics of TBI dysarthria. Chapter 8 provides a comprehensive overview of the treatments that can be applied to the dysarthrias manifest in persons who have suffered TBI.

Although, as in the case of communication impairments, it has been recognized for some time that individuals with TBI frequently experience swallowing disorders, it is only recently that speech-language pathologists have begun to incorporate dysphagia programs into their overall management of individuals with TBI. In a 1-year study of individuals admitted to a rehabilitation facility, Winstein (1983) found that approximately 27% of the TBI cases exhibited swallowing problems on admission, reflecting the need for initiation of appropriate interventions. The physiology of swallowing is described in Chapter 13 of the current book. Chapter 14 outlines procedures for assessing swallowing disorders in both adults and children, while Chapter 15 describes appropriate management and treatment programs for swallowing disorders in both groups.

Summary

Much of our current understanding of the communication disorders occurring subsequent to TBI has come from studies reported in the past 30 years. It is only in more recent years, however, that the importance of communication and swallowing abilities for the long-term quality of life of survivors of TBI has begun to be recognized. Several factors that appear to have minimized the perceived importance of speech, language, and swallowing deficits following TBI to various health professionals include: the failure of researchers to develop terminology to adequately describe the disorders; the lack of empirical data regarding the nature of speech, language, and swallowing disorders post-TBI; the failure of researchers to recognize the disorders as unique speech and language symptomatology; the perception that communicative disorders post-TBI resolve completely, especially in children; and an opinion that communication and swallowing disorders in TBI cases need only be treated as an accessory to medical management.

Advances, in recent years, in our understanding of the basic mechanisms involved in brain damage associated with TBI have enabled the introduction of important improvements in the medical management of TBI cases. This in turn has led to improved survival rates for persons with TBI. The improved survival rate, combined with the increasing incidence of TBI in most Western countries and the now recognized serious economic and social consequences of associated communicative and swallowing disorders, has necessitated greater research efforts aimed at developing more effective and long-lasting treatments for these disorders. Contemporary procedures for the assessment and treatment of communicative and swallowing disorders in both children and adults with TBI are detailed in subsequent chapters of this book. In addition, the following chapters provide an overview of recent research aimed at further delineating the nature of the various communicative and swallowing disorders occurring as sequelae to TBI in both children and adults.

References

Adams, J.H. (1975). The neuropathology of head injuries. In P.J. Vinken & G.W. Bruyn (Eds.), *Handbook of Clinical Neurology: Vol. 23 Injuries of the Brain and Skull: Part 1* (pp. 35–65). Amsterdam: North-Holland Publishing Company.

Adams, J.H., Graham, D.I., Gennarelli, T.A., & Maxwell, W.L. (1991). Diffuse axonal injury in non-missile head injury. *Journal of Neurology, Neurosurgery, and Psychiatry, 54*, 481–483.

Adams, J.H., Graham, D.I., Murray, L.S., & Scott, G. (1982). Diffuse axonal injury due to non-missile head injury in humans. An analysis of 45 cases. *Annals of Neurology, 12*, 557–563.

Adams, J.H., Graham, D.I., Scott, G., Parker, L.S., & Doyle, D. (1980). Brain damage in fatal non-missile head injury. *Journal of Clinical Pathology, 33*, 1132–1145.

Adams, J.H., Mitchell, D.E., Graham, D.I., & Doyle, D. (1977). Diffuse brain damage of immediate impact type: Its relationship to primary brainstem damage in head injury. *Brain, 100*, 489–502.

Auerbach, S.H. (1986). Neuroanatomical correlates of attention and memory disorder in traumatic brain injury: An application of neurobehavioral subtypes. *Journal of Head Trauma Rehabilitation, 3*, 1–12.

Bigler, E.D. (1990). Neuropathology of traumatic brain injury. In E. Bigler (Ed.), *Traumatic Brain Injury* (pp. 13–49). Austin, Texas: Pro-ed.

Bigler, E.D., Kurth, S., Blatter, D., & Abildskov, T. (1993). Day-of-injury CT as an index to pre-injury brain morphology: Degree of post-injury degenerative changes identified by CT and MR neuroimaging. *Brain Injury, 7*, 125–134.

Blumbergs, P.C., Jones, N.R., & North, J.B. (1989). Diffuse axonal injury in head trauma. *Journal of Neurology, Neurosurgery and Psychiatry, 52*, 838–841.

Breasted, J.H. (1930). *The Edwin Smith Surgical Papyrus Vol. 1* Chicago: University of Chicago Press.

Canter, G.J., Trost, J.E., & Burns, M.S. (1985). Contrasting speech patterns in apraxia of speech and phonemic paraphasia. *Brain and Language, 24*, 204–222.

Coloquhoun, I.R. & Rawlinson, J. (1989). The significance of hematomas of the basal ganglia in closed head injury. *Clinical Radiology, 40*, 619–621.

Craft, A.W. (1972). Head injury in children. In P.J. Vinken & G.W. Bruyn (Eds.), *Handbook of Clinical Neurology Vol. 23*. New York: Elsévier—North Holland.

Cullum, C.M. & Bigler, E.D. (1986). Ventricle size, cortical atrophy, and the relationship with neuropsychological status in closed head injury: A quantitative analysis. *Journal of Clinical Experimental Neuropsychology, 8*, 437–452.

Darley, F.L., Aronson, A.E., & Brown, J.R. (1969a). Differential diagnostic patterns of dysarthria. *Journal of Speech and Hearing Research, 12*, 246–269.

Darley, F.L., Aronson, A.E., & Brown, J.R. (1969b). Clusters of deviant speech dimensions in the dysarthrias. *Journal of Speech and Hearing Research, 12*, 462–496.

Darley, F.L., Aronson, A.E., & Brown, J.R. (1975). *Motor Speech Disorders*. Philadelphia: W.B. Saunders Company.

Dresser, A.C., Meirowsky, A.M., Weiss, G.J., McNeel, M.L., Simon, G.A., & Caveness, W.F. (1973). Gainful employment following head injury: Prognostic factors. *Archives of Neurology, 29*, 111–116.

Dworkin, J.P. & Abkarian, G.G. (1997). Treatment of phonation in a patient with apraxia and dysarthria secondary to severe closed head injury. *Journal of Medical Speech Language Pathology, 4*, 105–115.

Ewing-Cobbs, L., Fletcher, J.M., & Levin, H.S. (1986). Neurobehavioral sequelae following head injury in children: Educational implications. *Journal of Head Trauma Rehabilitation, 1*, 57–65.

Friede, R.L. (1973). *Developmental Neuropathology*. New York: Springer.

Gennarelli, T.A. (1993). Mechanisms of brain injury. *Journal of Emergency Medicine, 11*, 5–11.

Gennarelli, T.A., Thibault, L.E., Adams, H.J., Graham, D.I., Thompson, C.J., & Marcincin, R.P. (1982). Diffuse axonal injury. *Annals of Neurology, 12*, 212–223.

Gjerris, F. (1986). Head injuries in children: Special features. *Acta Neurochirurgica, Supplement 36*, 155–158.

Goldstein, K. (1948). *Language and Language Disturbances*. New York: Grune & Stratton.

Graham, D.J. & Adams, J.H. (1971). Ischaemic brain damage in fatal head injuries. *Lancet, 1*, 265–266.

Graham, D.J., Adams, J.H., & Doyle, D. (1978). Ischaemic brain damage in fatal nonmissile head injuries. *Journal of Neurological Science, 39*, 213–234.

Groher, M. (1977). Language and memory disorders following closed head trauma. *Journal of Speech and Hearing Research, 20*, 212–222.

Groher, M. (1983). Communication disorders. In M. Rosenthal, E. Griffith, M. Bond, & J.D. Miller (Eds.), *Rehabilitation of the Head Injured Adult*. Philadelphia: Davis.

Gurdijian, E.S. & Gurdijian, E.S. (1975). Re-evaluation of the biomechanics of blunt impact head injury. *Surgery, Gynecology and Obstetrics, 140*, 845–850.

Gurdijian, E.S. & Gurdijian, E.S. (1976). Cerebral contusions: Re-evaluation of the mechanism of their development. *Journal of Trauma, 16*, 35–51.

Guthrie, E., Mast, J., Richards, P., McQuaid, M., & Pavlakis, S. (1999). Traumatic brain injury in children and adolescents. *Child and Adolescent Psychiatric Clinics of North America, 8*, 807–826.

Hartley, L.L. & Levin, H.S. (1990). Linguistic deficits after closed head injury: A current appraisal. *Aphasiology, 4*, 353–370.

Hendrick, E.B., Hardwood-Nash, D., & Hudson, A.R. (1964). Head injuries in children: A survey of 4465 consecutive cases at the hospital of sick children, Toronto Canada. *Clinical Neurosurgery, 11*, 45–65.

Holbourn, A.H.S. (1943). Mechanics of head injuries. *Lancet, 2*, 438–441.

Javid, M. & Settlage, P. (1956). Effect of urea on cerebrospinal fluid pressure in human subjects: Preliminary report. *Journal of the American Medical Association, 160*, 943–949.

Jellinger, K. (1983). The neuropathology of pediatric head injuries. In K. Shapiro (Ed.), *Pediatric Head Trauma* (pp 87–115). Mount Kisco, New York: Futura.

Jellinger, K. & Seitelberger, F. (1970). Protracted post-traumatic encephalopathy: Pathology, pathogenesis, and clinical implications. *Journal of Neurological Sciences, 10*, 51–94.

Jennett, B. (1986). Head trauma. In A.K. Asbury, G.M. McKann, & W.I. McDonald (Eds.), *Diseases of the Nervous System* (pp. 1282–1297). Philadelphia: W.B. Saunders.

Katz, M.D. (1992). Neuropathology and neurobehavioral recovery from closed head injury. *Journal of Head Trauma Rehabilitation, 7*, 1–15.

Kelso, J.A.S. & Tuller, B. (1981). Toward a theory of apractic syndromes. *Brain and Language, 12*, 224–245.

Kent, R.D. & McNeil, M.R. (1987). Relative timing of sentence repetition in apraxia of speech and conduction aphasia. In J.H. Ryalls (Ed.), *Phonetic Approaches to Speech Production in Aphasia and Related Disorders* (pp. 181–220). Boston: College-Hill Press.

Kent, R.D., Netsell, R. & Bauer, L. (1975). Cineradiographic assessment of articulatory mobility in the dysarthrias. *Journal of Speech and Hearing Disorders, 40*, 467–480.

Kent, R.D. & Rosenbek, J.C. (1983). Acoustic patterns of apraxia of speech. *Journal of Speech and Hearing Research, 26*, 231–249.

Klauber, M.R., Barrett-Connor, E., Marshall, L.F., & Bowers, S.A. (1981) The epidemiology of head injury: A prospective study of an entire community—San Diego County, California 1978. *American Journal of Epidemiology, 113*, 500–509.

Kraus, J.F. (1995). Epidemiological features of brain injury in children: Occurrence, children at risk, causes and manner of injury, severity and outcomes. In S.H. Broman & M.E. Michel (Eds.), *Traumatic Head Injury in Children* (pp. 22–39). New York: Oxford University Press.

Kraus, J.F., Black, M.A., Hessal, N., Ley, P., Rokow, W., Sullivan, C., Bowers, S., Knowlton, S., & Marshall, L. (1984). The incidence of acute brain injury and serious impairment in a defined population. *American Journal of Epidemiology, 119*, 186–201.

Lebrun, Y. (1989). Apraxia of speech: The history of a concept. In P. Square-Storer (Ed.), *Acquired Apraxia of Speech in Aphasic Adults* (pp. 3–19). London: Taylor & Francis.

Lehiste, I. (1965). Some acoustic characteristics of dysarthric speech. *Biblotheca Phonetica, 2*, 1–124.

Letarte, P.B. (1999). Neurotrauma care in the new millennium. *Surgical Clinics of North America, 79*, 1449–1470.

Levin, H.S., Benton, A.L., & Grossman, M.D. (1982). *Neurobehavioural Consequences of Closed Head Injury*. New York: Oxford University Press.

Levin, H.S., Ewing-Cobbs, L., & Benton, A.L. (1983). Age and recovery from brain damage. In S.W. Scheff (Ed.), *Aging and the Recovery of Function in the Central Nervous System* (pp. 233–240). New York: Plenum Publishing.

Levin, H.S., Meyers, C.A., Grossman, R.G., & Sawer, M. (1981). Ventricular enlargement after closed head injury. *Archives of Neurology, 38*, 623–629.

Lezak, M. (1983). *Neuropsychological Assessment* (2nd ed.) New York: Oxford University Press.

Lichtheim, L. (1885). On aphasia. *Brain, 7*, 433–484.

Lindenberg, R. & Freytag, E. (1969). Morphology of brain lesions from blunt trauma in early infancy. *Archives of Pathology (Chicago), 87*, 298–305.

Lundberg, N. (1960). Continuous recording and control of ventricular fluid pressure in neurosurgical practice. *Acta Psychiatria Scandinavica, Suppl. 36*, 1–193.

Luria, A.R. (1970). *Traumatic Aphasia*. The Hague: Mouton.

MacPherson, P., Teasdale, E., Dhaker, S., Allerdyce, G., & Gailbraith, S. (1986). The significance of traumatic haematoma in the region of the basal ganglia. *Journal of Neurology, Neurosurgery and Psychiatry, 49*, 29–34.

Menkes, J.H. & Till, K. (1995). Postnatal trauma and injuries by physical agents. In J.H. Menkes (Ed.), *Textbook of Child Neurology* (pp. 557–597). Baltimore: Williams & Wilkins.

Miller, J.D., & Sweet, R.C. (1978). Early insults to the injured brain. *Journal of the American Medical Association, 240*, 439–442.

Murdoch, B.E. (1990). *Acquired Speech and Language Disorders: A Neuroanatomical and Functional Neurological Approach*. London: Chapman and Hall.

Murdoch, B.E., Theodoros, D.G., Stokes, P.D., & Chenery, H.J. (1993). Abnormal patterns of speech breathing in dysarthria following severe closed head injury. *Brain Injury, 7*, 295–308.

Najenson, T., Sazbon, L., Fiselzon, J., Becker, E., & Schecter, I. (1978). Recovery of communicative functions after prolonged traumatic coma. *Scandinavian Journal of Rehabilitation Medicine, 10*, 15–21.

National Head Injury Foundation. (1985). *An educator's manual: What educators need to know about students with traumatic brain injury*. Framingham, Massachusetts: Author.

Naugle, R.I. (1990). Epidemiology of traumatic brain injury in adults. In E.D. Bigler (Ed.), *Traumatic Brain Injury: Mechanisms of Damage, Assessment, Intervention, and Outcome* (pp. 69–103). Austin, Texas: Pro-ed.

Odell, K., McNeil, M., Rosenbek, J.C., & Hunter, L. (1990). Perceptual characteristics of consonant production by apraxic speakers. *Journal of Speech and Hearing Disorders, 55*, 345–359.

Ommaya, A.K. & Gennarelli, T.A. (1974). Cerebral concussion and traumatic unconsciousness. *Brain, 97*, 633–645.

Pang, D. (1985). Pathophysiologic correlates of neurobehavioural syndromes following closed head injury. In M. Ylvisaker (Ed.), *Head Injury Rehabilitation: Children and Adolescents* (pp. 3–70). Austin Texas: Pro-ed.

Pierce, R.S. (1991). Apraxia of speech versus phonemic paraphasia: Theoretical, diagnostic and treatment considerations. In M. Cannito & D. Vogel (Eds.), *Treating Disordered Speech Motor Control: For Clinicians by Clinicians* (pp. 185–216). Austin, Texas: Pro-ed.

Reilly, P.L. & Adams, J.H. (1975). Patients with head injury who talk and die. *Lancet, 2*, 375–377.

Rosner, M.J. (1995). Introduction to cerebral perfusion pressure management. *Neurosurgical Clinics of North America, 6*, 761–773.

Rosner, M.J. & Coley, I.B. (1986). Cerebral perfusion pressure, intracranial pressure and elevation. *Journal of Neurosurgery, 65*, 636–641.

Rosner, M.J. & Daughton, S. (1990). Cerebral perfusion pressure management in head trauma. *Journal of Trauma, 30*, 933–940.

Rusk, H., Block, J., & Lowmann, E. (1969). Rehabilitation of the brain-injured patient: A report of 157 cases with long-term follow-up of 118. In E. Walker, W. Caveness, & M. Critchley (Eds.), *The Late Effects of Head Injury* (pp. 327–332). Springfield: Charles C. Thomas.

Russell, W.R. (1932). Cerebral involvement in head injury: A study based on the examination of two hundred cases. *Brain, 55*, 549–603.

Russell, W.R. & Espir, M.L.E. (1961). *Traumatic Aphasia*. London: Oxford University Press.

Sarno, M.T., Buonaguro, A., & Levita, E. (1986). Characteristics of verbal impairment in closed head injured patients. *Archives of Physical Medicine and Rehabilitation, 67*, 400–405.

Sarno, M.T. & Levin, H.S. (1985). Speech and language disorders after closed head injury. In J.K. Darby (Ed.), *Speech and Language Evaluation in Neurology: Adult Disorders* (pp. 323–339). New York: Grune & Stratton.

Schiller, F. (1947). Aphasia studied in patients with missile wounds. *Journal of Neurology, Neurosurgery and Psychiatry, 10*, 183–197.

Strich, S.J. (1956). Diffuse degeneration of the cerebral white matter in severe dementia following head injury. *Journal of Neurology, Neurosurgery and Psychiatry, 19*, 163–185.

Strich, S.J. (1961). Shearing of nerve fibers as a cause of brain damage due to head injury. *Lancet, 2*, 443–448.

Strich, S.J. (1969). The pathology of brain damage due to blunt head injuries. In A.E. Walker, W.F. Caveness, & M. Critchley (Eds.), *The Late Effects of Head Injury* (pp. 501–524). Springfield, Illinois: Charles C. Thomas.

Tate, R.L., McDonald, S., & Lulham, J.L. (1998). Traumatic brain injury: Severity of injury and outcome in an Australian population. *Journal of Australia and New Zealand Public Health, 22*, 11–15.

Teasdale, G.M. & Graham, D.I. (1998). Craniocerebral trauma: protection and retrieval of the neuronal population after injury. *Neurosurgery, 43*, 723–738.

Teasdale, G. M. & Jennett, B. (1974). Assessment of coma and impaired consciousness: A practical scale. *Lancet, 2*, 81–84.

Teasdale, G.M. & Jennett, B. (1976). Assessment and prognosis of coma after head injury. *Acta Neurochirurgica, 34*, 45–55.

Theodoros, D.G. & Murdoch, B.E. (1994). Laryngeal dysfunction in dysarthric speakers following severe closed head injury. *Brain injury, 8*, 667–684.

Theodoros, D.G., Murdoch, B.E., & Chenery, H.J. (1994). Perceptual speech characteristics of dysarthric speakers following severe closed head injury. *Brain injury, 8*, 101–124.

Theodoros, D.G., Murdoch, B.E., & Stokes, P.D. (1995). A physiological analysis of articulatory dysfunction in dysarthric speakers following severe closed head injury. *Brain Injury, 9*, 237–254.

Theodoros, D.G., Murdoch, B.E., Stokes, P.D., & Chenery, H.J. (1993). Hypernasality in dysarthric speakers following severe closed head injury: A perceptual and instrumental analysis. *Brain Injury, 7*, 59–69.

Van Dongen, K.J. & Braakman, R. (1980). Late computed tomography in survivors of severe head injury. *Neurosurgery, 7*, 14–22.

Vernon-Levett, P. (1991). Head injuries in children. *Critical Care Nursing Clinics of North America, 3*, 411–421.

Wertz, R.T., LaPointe, L.L., & Rosenbek, J.C. (1991). *Apraxia of Speech in Adults: The Disorder and Its Management.* Austin, Texas: Pro-ed.

Winstein, C. (1983). Neurogenic dysphagia: Frequency, progression and outcome in adults following head injury. *Physical Therapy, 63*, 1992–1996.

Yorkston, K.M. & Beukelman, D.R. (1991). Motor speech disorders. In D.R. Beukelman & K.M. Yorkston (Eds.), *Communication Disorders Following Traumatic Brain Injury* (pp. 251–315). Austin, Texas: Pro-ed.

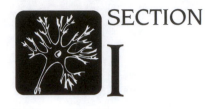

SECTION

I

Motor Speech Disorders Following Traumatic Brain Injury

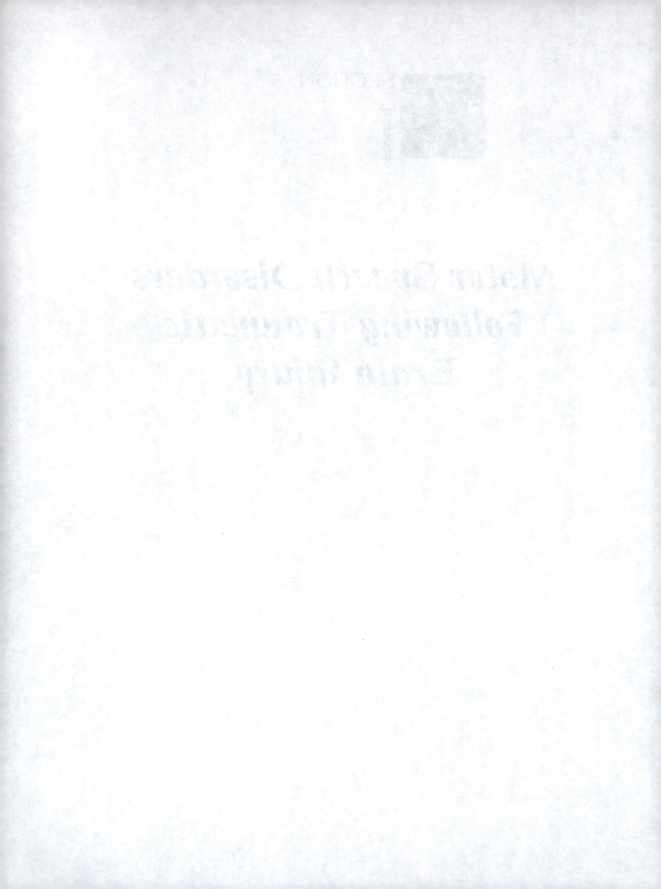

CHAPTER

Two

Dysarthria Following Traumatic Brain Injury: Incidence, Recovery, and Perceptual Features

Deborah G. Theodoros, Bruce E. Murdoch, Justine V. Goozée

Introduction

Dysarthria, a motor speech disorder, constitutes a substantial proportion of the communication impairment associated with traumatic brain injury (TBI). This speech disturbance is characterized by slurred, indistinct speech that impedes an individual's ability to communicate effectively with his/her family, friends, and members of the general community. The prevalence of TBI in modern society has reached epidemic proportions, with the greatest increase in frequency occurring during the age range from mid-adolescence to the mid-twenties. Consequently, the sudden development of a dysarthric speech disturbance following TBI has an enormous impact on the lives of many individuals during their most productive years, affecting various psychological, social, academic, and occupational aspects of life.

While the incidence, range of severity, and persistence of the dysarthric speech disturbance in the TBI population have been partially identified and reported in the literature, there has been a notable absence of comprehensive descriptions and analyses of this speech disorder in persons following TBI. The failure to obtain detailed and accurate knowledge of the perceptual and physiological features of this motor speech disorder may result in the development of therapy programs that are ineffective in the communicative rehabilitation of these individuals.

The dysarthria associated with TBI in adults is relatively common and is characterized by: variable and unpredictable recovery patterns and long-term outcomes, a wide range of severity, and an extensive variety of speech behaviors and deficits in neuromuscular control of the speech mechanism. As a result, the management of dysarthric speakers following TBI constitutes a major challenge to the speech clinician.

Incidence and Severity of Dysarthria Following TBI

In the majority of studies reporting on the incidence of communication impairment following TBI, dysarthria has been found to represent slightly more than one-third of the communicative dysfunction evident in TBI populations. An early study by Rusk, Block, and Lowmann (1969), revealed that dysarthria was present in approximately one-third of their subjects during the acute phase postinjury. In an investigation of the nature of verbal performance of 56 CHI subjects, Sarno (1980) identified dysarthria in 38% of her population, while in a replication study, 32% of the 69 subjects were found to exhibit dysarthric speech disturbances (Sarno, 1984). A comparable incidence of dysarthria (34%) was found in a group of 125 patients involved in a third study, by Taylor Sarno, Buonaguro, and Levita (1986). Similar incidence trends relating to the presence of dysarthria have been observed by other investigators (Luzzatti, Willmes, Taricco, Colombo, & Chiesa, 1989; Thomsen, 1975, 1984) while higher incidences of dysarthria following TBI and prolonged coma have been reported by Groher (1977) and Najenson, Sazbon, Fiselzon, Becker, and Schecter (1978).

The severity of dysarthric speech following TBI has been noted to cover the entire spectrum of dysfunction, ranging from mild articulatory imprecision to total unintelligibility of speech (Taylor Sarno et al., 1986). These clinical findings are supported by the known biomechanics and neuropathological consequences of TBI (as described in the previous chapter), in that damage may occur to any area of the brain with subsequent disturbances in the basic motor processes involved in speech production, either in isolation or in combination. Furthermore, the severity of the dysarthric speech disturbance following TBI has been found to be associated with the level of severity of cognitive deficits demonstrated by the individual. Yorkston, Honsinger, Mitsuda, and Hammen (1989) found that the prevalence and severity of dysarthria increased with more severe levels of cognitive deficit.

Neuropathological Bases of Dysarthria Following TBI

The nature of traumatic brain injury is such that multifocal abnormalities (Gentry, Godersky, & Thompson, 1988) are likely to occur, and potentially may result in a dysarthric speech disturbance. Despite the notable clinical prevalence of dysarthria following TBI (see "Incidence and Severity of Dysarthria Following TBI" in this chapter), little research concerning the specific neuropathological bases of the presenting dysarthric speech disturbances has been conducted. In a study by Netsell and Lefkowitz (1992), magnetic resonance imaging (MRI) was used to examine the anatomical lesions associated with dysarthria and other clinical speech-related deficits, in a group of 10 subjects following TBI. Each subject was rated according to the severity of dysarthria, lability, flatness, and delayed initiation of speech while the sites of lesion for each subject were identified on MRI scans. The study revealed an extensive range of multifocal lesions and speech disturbances of differing types and severity (Netsell & Lefkowitz, 1992). Almost 80% of the lesions identified by MRI were subcortical in nature and were associated with the more severe degrees of dysarthria. Netsell and Lefkowitz (1992) hypothesized that certain subcortical lesions are responsible for the most severe and persistent dysarthrias.

Furthermore, Netsell and Lefkowitz (1992) suggested that specific patterns of speech disturbances were related to different anatomical systems of the brain, according to the concept of a triune brain as espoused by MacLean (1970). The "triune brain" consists of the phylogenetically old reticular system, the more developed limbic system, and the more recently evolved neocortical system (MacLean, 1970). According to Netsell and Lefkowitz (1992), the reticular system is implicated in the initiation of speech, with the presumed sites of lesion being the periaquaductal gray and/or lateral tegmental area. While it has been suggested that this system of the brain may represent the deepest level of the mechanism that initiates speech (Botez & Barbeau, 1971), some limbic structures, such as the hippocampus and amygdala, may also be involved in the initiation of such action (Goldberg, 1985; Mesulam, 1990).

The frontal limbic system is considered to be associated with mediating feelings and emotions (affect; Mendez, Adams, & Lewandowski, 1989). Anatomical lesions of the right hemisphere (Kent & Rosenbek, 1982; Ley & Bryden, 1982), basal ganglia input to the anterior cingulate cortex, or the supplementary motor area of either hemisphere (Cancelliere & Kertesz, 1990) have been noted to result in impairments of the emotional aspects of communication. The neocortical system is thought to be responsible for the more refined sensorimotor control of speech movements involving the entire vocal tract. Anatomical areas involved in this neural system include the lower motor cortex, premotor cortex, Broca's Area, prefrontal cortex, supplementary motor area, somatosensory cortex, supramarginal gyrus, basal ganglia, neocerebellum, and ventral lateral thalamus. Netsell and Lefkowitz (1992) suggested that damage to areas in the neocortical system are responsible for the dysarthria associated with TBI. In their study of 10 TBI subjects, the subjects with the more severe degrees of dysarthria demonstrated lesions of the neocortical system, while those subjects with milder forms of dysarthria exhibited negligible involvement of this system (Netsell & Lefkowitz, 1992).

Further support for Netsell and Lefkowitz's hypothesis of distinct patterns of speech production resulting from damage to the reticular, limbic, and neocortical neural systems following TBI can be seen in reports of recovery of posttraumatic mutism. Von Cramon (1981) and Vogel and von Cramon (1982), in their studies of 11 TBI subjects, documented recovery along a continuum from mutism, to emotional vocalizations, to the production of propositional speech and more finely coordinated articulatory skills. The recovery pattern observed in these subjects was considered to reflect progressive improvement of the reticular, limbic, and neocortical systems, respectively.

In a later study, Lefkowitz and Netsell (1994) evaluated the same group of TBI subjects as reported in Netsell and Lefkowitz (1992), using five categories of structural correlation for each clinical deficit. The speech ratings of dysarthria, affective dysprosody (lability and flatness), and delayed initiation of speech for each subject were correlated with coexistent structural lesions: discrete lesion (identifiable area of increased or decreased signal intensity); atrophic lesion (not directly visualized, but inferred by atrophy of the structure in which it is located); afferent fiber lesion (suggested hypothetical condition when inconsistencies occur between structural and clinical deficits); nonrecognized lesion (lesion found in a structure or pathway not usually recognized as associated with speech); functional lesion (viable but malfunctioning tissues, and damage that occurs below the limits of MRI resolution) (Lefkowitz & Netsell, 1994). These specific lesion categories existed within a continuum, from discrete to functional lesions, in which there was a decreasing association between a particular clinical deficit and the observed MRI lesion or lack of lesion. The results of this study indicated that a variety of anatomical lesions were present in a group of subjects with shared clinical deficits. The majority (46%) of the clinical speech deficits corresponded to discrete lesions, 29% were associated with atrophic lesions, 11% were due to afferent fiber lesions, and 7% were related to nonrecognized lesions, while 14 % of the clinical deficits corresponded to functional lesions. Although these studies by Netsell and Lefkowitz (1992) and Lefkowitz and Netsell (1994) have provided a framework for the investigation of the neuropathological bases of dysarthric speech disturbances in persons following TBI, further studies involving larger sample sizes are required to pursue a greater understanding of this aspect of TBI.

Recovery of Speech and Long-Term Outcome Following TBI

The pattern of recovery of speech and long-term outcome following TBI has been noted to be as variable and unpredictable as the speech deficits exhibited by this clinical population. Some traumatically brain-injured individuals have been observed to remain as severely speech impaired over a long period of time as they were in the initial stages postinjury, while others have demonstrated significant and continuous improvement several years following the head injury (Netsell & Lefkowitz, 1992).

In the acute stage postinjury, mutism, or the inability or refusal to speak, has been found to persist in 3% of a TBI population for varying periods of time postcoma (Levin et al., 1983). In a study of 350 TBI cases with mutism following arousal from coma, Levin et al. (1983) found that those individuals who were mute following left focal basal ganglia lesions tended to recover consciousness more rapidly and demonstrated a better prognosis for linguistic outcome. Mutism resulting from severe diffuse TBI, however, was found to be more closely associated with residual linguistic deficits.

In a study of the recovery of functional speech following TBI, Dongilli, Hakel, and Beukelman (1992) found that of the 27 patients who entered an inpatient rehabilitation program, just over half of these individuals became functional speakers by the time they were discharged. It was noted, however, that functional speech was not regained until the person had reached the cognitive functioning of levels of V and VI on the Ranchos Los Amigos Scale of Cognitive Functioning (Hagen, Malkmus, & Durham, 1979). At these levels of cognitive functioning, improved control of language systems became evident, thus enabling functional speech to occur (Dongilli et al., 1992). In addition, Dongilli et al. (1992) found that the reduction or elimination of primitive oral reflexes in persons following TBI appeared to be related to the recovery of functional speech, in that once these reflexes were integrated, the patients' potential to achieve functional speech improved.

In relation to the recovery of more specific aspects of speech production, von Cramon (1981) found that in the initial stage of recovery from posttraumatic mutism, the patients demonstrated complete loss of voluntary control of the laryngeal muscles, which was followed by the use of nonverbal signals during the second stage of mutism. Nonspontaneous verbalization in response to stimuli was apparent in the final stage of mutism. Phonation during this period was characterized by a whispery and breathy vocal quality. In a follow-up study of the recovery of phonation in eight subjects following TBI, Vogel and von Cramon (1982) identified a progressive change in laryngeal function from a hypofunctional pattern of laryngeal activity to one consistent with hyperfunction (See Chapter 5, "Preceptual Features of Laryngeal Dysfunction Following TBI"). The recovery of articulatory function following TBI has also been documented and suggests that the phonetic inventory is gradually restored with speech production being phonetically sensitive to articulation requiring posterior closure of the tongue, stricture for fricative production, and gross displacement of the tongue for the production of vowels (Vogel and von Cramon, 1983) (See Chapter 3, "Recovery of Articulatory Function Following TBI").

Yorkston and Beukelman (1991) stressed the importance of distinguishing mutism following TBI from other forms of speechlessness, such as a persistent vegetative state and the locked-in syndrome, which may also occur in the TBI population. Persistent vegetative state is used to describe individuals following TBI who do not demonstrate any cognitive interaction with their environment (Jennet & Plum, 1972). The locked-in syndrome, however, relates to those persons with relatively preserved language comprehension who are unable to speak due to a profound movement disorder (Bauer, Gerstenbrand, & Rump, 1979).

One of the most typical characteristics of dysarthria following TBI is the long-term persistence of the speech disorder. While it frequently accompanies a language impairment initially, dysarthria has been found to persist long after the language deficit has resolved (Levin, 1981; Najenson et al., 1978; Rusk et al., 1969; Sarno & Levin, 1985; Thomsen, 1984). Rusk et al. (1969) found that, of their 30 head-injured subjects diagnosed as being dysarthric 5 to 15 years earlier, half of these subjects remained unimproved, while the remaining half had improved significantly. In contrast, Thomsen (1984), in a follow-up study of 40 CHI patients, found that all 15 individuals who exhibited dysarthria at the time of the initial examination, continued to demonstrate a dysarthric speech disturbance 10 to 15 years postinjury.

These previous findings suggest that the prognosis for resolution of the speech disturbance following TBI is poor in this population (Hartley & Levin, 1990). The more recent literature, however, does suggest that notable improvements in physiological deficits, speech, and functional communication can be achieved for dysarthric speakers following TBI, using a variety of treatment techniques (Aten, 1988;

Beukelman & Yorkston, 1977; Brand, Matsko, & Avart, 1988; Enderby & Crow, 1990; Kuehn & Wachtel, 1994; Light, Beesley, & Collier, 1988; Nemec & Cohen, 1984; Netsell & Daniel, 1979; Simmons, 1983; Workinger & Netsell, 1992). There is also evidence to suggest that, with treatment, improvements in speech and communication may occur many years post-TBI (Aten, 1988; Beukelman & Garrett, 1988; Enderby & Crow, 1990; Harris & Murry, 1984; Keatley & Wirz, 1994; Keenan & Barnhart, 1993; Light et al., 1988; Workinger & Netsell, 1992). Indeed, the restoration of functional verbal communication has been reported in subjects 13 years (Workinger & Netsell, 1992), 9 years (Beukelman & Garrett, 1988), and 3 years post head injury (Light et al., 1988). Despite the fact that the recovery of speech and functional communication may be slow for many individuals following TBI (Groher, 1977, 1989), the rehabilitation of communicative function in these individuals should remain ongoing and proactive, albeit at different stages of recovery (Enderby & Crow, 1990). In particular, those persons with severe dysarthria warrant long-term follow-up (Yorkston, 1996).

Perceptual Assessment of Dysarthria Following TBI

Clinically, perceptual assessment of the dysarthric speech disturbances evident in persons following TBI constitutes the core component of evaluation of the speech output in this population. A perceptual analysis of speech production readily provides the clinician with a basis for diagnosis and treatment of these individuals during the acute and chronic stages of rehabilitation. This method of assessment is not only economical with respect to time and financial outlay, but is also readily adopted by clinicians and applicable to most clinical environments in which TBI individuals may be managed.

Perceptual assessments utilized with dysarthric speakers following TBI have mainly included the use of perceptual ratings scales in the analysis of speech samples, perceptual evaluation of motor speech subsystem function, quantifiable measures of speech intelligibility and rate of speech, and articulatory error analysis. A study by Frank and Barrineau (1996), in which speech assessment protocols being utilized by speech-language pathologists for adult TBI individuals were identified, revealed that the five most frequently used assessment measures for dysarthria were the Assessment of Intelligibility of Dysarthric Speech (ASSIDS; Yorkston & Beukelman, 1981a), informal assessment, the Frenchay Dysarthria Assessment (Enderby, 1983), oral-motor examination, and the Dysarthria Profile (Robertson, 1982).

Perceptual Analyses of Speech Samples

The most frequently used perceptual rating scale to assess dysarthric speech disturbances, in both clinical and research environments, was devised by Darley and colleagues (Darley, 1984; Darley, Aronson, & Brown, 1969a, b, 1975). Thirty-eight speech dimensions relating to five aspects of speech production (prosody, respiration, phonation, resonance, articulation), and overall intelligibility are rated according to a seven-point equal-appearing interval scale of severity, during the reading of a standard passage (The Grandfather Passage). A modified version of this scale was developed by FitzGerald, Murdoch, and Chenery (1987), in which 32 speech dimensions were rated according to a 1–4, a 1–5, or a 1–7 equal interval scale. Each rater was provided with a description of each dimension and the appropriate rating scale. The speech dimensions indicating the severity of a dysfunction were rated on a four-point scale (e.g., overall intelligibility), while those speech dimensions rated according to the frequency of occurrence in the speech sample (e.g., excessive loudness variation) were rated on a five-point scale. A seven-point scale was used for those speech dimensions that could be rated on the same scale as either too high or too low (e.g., loudness level). This modified perceptual rating scale was used by Theodoros, Murdoch, and Chenery (1994) to assess the speech output of TBI dysarthric speakers and to diagnose the type of dysarthria evident in these subjects. The perceptual analysis in this instance was effective in identifying impairments in all processes of speech production in their group, as well as a variety of different forms of dysarthria.

Perceptual Evaluation of Motor Speech Subsystem Function

Perceptual assessment of motor speech subsystem function in TBI dysarthric speakers may be readily performed using standardized assessment tools and informal clinical assessments. The Frenchay Dysarthria Assessment (FDA; Enderby, 1983) provides a standarized assessment of motor speech function, involving respiration, articulation, resonance, phonation, and reflex activity. The 28 aspects of motor speech function assessed using this tool are grouped according to the following sections: reflex, respiration, lips, jaw, palate, laryngeal, tongue, and intelligibility. Each feature is rated according to a nine-point rating scale (9 = normal function, 1 = severe dysfunction) based on specific descriptors. In a survey of 237 speech-language pathologists in the United States, the FDA was found to be used by approximately 25% of clinicians to identify motor speech subsystem impairments in persons following TBI (Frank & Barrineau, 1996).

A similar tool for assessing motor speech subsystem function is the Dysarthria Profile (Robertson, 1982), designed to evaluate various aspects of respiration, phonation, facial musculature, diadochokinesis, reflexes, articulation, intelligibility, and prosody. The profile utilizes a descriptive rating scale reflecting normal, good, fair, poor, or nil performance, which may also be quantified (0 = nil, 1 = poor, 2 = fair, 3 = good, 4 = normal performance). In comparison to the FDA, the Dysarthria Profile was found to be used less frequently by clinicians (9%) in the assessment of TBI adults with dysarthria (Frank & Barrineau, 1996). This finding may reflect the fact that the Dysarthria Profile provides less detailed behavioral descriptors, compared to those used in the FDA.

Clinically, it is frequently the case that the speech mechanism in persons following TBI is evaluated using nonstandardized "bedside" screening assessments, which are used in the formulation of an initial diagnosis and the identification of immediate treatment directions. Such evaluations usually involve a restricted battery of tests from which the clinician is able to observe and rate the status of motor speech function. These informal assessments are useful in the short-term, particularly in the acute stage of the rehabilitative process. These procedures, however, lack consistency in assessment tasks and rating of the individual's performance.

Despite these inadequacies, Frank and Barrineau (1996) found that approximately one-third (32.9%) of clinicians continued to utilize informal assessments to evaluate dysarthria in adults following TBI.

Perceptual Evaluation of Speech Intelligibility

Although an evaluation of overall intelligibility may be obtained through the speech sample analysis procedures as used by Darley et al. (1975) and FitzGerald et al. (1987), this measure merely reflects the functional impact of the individual's speech on the listener. Defining levels of impairment in specific parameters of speech intelligibility, such as rate of speech and the degree of intelligibility at word and sentence level, however, would provide the clinician with more specific treatment directions to enhance speech intelligibility.

The most commonly used standardized and detailed assessment of speech intelligibility in dysarthric speakers following TBI is the Assessment of Intelligibility of Dysarthric Speech (ASSIDS) by Yorkston and Beukelman (1981a) and its computerized counterpart (CAIDS) (Yorkston, Beukelman, & Traynor, 1984). Frank and Barrineau (1996) found that 33% of clinicians used this particular assessment with the TBI population. The ASSIDS quantifies both single-word and sentence intelligibility as well as overall speaking rate and rate of intelligible speech. The test requires the dysarthric speaker to read or imitate 50 randomly selected single words and 22 randomly selected sentences, ranging in length from 5 to 15 words. The individual's responses are recorded and later transcribed by naïve listeners. Five separate measures are obtained from the recordings: percent intelligibility for single words; percent intelligibility for sentences; a total speaking rate in words per minute (WPM); the rate of intelligible words per minute (IWPM); and a communication efficiency ratio (CER), which is determined by dividing the rate of intelligible speech by the mean rate of intelligible speech produced by normal speakers (190 IWPM) (Yorkston et al., 1984).

Articulatory Error Analysis

Specific evaluation of articulatory errors produced by dysarthric speakers following TBI may be performed using standard articulatory inventories and/or specific tests of phonetic contrasts. The Fisher-Logemann Test of Articulation Competence (Fisher & Logemann, 1971) may be used to identify, quantify, and determine the type of articulation errors in this population. Although this test is more frequently used with the pediatric population, it has application for use with adult dysarthric speakers. The test requires the individual to read or name pictures of single words, as well as read a number of sentences. The place and manner of articulation is determined from these responses.

A specific analysis of articulatory errors relating to phonetic contrasts has been developed by Kent, Weismer, Kent, and Rosenbek (1989) for use with dysarthric speakers and may be readily applied to those persons following TBI. The test requires the speaker to read or imitate 70 single words, which have been selected to illustrate 19 phonetic contrasts. A single-word intelligibility measure is obtained from the speech samples, as well as the frequency and type of phonetic errors produced by the speaker.

Perceptual Features of Dysarthria Following TBI

Although the diversity of the dysarthric speech characteristics associated with TBI is clearly evident in clinical practice, there has been limited documentation of these abnormal perceptual speech features. While a few investigations have focused on specific perceptual characteristics such as articulation and dysphonia (Vogel & von Cramon, 1982, 1983), there remains only one study in the literature to date, that has comprehensively examined the perceptual speech characteristics of dysarthric speakers following TBI. Theodoros et al. (1994) investigated the perceptual speech features, motor speech subsystem function, and overall intelligibility of a group of 20 subjects following severe closed head injury (CHI). The study revealed that the CHI subjects were significantly less intelligible than their matched controls for both single words and sentences, slower in their rate of production of intelligible speech, and less communicatively efficient. The CHI subjects were found to exhibit deficits in the prosodic, resonatory, articulatory, respiratory, and phonatory aspects of speech production, with the most frequently occurring deviant speech dimensions being related to disturbances of prosody, resonance, and articulation. Perceptual assessment of motor speech function, using the FDA revealed that these subjects, as a group, demonstrated moderate to severe impairment of laryngeal function, moderate impairment of palatal competence and tongue movement during speech, mild to moderate dysfunction in respiration and lip movements during speech and nonspeech-related tongue movements, and a mild impairment of nonspeech lip movements.

The TBI subjects investigated in the Theodoros et al. (1994) study were combined with an additional cohort of similar subjects who have recently been examined in our laboratory to provide a more comprehensive profile of the overall intelligibility, perceptual speech features, and motor speech function exhibited by a group of dysarthric speakers following TBI. The group consisted of 43 subjects with a mean age of 28.93 years (SD = 7.84). Thirty-eight of the subjects were male (M = 27.95 years, SD = 7.23) and five were female (M = 39.0 years, SD = 8.04). All subjects had suffered a severe head injury with Glasgow Coma Scores of eight or less on admission to hospital. The biographical details of the 43 TBI subjects are outlined in Table 2-1.

Table 2-1. Biographical and clinical details of TBI subjects in the combined group (N = 43).

Subject	Age at Assessment (Years)	Sex	Years Postinjury	Nature of Accident	GCS	Severity of TBI
1	26	M	0.5	Fall	3	Severe
2	21	M	2.5	MVA	4	Severe
3	34	F	0.3	Fall	4	Severe
4	28	M	3.0	STL	3	Severe
5	18	M	0.5	MVA	4	Severe
6	39	M	21.5	MVA	3	Severe
7	21	M	0.3	MCA	3	Severe
8	32	M	8.0	Fall	4	Severe
9	35	F	9.0	MVA	4	Severe

(continues)

Table 2-1. (*continued*)

Subject	Age at Assessment (Years)	Sex	Years Postinjury	Nature of Accident	GCS	Severity of TBI
10	25	M	7.0	MVA	4	Severe
11	26	F	6.4	MVA	4	Severe
12	26	M	7.0	MVA	4	Severe
13	27	M	8.7	MCA	6	Severe
14	25	M	0.3	AC	8	Severe
15	55	M	2.0	MVA	4	Severe
16	33	M	8.3	RA	5	Severe
17	23	M	0.3	MCA	3	Severe
18	23	M	1.9	AS	3	Severe
19	30	M	0.3	WSA	3	Severe
20	28	M	2.0	MVA	5	Severe
21	25	M	0.6	MVA	3	Severe
22	31	M	16.0	FBI	3	Severe
23	25	M	8.7	MCA	5	Severe
24	36	M	7.4	MVA	6	Severe
25	32	M	0.4	Fall	5	Severe
26	41	M	23.0	Fall	3	Severe
27	34	M	5.2	MVA	3	Severe
28	17	M	2.6	RA	4	Severe
29	18	M	8.4	CA	3	Severe
30	19	M	1.8	MVA	NDA	Severe
31	22	M	0.8	MVA	3	Severe
32	23	M	4.0	MVA	4	Severe
33	26	M	9.3	CA	4	Severe
34	27	M	3.7	AS & MVA	3	Severe
35	27	M	7.2	MVA	4	Severe
36	27	M	5.0	AS	4	Severe
37	27	M	8.5	MVA	4	Severe
38	28	M	1.6	MVA	3	Severe
39	29	M	1.0	SI	3	Severe
40	32	M	1.9	MVA	NDA	Severe
41	36	M	2.2	SI	3	Severe
42	36	F	2.0	MVA	6	Severe
43	51	F	11.6	AS	NDA	Severe

AC = Aircraft crash; AS = assaulted; CA = Cyclist accident; FBI = Football injury; GCS = Glasgow Coma score; MCA = Motor cycle accident; MVA = Motor vehicle accident; NDA = No details available; RA = Railway accident; SI = Sports injury; STL = Struck by tree limb; WSA = Water-skiing accident

Intelligibility, Rate, and Efficiency of Dysarthric Speech Following TBI

The dysarthric speech output of individuals following TBI has been identified as significantly less intelligible, slower in rate, and less communicatively efficient than normal speakers. When the speech intelligibility of the group of 43 TBI subjects studied in our laboratory was measured using The Assessment of Intelligibility of Dysarthric Speech (ASSIDS, Yorkston & Beukelman, 1981a), it was found that these individuals demonstrated significantly poorer word and sentence intelligibility than a group of control subjects matched for age and sex. Indeed, the word and sentence intelligibility of the TBI dysarthric speakers was found to be 25% and 20% lower than the normal speakers, respectively (See Table 2-2). Furthermore, the TBI subjects produced an overall rate of speech (words per minute) that was approximately half that of the control group, while the rate of intelligible speech (intelligible words per minute) produced by this group was found to be less than half the speed of the control subjects (See Table 2-2). Due to the reduced rate of intelligible speech, the communicative effectiveness of the TBI subjects' speech output was found to be approximately half of the level of effectiveness of their normal counterparts (See Table 2-2).

Deviant Speech Features in Dysarthria Following TBI

Perceptual analysis of the speech output of dysarthric speakers following TBI has revealed deviant speech features in all aspects of speech production, including prosody, resonance, phonation, articulation, respiration, and overall speech intelligibility. In general, the majority of these deficits are exhibited by the dysarthric TBI individuals to a mild to moderate degree.

Compared to a matched control group, TBI dysarthric speakers have been found to demonstrate significantly greater impairment or abnormality in the majority of speech dimensions evaluated during perceptual analysis of a standardized speech sample (Theodoros et al., 1994). A recent study of the 43 TBI dysarthric speakers listed in Table 2-1, using the same perceptual speech analysis, similarly identified 24 out of a possible 32 speech dimensions as being significantly impaired compared to a control group. Of these 24 deviant speech features, 10 dimensions (pitch variation,

Table 2-2. Intelligibility, rate, and efficiency of dysarthric speech following TBI, as assessed on the ASSIDS (Yorkston & Beukelman, 1981a).

	TBI Subjects (N = 43)		Control Subjects (N = 43)	
	M	SD	M	SD
% Word intelligibility	69.03	19.63	94.97	3.63
% Sentence intelligibility	79.89	23.32	99.37	0.59
Total words per minute (WPM)	127.31	45.68	240.08	35.02
Intelligible words per minute (IWPM)	106.32	56.24	238.71	34.50
Communication efficiency ratio (CER)	0.55	0.29	1.25	0.18

pitch steadiness, loudness variation, loudness maintenance, phrase length, general rate, general stress pattern, abnormal rate fluctuations, prolonged intervals, short rushes of speech) related to prosody, two (hypernasality, mixed nasality) pertained to resonance, three (precision of consonants and vowels, length of phonemes) to articulation, three (breath support for speech, forced inspiration/expiration) to respiration, five (harshness, strained-strangled vocal quality, intermittent breathiness, hoarseness, glottal fry) to phonation, and one to overall intelligibility (See Table 2-3).

Table 2-3. Speech dimensions significantly impaired/abnormal in dysarthric TBI subjects, compared to normal speakers.

A   OVERALL INTELLIGIBILITY

B   PROSODY

  • Normal pitch variation
  • Pitch steadiness
  • Normal loudness variation
  • Maintenance of loudness
  • Phrase length
  • Rate of speech
  • General stress pattern
  • Rate fluctuations
  • Prolonged intervals
  • Short rushes of speech

C   RESPIRATION

  • Breath support for speech
  • Forced inspiration/expiration
  • Audible inspiration

D   PHONATION

  • Harshness
  • Strained-strangled vocal quality
  • Intermittent breathiness
  • Hoarseness
  • Glottal fry

E   RESONANCE

  • Hypernasality
  • Mixed nasality

F   ARTICULATION

  • Precision of consonants
  • Precision of vowels
  • Length of phonemes

The most frequently occurring deviant speech dimensions related to impairments in prosody, resonance, articulation, respiratory support for speech, and overall speech intelligibility, with those deviant speech dimensions pertaining to phonation (vocal quality) being less apparent in the speech of the TBI subjects. Abnormal prosodic features, including impairments in rate, pitch and loudness variation, stress patterning, phrase length, and interval duration, were the most predominant deviant aspects of speech production identified in the TBI speakers. These prosodic disturbances constituted 60% of the most frequently occurring deviant speech dimensions. The 10 most frequently occurring deviant speech dimensions identified in this group were hypernasality, impaired rate of speech, imprecise consonant production, reduced normal pitch variation, reduced breath support for speech, abnormal stress, reduced phrase length, impaired overall intelligibility, prolonged intervals, and reduced normal loudness variation (See Table 2-4). The prosodic disturbances identified in this group of TBI dysarthric speakers are consistent with previous reports of prosodic impairment in head-injured individuals (Bellaire, Yorkston, & Beukelman, 1986; McHenry, 1998; Vogel & von Cramon, 1983; Yorkston, Beukelman, Minifie, & Sapir, 1984; Ziegler, Hoole, Hartmann, & von Cramon, 1988).

Hypernasality was identified as the most frequently occurring deviant speech dimension, evident in 98% of the TBI subjects. The majority of these subjects demonstrated mild to moderate degrees of hypernasality (33%–43%), with 24% of the subjects exhibiting severe hypernasality (See Table 2-5). A disturbance in the general rate of speech was perceived to be present in 95% of the TBI subjects, with the majority (79%) of these speakers demonstrating a reduction in rate. Abnormal speech rate was apparent to a mild-to-moderate degree in the majority of subjects, with only four (9%) individuals exhibiting a severe impairment in this speech dimension. Articulatory disturbance, in the form of imprecise consonant production, was found to be present in 91% of the TBI subjects, with 54% of these subjects demonstrating mild consonant imprecision, 33% exhibiting a moderate impairment, and the remaining 13% of the subjects rated as exhibiting severe consonant imprecision.

***Table* 2-4.** The 10 most frequently occurring deviant speech features in 43 dysarthric speakers following TBI.

Deviant Speech Feature	Frequency of Occurrence
Hypernasality	98%
Impaired rate	95%
Imprecise consonants	91%
Reduced normal pitch variation	88%
Reduced breath support for speech	88%
Abnormal stress pattern	86%
Reduced phrase length	84%
Impaired overall intelligibility	79%
Prolonged intervals	79%
Reduced normal loudness variation	77%

Both reduced normal variation of pitch and breath support for speech were identified in 88% of the TBI subjects, with the majority of these subjects (84% to 85%) mild-to-moderately impaired in their ability to vary pitch levels normally and to generate adequate breath support for speech.

Table 2-5. Frequency of occurrence and severity of deviant speech dimensions identified in dysarthric speakers following TBI (N = 43).

Deviant Speech Dimension	Frequency of Deviation in Total Sample of TBI Subjects		Severity of Deviation					
			Mild		Moderate		Severe	
	n	%	n	%	n	%	n	%
Hypernasality	42	98	18	43	14	33	10	24
General rate	41	95	22	54	15	37	4	9
Consonant precision	39	91	21	54	13	33	5	13
Pitch variation	38	88	16	42	16	42	6	16
Breath support	38	88	20	53	12	32	6	15
General stress	37	86	19	51	13	35	5	14
Phrase length	36	84	16	44	11	31	9	25
Overall intelligibility	34	79	17	50	14	41	3	9
Prolonged intervals	34	79	16	48	9	26	9	26
Loudness variation	33	77	12	36	15	46	6	18
Length phonemes	30	70	18	60	10	33	2	7
Rate maintenance	30	68	20	67	10	33	0	0
Pitch level	28	65	21	75	7	25	0	0
Vowel precision	25	58	14	56	9	36	2	8
Rate fluctuations	24	56	15	63	4	17	5	20
Harshness	23	53	14	61	8	35	1	4
Loudness maintenance	22	51	17	77	4	18	1	5
Hoarseness	21	49	10	48	10	48	1	4
Loudness level	20	46	16	80	3	15	1	5
Mixed nasality	19	44	15	79	3	16	1	5
Strain-strangled	18	42	13	72	4	22	1	6
Audible inspiration	18	42	10	55	3	17	5	28
Pitch steadiness	17	39	15	88	2	12	0	0
Short rushes	17	39	10	59	3	18	4	23
Intermittent breathiness	16	37	8	50	8	50	0	0
Glottal fry	15	35	11	73	4	27	0	0
Forced Insp/Exp	12	28	6	50	2	17	4	33
Ex. Pitch fluctuation	8	19	6	75	0	0	2	25

(continues)

Table 2-5. (continued)

Deviant Speech Dimension	Frequency of Deviation in Total Sample of TBI Subjects		Severity of Deviation					
			Mild		Moderate		Severe	
Ex. Loudness variation	7	16	5	71	0	0	2	29
Pitch breaks	5	12	4	80	1	20	0	0
Wetness	5	12	4	80	0	0	1	20
Grunt	0	0	0	0	0	0	0	0

Insp/Exp. = Inspiration/Expiration; Ex. = Excessive

The sixth most frequently occurring abnormal speech feature in the TBI subjects was an impaired stress pattern during speech, evident in 86% of the dysarthric speakers. Approximately half of the subjects were found to demonstrate a mild excess of stress on usually unstressed parts of speech, one-third exhibited a moderate excess of stress, and the remaining 14% of subjects were found to demonstrate a severe degree of excess and equal stress on syllables in all words. Eighty-four percent (84%) of the TBI subjects demonstrated a reduction in phrase length, which was evident to a mild-to-moderate degree in 75% of the subjects. Overall intelligibility was found to be affected in 79% of the TBI subjects, with half of the subjects requiring the listener to exert some effort to understand their speech. For 41% of the speakers, the listener was required to exert great effort to comprehend their speech output. Speech was barely recognizable in only three (9%) subjects. The reduction in overall intelligibility would appear to be the result of the combined effects of deficits in all aspects of speech production identified through perceptual analysis. The ninth most frequently occurring deviant speech dimension perceived to be present in the TBI subjects was prolonged intervals during speech, which occurred to a mild-to-moderate degree in 74% of the subjects who exhibited this feature, and to a severe degree in 26% of this group. Finally, a reduction in the normal variation of loudness was apparent in the speech of 77% of the TBI subjects, with the majority of the subjects exhibiting a mild-to-moderate impairment in loudness variation and 18% of the speakers demonstrating a severe loss of normal loudness variation.

Abnormal phonatory speech dimensions were not perceived to be present in the speech of dysarthric TBI subjects as frequently as other features, occurring in slightly more than 50% or less of the subjects (See Table 2-5). Harshness, hoarseness, and strained-strangled vocal qualities, intermittent breathiness, and glottal fry were perceived to be present in 35% to 53% of the TBI subjects. While these reduced frequencies of occurrence of abnormal phonatory features may indicate the true status of phonatory dysfunction in the speech of persons following TBI, these values may also reflect the inadequacies of perceptual analysis, in that vocal features such as these are often difficult to discriminate against a background of other deviant speech features. Physiological assessment of laryngeal function, therefore, is required to further elucidate the underlying bases of these deviant vocal qualities and possibly to identify other laryngeal deficits not apparent through perceptual analysis.

The range of disturbances identified in the speech production of the 43 dysarthric TBI speakers is consistent with the diffuse neurological damage that can occur with TBI. The speech mechanism is likely to be affected across all subsystems to some degree, with a combined effect of a marked reduction in the intelligibility of speech.

Motor Speech Subsystem Function Following TBI

Clinical assessment of the motor speech subsystem function of TBI subjects, using the Frenchay Dysarthria Assessment (FDA) (Enderby, 1983) has identified impairment in respiratory, lip, palatal, laryngeal, and tongue function, as well as deficits in reflexes such as coughing, swallowing, and saliva control (Theodoros et al., 1994). In the group of 43 TBI subjects evaluated in our laboratory, laryngeal function was found to be the most impaired aspect of the speech mechanism, with moderate to severe deficits in pitch variation and vocal quality during speech evident in these individuals (See Figure 2-1). Laryngeal function was also impaired to a moderate degree in relation to phonation time and volume variation. Palatal function in the TBI subjects was rated as being moderately impaired during speech due to the perception of hypernasality in the subjects' speech output. This finding was supported by an observed impairment in palatal maintenance to a mild-to-moderate degree in this group. A moderate degree of tongue dysfunction during speech was observed in the TBI subjects with mild-to-moderate impairments in specific nonspeech tongue movements (lateral, elevation, and alternate movements) apparent on testing. The appearance of the tongue at rest and protrusion movements were also noted to be mildly abnormal in this group. Lip function was rated as being mildly impaired for specific nonspeech movements (lip spread, seal, and alternate movements), with a further reduction in lip function to a mild to moderate degree during speech. The TBI subjects were also found to exhibit a mild to moderate reduction in breath support for speech. Neurological impairment of basic oromotor reflexes was evident in the TBI subjects in the form of mild impairments in coughing, swallowing, and saliva control.

Type and Severity of Dysarthria Following TBI

The type and severity of dysarthria evident in persons following TBI is dependent upon the site and extent of the lesion(s) induced by the TBI. The nature of TBI is such that the subsequent brain damage may result in heterogeneous disturbances in the neuromuscular control of the speech production mechanism. As a result, it is possible for any type and degree of severity of dysarthria, or combinations thereof, to manifest in this population.

Various types of dysarthria have been observed in individuals following TBI. Marquardt, Stoll, and Sussman (1990) have suggested that the most frequently occurring dysarthria following CHI would appear to be spastic dysarthria resulting from bilateral upper motor neuron damage and lesions affecting pyramidal and extrapyramidal fiber tracts. In that the upper motor neurons, which convey impulses from the motor areas of the cerebral cortex, are located in the frontal lobes, radiological findings indicating a common occurrence of anterior and frontal lobe lesions following CHI (Langfitt et al., 1986; Netsell & Lefkowitz, 1992; Wilson, Hadley, Weidmann, & Teasdale, 1992)

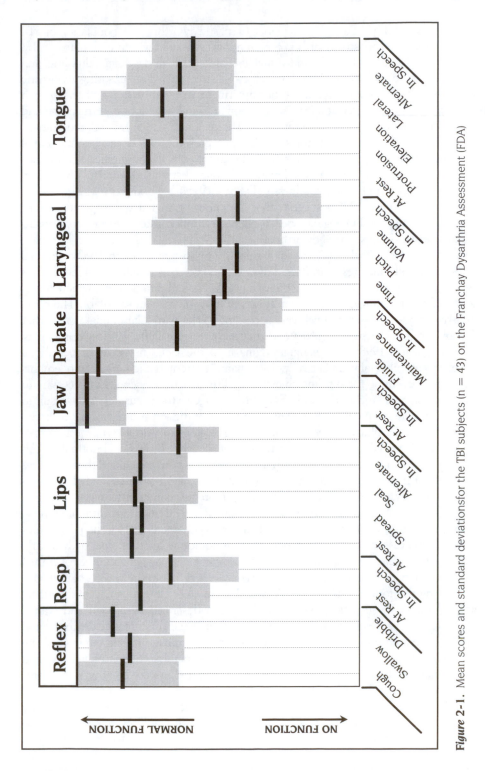

Figure 2-1. Mean scores and standard deviations for the TBI subjects (n = 43) on the Franchay Dysarthria Assessment (FDA)

support the suggestion of a higher incidence of spastic dysarthria in a population of TBI dysarthric speakers. Spastic dysarthria is commonly associated with pseudobulbar palsy, a clinical syndrome in which the individual also presents with dysphagia, drooling, and emotional lability (Duffy, 1995a; Thompson-Ward, 1998). The ensuring dysarthric speech disturbance is a consequence of impairment in all subsystems of the speech mechanism to some degree and is related to slowness and a reduction in the range and force of movement, and excessive muscle spasticity (Duffy, 1995a). The predominant characteristics of spastic dysarthria include both prosodic excess (excess and equal stress)and insufficiency (reduced stress), a reduced rate of speech, imprecise consonant and vowel production, hypernasality, harshness, strained-strangled, effortful phonation, and monopitch and monoloudness (Duffy, 1995a; Thompson-Ward, 1998). Diagnostically, Duffy (1995a) suggests that a strained-strangled vocal quality, a slow speech rate, and slow but regular speech alternate motion rates are the most distinguishing features of this type of dysarthria.

Damage to the cranial nerve nuclei within the brainstem or to the bulbar cranial nerves specifically, may result in flaccid dysarthria. The speech deficits evident in this type of dysarthria are due to reduced muscle weakness and muscle tone, which subsequently affects the range, speed, and accuracy of movement (Duffy, 1995b). The characteristics of flaccid dysarthria will vary according to the particular cranial nerves that are damaged and the speech subsystems that are affected (Duffy, 1995b; Murdoch & Thompson-Ward, 1998). For example, damage to the facial nerve in its peripheral course, either unilaterally or bilaterally, will impair the strength and range of movements of the lips, preventing them from achieving the firm articulatory contacts necessary to produce plosive and fricative sounds. Similarly, damage to the vagus nerve can result in unilateral or bilateral paralysis of the levator muscles of the soft palate and the constrictor muscles of the pharynx, resulting in varying degrees of velopharyngeal incompetence, causing nasal emission and hypernasality of speech. Clusters of abnormal speech characteristics identified in persons with flaccid dysarthria have included those features associated with phonatory incompetence (breathiness, short phrases, audible inspiration), resonatory incompetence (hypernasality, imprecise consonants, nasal emission, short phrases), and phonatory-prosodic insufficiency (harshness, monoloudness, monopitch; Darley et al., 1975). Flaccid dysarthria is characterized by the presence of phonatory and resonatory incompetence, which is not found in other types of dysarthria (Duffy, 1995b). As a TBI may result in the simultaneous damage of a number of cranial nerves, a variety of flaccid dysarthric features may be evident in the speech of individuals following this form of brain insult. A typical example of a range of flaccid dysarthric features in a single subject following TBI has been described by Netsell and Daniel (1979). This 20-year-old man with a severe dysarthric speech disturbance demonstrated markedly impaired respiratory and laryngeal function, complete flaccid paralysis of the velopharyngeal muscles, and moderate to severe flaccid paralysis of the tongue, jaw, and lip musculature. These physiological impairments resulted in very breathy, soft, hypernasal speech, which was minimally intelligible.

A TBI may also cause bilateral or generalized damage to the cerebellum, resulting in ataxic dysarthria. Several studies have reported on the presence of predominantly ataxic dysarthria in TBI subjects (Simmons, 1983;Yorkston& Beukelman, 1981b; Yorkston et al., 1984). This form of dysarthria is characterized by impairments predominantly in articulation and prosody, resulting from the effects of incoordination and reduced muscle tone in the speech musculature (Duffy, 1995c; Murdoch & Theodoros, 1998). Speech movements are slow, and typically inaccurate in force, range, timing, and direction (Duffy, 1995c). According to Brown, Darley, and Aronson (1970), the abnormal speech features evident in ataxic dysarthria are associated with articulatory inaccuracy (imprecise consonants and distorted vowel production, irregular articulatory breakdowns), prosodic excess (excess and equal stress, prolongation of phonemes and intervals, slow rate), and phonatory-prosodic insufficiency (harshness, monopitch, monoloudness).

Forms of hypokinetic and hyperkinetic dysarthria may also become evident in the speech of TBI individuals following damage to the extrapyramidal system, involving such subcortical structures as the basal ganglia, the substantia nigra, the red nuclei, and the subthalamic nuclei of the upper brainstem (Murdoch, 1990). Marquardt et al. (1990) suggested that hypokinetic and hyperkinetic dysarthia were less common in dysarthric speakers following TBI than the previously described dysarthric speech patterns.

Hypokinetic dysarthria is typified by the presence of deviant phonatory, articulatory, and prosodic deficits that reflect the effects of rigidity, reduced force and range of movement, and variable speed of movement, associated with basal ganglia pathology, on speech production (Duffy, 1995d; Theodoros & Murdoch, 1998a). Specifically, the deviant perceptual features evident in hypokinetic speech include monopitch, monoloudness, reduced stress, imprecise articulation, inappropriate silences, short rushes of speech, harsh/hoarse and breathy vocal quality, low pitch, repetition of phonemes, increased rate of speech, impaired control of volume, and variable rate (Darley, Aronson, & Brown, 1969b; Duffy, 1995d; Theodoros & Murdoch, 1998a). While the presence of a rapid rate of speech is diagnostic of this type of dysarthria, some perceptual features, such as monopitch, reduced stress, monoloudness, inappropriate silences, short rushes of speech, and variable rate, are also usually more distinctive in hypokinetic dysarthria than in any other single type (Duffy, 1995d).

Hyperkinetic dysarthria is characterized by the presence of highly variable deviant speech features, resulting from unpredictable, involuntary movements and variations in muscle tone (Duffy, 1995e; Theodoros & Murdoch, 1998b). These abnormal involuntary movements disturb the rhythm and rate of speech movements and may involve any or all subsystems of the speech mechanism, although this form of dysarthria may result from disruption to only one component, or part thereof (e.g., tongue, palate etc.; Duffy, 1995e; Theodoros & Murdoch, 1998b). There are a variety of movement disorders that may result in a form of hyperkinetic dysarthria, and these include dyskinesia, myoclonus, tics, chorea, ballism, athetosis, dystonia, spasm, and tremor. Descriptions of these movement disorders and their effects on speech are detailed in Duffy (1995e) and Theodoros and Murdoch (1998b). Although the prosodic aspects of speech involving variations in pitch and loudness, stress, rate, phrase and phoneme length, and interval duration between words are often the most affected in hyperkinetic dysarthria due to the involuntary movements, other deviant speech features may include abrupt inhalations and exhalations, momentary voice arrests, strained-strangled vocal quality, imprecise articulation, irregular articulatory breakdowns, and hypernasality (Darley et al., 1975; Duffy, 1995e; Theodoros & Murdoch, 1998b; Zraick & LaPointe, 1997).

Since a TBI frequently involves simultaneous damage to several areas of the brain, it is not unusual for a pattern of mixed dysarthria involving combinations of the various types of dysarthria, to prevail as the speech disorder (Marquardt et al., 1990; Murdoch, 1990; Yorkston & Beukelman, 1981a). The specific speech deficits exhibited by the speaker are dependent on the site(s) and extent of the brain damage.

Although the previously mentioned types of dysarthria have been identified in isolated cases of TBI dysarthric speakers, there have been few group studies that have sought to document the incidence and severity of the different dysarthria types in a TBI population. A recent study by Theodoros et al. (1994) identified the presence of four specific types of dysarthria (spastic, hypokinetic, ataxic, and flaccid dysarthria) and four mixed forms of dysarthria (spastic-ataxic, spastic-hypokinetic, spastic-flaccid, and flaccid-ataxic dysarthria) in a group of 20 CHI dysarthric speakers. Within this group, spastic-ataxic dysarthria was found to be the most prevalent form of dysarthria, occurring in 25% of the subject group. The various types of dysarthria identified in this group ranged in severity from mild to severe, with the majority of the subjects exhibiting a mild-to-moderate degree of speech impairment.

In an investigation of a larger sample of dysarthric speakers (N= 43) in our laboratory, including the subject cohort in the Theodoros et al. (1994) study, a similar pattern of type and severity of dysarthria was apparent (See Table 2-6). In this particular group of TBI subjects, the mixed forms of dysarthria (spastic-ataxic, spastic-hypokinetic, spastic-flaccid, flaccid-ataxic, spastic-flaccid-ataxic) were found to be more prevalent in the speech of the TBI subjects (53%), compared to specific types of dysarthria (spastic, ataxic, flaccid, hypokinetic; 45%). The most frequently occurring types of dysarthria evident in this group were spastic-ataxic, spastic, hypokinetic, and flaccid dysarthria.

Approximately half of the 43 persons with dysarthria following TBI demonstrated a mild to mild-moderate degree of severity of dysarthria (51%), while the remaining individuals exhibited dysarthric speech disturbances that were considered to be moderately-to-severely impaired (49%) (See Table 2-6). The most severe dysarthric impairments in the TBI subjects were evident in those individuals with spastic-ataxic, spastic-hypokinetic, flaccid, and flaccid-ataxic types of dysarthria. The increased level of severity in the mixed types of dysarthria is consistent with the widespread neurological damage underlying the manifestation of these forms of dysarthria. The severe level of impairment associated with flaccid dysarthria in this group of TBI subjects would appear to be due to the effects of sudden acceleration/deceleration forces on the head and neck, resulting in damage to the brainstem and the cranial nerves involved in speech production.

Summary

Dysarthria has been found to occur in approximately one-third of the TBI population. The speech disorder in these cases is characterized by marked variability in relation to neuropathology, recovery patterns and long-term outcomes, the type of dysarthria, and the specific perceptual speech abnormalities evident in an individual's speech production. Perceptually, the speech output of dysarthric speakers following TBI features deficits in all aspects of speech production. The most frequently

Table 2-6. Type and severity of dysarthria following TBI (N = 43).

Type of Dysarthria	n	%	Mild	Mild-Moderate	Moderate	Moderate-Severe
Spastic	7	16	4	1	2	
Hypokinetic	5	12	3	2		
Flaccid	5	12	1		2	2
Ataxic	2	5	2			
Spastic-ataxic	13	30	5	2	3	1
Spastic-hypokinetic	3	7		1	1	
Spastic-flaccid	2	5			1	1
Spastic-flaccid-Ataxic	1	2			1	
Flaccid-ataxic	4	9			1	2
Non-classifiable	1	2	1			

occurring deviant speech dimensions are related to resonance, prosody, articulation, and respiration. Speech intelligibility and rate of speech in these individuals are significantly reduced as compared to normal speakers. A variety of different types of dysarthria may be present in this population, with the mixed forms of the speech disturbance being the most prevalent. The level of severity of dysarthria spans a continuum from mild to severe across a group of TBI individuals, with mild to mild-moderate dysarthria occurring in approximately one-half of the population, and moderate-to-severe dysarthric speech disturbances evident in the remaining individuals. The diverse classifications of dysarthria and the varying degrees of impairment identified in dysarthric speakers following TBI reflect a wide distribution and extent of lesion sites, as well as extensive variation in the deviant speech features exhibited by these subjects. Perceptual assessment of the dysarthric speech disturbance in persons following TBI, therefore, requires careful consideration of each individual, with the underlying assumption that a number of possible combinations of abnormal perceptual features may be present in the speech output. Furthermore, the findings of the perceptual assessments of the dysarthric speech disturbances in individuals following TBI should be confirmed through physiological analyses of the motor speech subsystems. A comprehensive perceptual and physiological evaluation of each person's speech mechanism will provide clearer directions for the development of effective treatment programs. Reports of comprehensive studies of physiological analyses of each of the major motor subsystems of the speech production mechanism in dysarthric speakers following TBI will follow in Chapters 3, 4, 5, and 6 in this book.

Although the perceptual features of the dysarthric speech disturbance in persons following TBI may be obvious, and the basic physiological impairments identified instrumentally, the degree of disability experienced by the individual in communicating effectively in social contexts is not as readily apparent, nor routinely targeted in therapy. Furthermore, enhancing the opportunities for the individual to participate in society in a meaningful and productive manner is frequently overlooked, and is generally outside the therapeutic arena of the speech pathologist. A model for intervention which encompasses this broader management perspective is required to facilitate successful reintegration of the TBI individual with dysarthria into society. Such a framework for intervention is presented in Chapter 8.

References

Aten, J. L. (1988). Spastic dysarthria: Revising understanding of the disorder and speech treatment procedures. *Journal of Head Trauma Rehabilitation, 3,* 63–73.

Bauer, B., Gerstenbrand, R., & Rump, E. (1979). Varieties of locked-in syndrome. *Journal of Neurology, 221,* 77–91.

Bellaire, K., Yorkston, K.M., & Beukelman, D.R. (1986). Modification of breathing pattern to increase naturalness of a mildly dysarthric speaker. *Journal of Communication Disorders, 19,* 271–280.

Beukelman, D.R., & Garrett, K. (1988). Augmentative and alternative communication for adults with acquired severe communication disorders. *Augmentative and Alternative Communication, 4,* 104–121.

Beukelman, D.R. & Yorkston, K.M. (1977). A communication system for the severely dysarthric speaker with an intact language system. *Journal of Speech and Hearing Disorders, 42,* 265–270.

Botez, M. & Barbeau, A. (1971). Role of subcortical structures, and particularly of the thalamus, in the mechanisms of speech and language. *International Journal of Neurology, 8,* 300–320.

Brand, H.A., Matsko, T.A., & Avart, H.N. (1988). Speech prosthesis retention problems in dysarthria: Case report. *Archives of Physical Medicine and Rehabilitation, 69,* 213–214.

Brown, J.R., Darley, F.L., & Aronson, A.E. (1970). Ataxic dysarthria. *International Journal of Neurology, 7,* 302–318.

Cancelliere, A., & Kertesz, A. (1990). Lesion localization in acquired deficits of emotional expression and comprehension. *Brain and Cognition, 13,* 133–147.

Darley, F.L. (1984). Perceptual analysis of the dysarthrias. *Seminars in Speech and Language, 5,* 267–268.

Darley, F.L., Aronson, A.E., & Brown, J.R. (1969a). Differential diagnostic patterns of dysarthria. *Journal of Speech and Hearing Research, 12,* 246–269.

Darley, F.L., Aronson, A.E., & Brown, J.R. (1969b). Clusters of deviant speech dimensions in the dysarthrias. *Journal of Speech and Hearing Research, 12,* 462–496.

Darley, F.L., Aronson, A.E., Brown, J.R. (1975). *Motor Speech Disorders.* Philadelphia: W.B. Saunders Company.

Dongilli, P.A., Hakel, M.E., & Beukelman, D.R. (1992). Recovery of functional speech following traumatic brain injury. *Journal of Head Trauma Rehabilitation, 7,* 91–101.

Duffy, J.R. (1995a). Spastic dysarthria. In J.R. Duffy, *Motor Speech Disorders: Substrates, Differential Diagnosis, and Management* (pp.128–144). St. Louis: Mosby.

Duffy, J.R. (1995b). Flaccid dysarthria. In J.R. Duffy, *Motor Speech Disorders: Substrates, Differential Diagnosis, and Management* (pp.99–127). St. Louis: Mosby.

Duffy, J.R. (1995c). Ataxic dysarthria. In J.R. Duffy, *Motor Speech Disorders: Substrates, Differential Diagnosis, and Management* (pp.145–165). St. Louis: Mosby.

Duffy, J.R. (1995d). Hypokinetic dysarthria. In J.R. Duffy, *Motor Speech Disorders: Substrates, Differential Diagnosis, and Management* (pp.166–188). St. Louis: Mosby.

Duffy, J.R. (1995e). Hyperkinetic dysarthria. In J.R. Duffy, *Motor Speech Disorders: Substrates, Differential Diagnosis, and Management* (pp.189–221). St. Louis: Mosby.

Enderby, P.M. (1983). *Frenchay Dysarthria Assessment.* San Diego: College-Hill Press.

Enderby, P. & Crow, E. (1990). Long-term recovery patterns of severe dysarthria following head injury. *British Journal of Disorders of Communication, 25,* 341–354.

Fisher, H.B., & Logemann, J.A. (1971). *The Fisher-Logemann Test of Articulation Competence.* Boston: Houghton Mifflin.

FitzGerald, F.J., Murdoch, B.E., & Chenery, H.J. (1987). Multiple sclerosis: Associated speech and language disorders. *Australian Journal of Human Communication Disorders, 15,* 15–33.

Frank, E.M., & Barrineau, S. (1996). Current speech-language assessment protocols for adults with traumatic brain injury. *Journal of Medical Speech-Language Pathology, 4,* 81–101.

Gentry, L., Godersky, J., & Thompson, B. (1988). MR imaging of head trauma: Review of the distribution and radiopathologic features of traumatic lesions. *American Journal of Nuclear Medicine, 150,* 663–672.

Goldberg, G. (1985). Supplementary motor area structure and function: review and hypotheses. *Behavioural Brain Science, 8,* 567–616.

Groher, M. (1977). Language and memory disorders following closed head trauma. *Journal of Speech and Hearing Research, 20,* 212–223.

Groher, M. (1989). Communication disorders in adults. In M. Rosenthal, E. Griffith, M. Bond, & J.D. Miller (Eds.), *Rehabilitation of the Adult and Child with Traumatic Brain Injury* (pp. 148–162). Philadelphia: F.A. Davis.

Hagen, C., Malkmus, D., & Durham, P. (1979). *Rehabilitation of the Head Injured Adult: Comprehensive Physical Management.* Downey: Professional Staff Association of Rancho Los Amigos Hospital.

Harris, B. & Murry, T. (1984). Dysarthria and asphagia: A case study of neuromuscular treatment. *Archives of Physical Medicine and Rehabilitation, 65,* 408–412.

Hartley, L.L., & Levin, H.S. (1990). Linguistic deficits after closed head injury: A current appraisal. *Aphasiology, 4,* 353–370.

Jennet, W.B., & Plum, F. (1972). The persistent vegetative state: A syndrome in search of a name. *Lancet, 1,* 734.

Keatley, A. & Wirz, S. (1994). Is 20 years too long? Improving intelligibility in long-standing dysarthria: A single case treatment study. *European Journal of Disorders of Communication, 29,* 183–202.

Keenan, J.E. & Barnhart, K.S. (1993). Development of yes/no systems in individuals with severe traumatic brain injuries. *Augmentative and Alternative Communication, 9,* 184–190.

Kent, R. & Netsell, R. (1978). Articulatory abnormalities in athetoid cerebral palsy. *Journal of Speech and Hearing Disorders, 42,* 353–373.

Kent, R. & Rosenbek, J. (1982). Prosodic disturbance and neurologic lesion. *Brain and Language, 15,* 259–291.

Kent, R.D., Weismer, G., Kent, J.D., & Rosenbek, J.R. (1989). Toward phonetic intelligibility testing in dysarthria. *Journal of Speech and Hearing Disorders, 54,* 482–499.

Kuehn, D.P. & Wachtel, J.M. (1994). CPAP therapy for treating hypernasality following closed head injury. In J.A. Till, K.M. Yorkston & D.R. Beukelman (Eds.), *Motor Speech Disorders: Advances in Assessment and Treatment* (pp. 207–212). Baltimore: Paul H. Brookes Publishing.

Langfitt, T.W., Obrist, W.D., Alavi, A., Grossman, R.I., Zimmerman, R., Jaggi, J., Uzell, B., Reivich, M., & Patton, D.R. (1986). Computerized tomography, magnetic resonance imaging, and positron emission tomography in the study of head trauma. *Journal of Neurosurgery, 64,* 760–767.

Lefkowitz, D. & Netsell, R. (1994). Correlation of clinical deficits with anatomical lesions, post-traumatic speech disorders, and MRI. *Journal of Medical Speech-Language Pathology, 2,* 1–15.

Levin, H.S. (1981). Aphasia in closed head injury. In M.T. Sarno (Ed.), *Acquired Aphasia* (pp. 427–463). New York: Academic Press.

Levin, H.S., Madison, C.F., Bailey, C.B., Meyers, C.A., Eisenberg, H.M., & Faustino, C.G. (1983). Mutism after closed head injury. *Archives of Neurology, 40,* 601–606.

Ley, R. & Bryden, M. (1982). A dissociation of right and left hemispheric effects for reorganizing emotional tone and verbal content. *Brain and Cognition, 1,* 3–9.

Light, J., Beesley, M., & Collier, B. (1988). Transition through multiple augmentative communication systems: A three-year case study of a head injured adolescent. *Augmentative and Alternative Communication, 4,* 2–14.

Luzzatti, C., Willmes, K., Taricco, M., Colombo, C., & Chiesa, G. (1989). Language disturbances after severe head injury: Do neurological or other associated cognitive disorders influence type, severity, and evolution of the verbal impairment? A preliminary report. *Aphasiology, 3,* 643–653.

MacLean, P. (1970). The triune brain, emotion, and scientific bias. In F. Schmitt (Ed.), *The Neurosciences Second Study Program.* New York: Rockefeller University Press.

Marquardt, T.P., Stoll, J., & Sussman, H. (1990). Disorders of communication in traumatic brain injury. In E.D. Bigler (Ed.), *Traumatic Brain Injury: Mechanisms of Damage, Assessment, Intervention, and Outcome* (pp. 181–205). Austin:Pro-Ed.

McHenry, M. (1998). The ability to effect intended stress following traumatic brain injury. *Brain Injury, 12,* 495–503.

Mendez, M., Adams, N., & Lewandowski, K. (1989). Neurobehavioural changes associated with caudate lesions. *Neurology, 39,* 349–454.

Mesulam, M. (1990). Large-scale neurocognitive networks and distributed processing for attention, language, and memory. *Annals of Neurology, 28,* 597–613.

Murdoch, B.E. (1990). *Acquired Speech and Language Disorders: A Neuroanatomical and Functional Neurological Approach.* London: Chapman and Hall.

Murdoch, B.E. & Theodoros, D. G. (1998). Ataxic dysarthria. In B.E. Murdoch (Ed.), *Dysarthria: A Physiological Approach to Assessment and Treatment* (pp.241–265). Cheltenham: Stanley Thornes (Publishers) Ltd.

Murdoch, B.E. & Thompson-Ward, E.C. (1998). Flaccid dysarthria. In B.E. Murdoch (Ed.), *Dysarthria: A Physiological Approach to Assessment and Treatment* (pp. 176–204). Cheltenham: Stanley Thornes (Publishers) Ltd.

Najenson, T., Sazbon, L., Fiselzon, J., Becker, E., & Schecter, I. (1978). Recovery of communicative functions after prolonged traumatic coma. *Scandanavian Journal of Rehabilitation Medicine, 10,* 15–21.

Nemec, R.E. & Cohen, K. (1984). EMG biofeedback in the modification of hypertonia in spastic dysarthria: Case report. *Archives of Physical Medicine and Rehabilitation, 65,* 103–104.

Netsell, R. & Daniel, B. (1979). Dysarthria in adults: Physiologic approach in rehabilitation. *Archives of Physical Medicine and Rehabilitation, 60,* 502–508.

Netsell, R. & Lefkowitz, D. (1992). Speech production following traumatic brain injury: Clinical and research implications. *American Speech-Language-Hearing Association Special Interests Division: Neurophysiology and Neurogenic Speech and Language Disorders, 2,* 1–8.

Robertson, S.J. (1982). *Dysarthria Profile.* San Antonio: Communication Skill Builders.

Rusk, H., Block, J., & Lowmann, E. (1969). Rehabilitation of the brain-injured patient: A report of 157 cases with long-term follow-up of 118. In E. Walker, W. Caveness, & M. Critchley (Eds.), *The Late Effects of Head Injury* (pp. 327–332). Springfield: Charles C. Thomas.

Sarno, M.T. (1980). The nature of verbal impairment after closed head injury. *Journal of Nervous and Mental Disease, 168,* 685–692.

Sarno, M.T. (1984). Verbal impairment after closed head injury: Report of a replication study. *Journal of Nervous and Mental Disease, 172,* 475–479.

Sarno, M.T., & Levin, H. S. (1985). Speech and language disorders after closed head injury. In J. K. Darby (Ed.), *Speech Evaluation in Neurology: Adult Disorders* (pp. 323–339). New York: Grune and Stratton.

Simmons, N. (1983). Acoustic analysis of ataxic dysarthria: An approach to monitoring treatment. In W. Berry (Ed.), *Clinical Dysarthria* (pp. 283–294). San Diego: College-Hill Press.

Taylor Sarno, M., Buonaguro, A., & Levita, E. (1986). Characteristics of verbal impairment in closed head injured patients. *Archives of Physical Medicine and Rehabilitation, 67,* 400–405.

Theodoros, D.G. & Murdoch, B.E. (1998a). Hypokinetic dysarthria. In B.E. Murdoch (Ed.), *Dysarthria: A Physiological Approach to Assessment and Treatment* (pp. 266–313). Cheltenham: Stanley Thornes (Publishers) Ltd.

Theodoros, D.G. & Murdoch, B.E. (1998b). Hyperkinetic dysarthria. In B. E. Murdoch (Ed.), *Dysarthria: A Physiological Approach to Assessment and Treatment* (pp. 314–336). Cheltenham: Stanley Thornes (Publishers) Ltd.

Theodoros, D.G., Murdoch, B.E., & Chenery, H J. (1994). Perceptual speech characteristics of dysarthric speakers following severe closed head injury. *Brain Injury, 8,* 101–124.

Thompson-Ward, E.C. (1998). Spastic dysarthria. In B. E. Murdoch (Ed.), *Dysarthria: A Physiological Approach to Assessment and Treatment* (pp. 205–241). Cheltenham: Stanley Thornes (Publishers) Ltd.

Thomsen, I.V. (1975). Evaluation and outcome of aphasia in patients with severe closed head trauma. *Journal of Neurology, Neurosurgery, and Psychiatry, 38,* 713–718.

Thomsen, I.V. (1984). Late outcome of very severe blunt head trauma: A 10–15 year second follow-up. *Journal of Neurology, Neurosurgery, and Psychiatry, 47,* 260–268.

Vogel, M. & von Cramon, D. (1982). Dysphonia after traumatic midbrain damage: A follow-up study. *Folia Phoniatrica, 34,* 150–159.

Vogel, M. & von Cramon, D. (1983). Articulatory recovery after traumatic midbrain damage: A follow-up study. *Folia Phoniatrica, 35,* 294–309.

Von Cramon, D. (1981). Traumatic mutism and the subsequent reorganization of speech functions. *Neuropsychology, 19,* 801–805.

Wilson, J.T.L., Hadley, D. M., Weidmann, K. D., & Teasdale, G.M. (1992). Intercorrelations of lesions detected by magnetic resonance imaging after closed head injury. *Brain Injury, 6,* 391–399.

Workinger, M. & Netsell, R. (1992). Restoration of intelligible speech 13 years post-head injury. *Brain Injury, 6,* 183–187.

Yorkston, K.M. (1996). Treatment efficacy: Dysarthria. *Journal of Speech and Hearing Research, 39.* S46-S57.

Yorkston, K.M., & Beukelman, D.R. (1981a). *Assessment of Intelligibility of Dysarthric Speech.* Austin: Pro-Ed.

Yorkston, K.M., & Beukelman, D.R. (1981b). Ataxic dysarthria: Treatment sequence based on intelligibility and prosodic considerations. *Journal of Speech and Hearing Disorders, 46,* 398–404.

Yorkston, KM., & Beukelman, D.R., (1991). Motor speech disorders. In D.R. Beukelman and K.M. Yorkston (Eds.), *Communication Disorders Following Traumatic Brain Injury: Management of Cognitive, Language, and Motor Impairments* (pp. 251–316). Austin: Pro-Ed.

Yorkston, K.M., Beukelman, D. R., Minifie, F.D., & Sapir, S. (1984). Assessment of stress patterning in dysarthric speakers. In M. McNeil, A. Aronson, & J. Rosenbek (Eds.), *The Dysarthrias: Physiology, Acoustics, Perception, Management* (pp. 131–162). San Diego: College-Hill Press.

Yorkston, K.M., Beukelman, D.R., & Traynor, D. (1984). *Computerized Assessment of intelligibility of dysarthric speech.* Tigard: C.C. Publications.

Yorkston, K.M., Honsinger, M.J., Mitsuda, P.M., & Hammen, V. (1989). The relationship between speech and swallowing disorders in head injured patients. *Journal of Head Trauma Rehabilitation, 4,* 1–16.

Ziegler, W., Hoole, P., Hartmann, E., & von Cramon, D. (1988). Accelerated speech in dysarthria after acquired brain injury: Acoustic correlates. *British Journal of Disorders of Communication, 23,* 215–228.

Zraick, R.I. & LaPointe, L.L. (1997). Hyperkinetic dysarthria. In M.R. McNeil (Ed.), *Clinical Management of Sensorimotor Speech Disorders* (pp. 249–260). New York: Thieme.

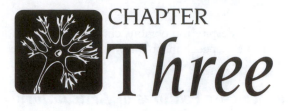

CHAPTER
Three

Articulatory Dysfunction Following Traumatic Brain Injury

Deborah G. Theodoros, Bruce E. Murdoch, Justine V. Goozée

Introduction

The articulatory subsystem of the speech production mechanism plays a crucial role in the final execution of speech, with the articulators (lips, tongue, and jaw) impeding the expiratory breath stream at various target positions to produce specific phonemes. The dysarthric speech disturbance associated with traumatic brain injury (TBI) can be directly related to impairment of the specific articulators of speech. Indeed, the neurological impairment that occurs following TBI may have substantial effects on the accuracy, rate, timing, strength, endurance, and range of movement of the articulators of speech, resulting in impaired speech intelligibility. The diversity of neurological impairment following TBI suggests that the effects on the articulators are likely to be extremely variable. A range of articulatory disturbances would therefore be expected to occur in individuals following TBI. To date, only a limited number of studies have been reported that have investigated the perceptual, acoustic, and underlying pathophysiological bases of the articulatory dysfunction following TBI, despite the obvious clinical manifestations of dysfunction in this component of the speech mechanism.

Perceptual and Acoustic Features of Articulatory Dysfunction Following TBI

Perceptual analyses of dysarthric speech following TBI have identified high incidences of articulatory disturbance in this population. Theodoros, Murdoch, & Chenery (1994) identified the presence of abnormal articulatory speech features (imprecise vowels and consonants and prolonged phonemes) in 65% to 95% of their group of 20 TBI subjects. A perceptual investigation of the speech production of a group of 43 TBI subjects completed by the current authors (See Chapter 2), indicated that 91% of the subjects exhibited consonant imprecision to a mild (54%), moderate (33%), and severe (13%) degree. The length of phonemes was considered to be prolonged in 70% of the subjects to a mild-to-moderate degree in the majority of cases. Vowel imprecision was evident in more than half (58%) of the dysarthric speakers, with 92% of these subjects producing vowels that were mild or moderately imprecise. These perceptual findings of articulatory disturbance were supported by the clinical assessment of the subjects' articulatory subsystem, using the Frenchay Dysarthria Assessment (FDA; Enderby, 1983), which identified mild-to-moderate impairments in nonspeech tongue movements, and a moderate degree of tongue dysfunction during speech. Similarly, lip function was noted to be mildly impaired for nonspeech lip movements, and mildly to moderately impaired during speech. Associated with these deficits in lip and tongue movements was the finding of a significant reduction in the rate of speech for the TBI subjects as determined by the Assessment of Intelligibility of Dysarthric Speech (ASSIDS; Yorkston & Beukelman, 1981; See Chapter 2, "Perceptual Assessment of Dysarthria Following TBI").

In general, the findings of acoustic studies of articulatory disturbance in individuals following TBI support those of the perceptual analyses. Acoustic features, including increased word and syllable durations; centralization of vowel formants resulting in vowel reduction and distortion (consistent with articulatory undershoot); spirantization; and the presence of slow, large amplitude cycles in the formant trajectories consistent with slow, exaggerated protrusions and retractions of the tongue, have been identified in TBI dysarthric speakers (Ziegler & von Cramon, 1983a, b, 1986). Reduced diadochokinetic speech rates in individuals following TBI have also been identified acoustically. Blumberger, Sullivan, and Clément (1995) found that the performance of a group of 28 TBI subjects (nine of whom were dysarthric) on a series of diadochokinetic rate tasks was significantly impaired, compared to that of a control group. In addition, these investigators found that the diadochokinetic rate tasks most effective in discriminating between the TBI subjects and the controls included the rapid repetition of /ta/, /ba/, /da/, and /cha/.

Recovery of Articulatory Function Following TBI

The recovery of articulatory function in TBI subjects following mutism has been documented both perceptually and acoustically. In a study of five subjects following TBI with traumatic midbrain syndrome, Vogel and von Cramon (1983) provided a detailed report of the recovering articulatory features and the corresponding spectrographic findings of this process. While mute, these patients were unable to produce individual speech sounds or perform simple nonspeech lip and tongue movements, such as spreading, rounding, protrusion, and elevation, with normal speed and accuracy. Individual vowels could not be easily distinguished as all vowels were perceived as a "schwa." Spectrographic analysis of this stage of recovery identified a gap in the upper frequency range where consonant production should have occurred, while the frequency values for the first and second formants were consistent with the production of a "schwa" vowel. During stage two of recovery, the patients began to produce individual speech sounds, the first of which was the bilabial /m/. The subjects began to approximate the labial and alveopalatal zone with their tongue, although stricture was inadequate for stop and fricative consonants. All patients were noted to have difficulty elevating the tongue to achieve the closure necessary for palatal and velar consonants. The subjects demonstrated impaired voiced-voiceless distinction, with a tendency to phonate throughout the entire utterance. The vowel distortion evident was due to centralization of high, mid and low vowels. These findings were supported acoustically, with no visible evidence of fricative or stop articulation, although the tendency to phonate indiscriminately throughout an utterance was apparent.

At the third stage of recovery, the patients were able to achieve the target of oral closures and strictures for continuants and stops, although the normally tense stops remained laxly articulated (e.g., velar plosives were affricated or produced as fricatives). Fricative articulation was usually achieved at this stage, with the normal production of labial, palatal, and velar fricatives. Lingual fricatives /s/ and /sh/, however, remained poorly differentiated. The subjects continued to demonstrate difficulties with the affricates and the /r/ phoneme. Voicing errors were noted to have reduced at this stage, with the most frequent error type being devoicing of normally voiced segments. With recovery to this stage, all vowels could now be identified, although the high vowels required greater approximation. Acoustically, a gap and a small spike for stop articulation were now visible on the sonogram, consistent with the emergence of complete oral closures for stop productions. Lax articulation, however, was evident in the weak or missing vertical striations following the spike. The evolving fricative production was apparent in the appearance of irregular vertical striations, which were decreased in color and number.

In the final stage four of recovery, the majority of the consonant distortions had disappeared, although difficulties with the production of alveolar and alveopalatal fricatives and affricates, and the phoneme /r/ remained. High vowel approximation remained insufficient. Consistent with these perceptual findings, the resonant bars of the fricatives continued to demonstrate decreased energy. In addition, although the spike for the velar stop /k/ had become sharper, aspiration was still absent, indicating lax velar stop articulation. Overall, spectrograms were found to be one-third longer for the TBI patients, compared to the control subjects, a finding consistent with a slower articulation rate noted to be present in this population.

In the very small sample of subjects studied by Vogel and von Cramon (1983), four of the five patients demonstrated recovery of articulatory function to near normal levels in just over 3 months. The investigators suggested that the characteristics of dysarthria following TBI were consistent with spastic dysarthria due to weakness, and a restricted range and velocity of articulatory movements. Vogel and von Cramon (1983) concluded that the recovery of articulatory function postmutism involved the gradual restoration of the phonetic inventory, with speech production being phonetically sensitive to articulation requiring closure with the back portion of the tongue, specific stricture to maintain turbulent air flow, and gross displacement of the tongue for vowel production. They hypothesized an order of recovery of phoneme production that began with nasal sounds, followed by /b/, /p/, /j/, /v/, and /f/, lingual sounds, and fricatives. This progression of recovery was based on the assumption that the primary articulators were more or less equally affected by the injury.

Despite the identification of abnormal perceptual and acoustic features of articulatory function in persons following TBI, the underlying bases of these disturbances have not yet been fully investigated. Indeed, Vogel and von Cramon's (1983) assumption of the primary articulators being similarly affected post-TBI is tenuous given the evidence of a number of studies that have identified differential impairment of oromotor function following neurological impairment (Abbs, Hartman, & Vishwanat, 1987; Abbs, Hunker, & Barlow, 1983; Barlow & Abbs, 1983, 1984, 1986; DePaul, Abbs, Caligiuri, Gracco, & Brooks, 1988; Hunker, Abbs, & Barlow, 1982). These studies provide compelling evidence to argue that a comprehensive physiological evaluation of the articulatory components of the speech mechanism is essential in determining the exact nature of the pathophysiology associated with articulatory disturbances in persons following TBI.

Physiological Assessment of Articulatory Function Following TBI

Physiological evaluation of articulatory function following TBI may involve the use of a range of instruments designed to assess both the static and dynamic aspects of the articulatory components of the speech mechanism. Such instrumentation has included strain-gauge, pressure and force transduction systems, dynamic imaging techniques (ultrasound, cineradiography, electromagnetic articulography [EMA], and electropalatography [EPG]), and electromyography (EMG). Parameters of articulatory function measured using these techniques have included: maximum and submaximal compression force exerted by each articulator during speech and nonspeech tasks, force control, rate and consistency of articulatory movement, endurance capacities of each articulator, movement patterns of individual articulators during speech, and degree of muscle tone and type of muscle activity.

Strain-gauge, Pressure, and Force Transduction Systems

Strain-gauge transduction systems utilized in the assessment of articulatory function are usually comprised of strain-gauges mounted to either side of a flexible metal strip, which is anchored to a stable support at one end, forming a cantilever (Thompson-Ward & Murdoch, 1998). The force produced by the action of either the lips, tongue, or jaw on the free end of the cantilever alters the shape of the metal strip, causing various degrees of tension on the strain-gauges. A number of investigators have used strain-gauge transduction systems to measure an individual's ability to generate and control the force of each lip, the tongue, and the jaw independently (Amerman, 1993; Barlow & Abbs, 1983, 1984, 1986; Barlow, Cole, & Abbs, 1983; Barlow & Netsell, 1986; Barlow & Rath, 1985; McNeil, Weismer, Adams, & Mulligan, 1990; Theodoros, Murdoch, & Stokes, 1995), while other systems have been designed that allow simultaneous measurement of the upper and lower lips and the jaw during speech (Abbs & Gilbert, 1973; Abbs & Netsell, 1973; Folkins & Abbs, 1975; Hughes & Abbs, 1976; Muller & Abbs, 1979). Although there are some limitations in the use of strain-gauge transduction systems for the assessment of articulatory function (Thompson-Ward & Murdoch, 1998), strain-gauge transducers are a valuable component of a physiological assessment battery as they are highly sensitive to force changes, relatively inexpensive, noninvasive, and may be utilized during both speech and nonspeech activities.

A pressure transduction system, designed to measure interlabial contact pressures during speech and nonspeech activities was developed by Hinton and Luschei (1992). The miniature transducer (Entran Flatline®, Entran Devices Inc., Model EPL-20001-10) utilized in this system is positioned on the upper or lower lip, and unlike some of the strain-gauge systems, does not interfere with articulatory movements during speech. The pressure transducer is 10.2 mm in length and 1.02 mm thick, with a circular stainless steel sensor surface 5.08 mm in diameter. The transducer responds linearly to external pressure in the range of 0–70 kilopascals. In our laboratory, the transducer is mounted on a thin aluminium strip, tapered at one end to form a tip upon which the transducer is attached. The apparatus, interfaced with a dedicated software package, has been used by the authors of the present chapter to assess interlabial contact pressure, pressure control, lip endurance, and lip pressures during speech in both normal and neurologically impaired individuals (Theodoros, Murdoch, & Horton, 1999; Thompson, Murdoch, Theodoros, & Stokes, 1996; Murdoch, Spencer, Theodoros, & Thompson, 1998).

Tongue strength, endurance, and fine force control have been measured using different versions of tongue pressure/force transducers. A miniature force transducer, attached to the end of a rigid stem, was designed by Dworkin and colleagues (Dworkin & Aronson, 1986; Dworkin, Aronson, & Mulder, 1980) to record maximum anterior and lateral tongue forces when positioned accordingly. A more widely used tongue pressure transducer is the Iowa Oral Performance Instrument (IOPI), described by Robin and colleagues (Robin, Somodi, & Luschei, 1991; Robin, Goel, Somodi, & Luschei, 1992) to measure tongue strength and endurance. This instrument consists of an air-filled rubber bulb attached to a pressure transducer. When placed on top of the tongue, the subject is required to squeeze the bulb against the roof of the mouth using the front of the tongue. A similar system developed in our laboratory has been used to evaluate tongue strength, endurance, fine force control, and rate and force of repetitive tongue movements in normal and neurologically impaired individuals, including persons with a TBI (Goozée, Murdoch, & Theodoros, In press, a; Murdoch et al., 1998; Theodoros et al., 1995; Thompson, Murdoch, & Stokes, 1995; Ward, Theodoros, & Murdoch, In press).

Ultrasonic and Radiological Imaging Techniques

While strain-gauge, pressure, and force transducers enable the clinician to obtain data pertaining to the static and force related features of articulatory function, imaging techniques have provided a means for examining the dynamic aspects of speech production through representation of the real-time movement and coordination of the articulators. Imaging techniques, such as ultrasound and cineradiography, have been found to be useful in displaying a number of articulatory parameters during speech.

Ultrasound, which involves the transmission of high-frequency sound waves that are reflected back when passing through body tissues, is capable of identifying surface displacement and changes in soft tissue organization of the tongue. This technique has been found to be useful in recording lingual movements during vowel and consonant production (Stone, 1991). Despite the fact that tongue tip movements and movements of other orofacial structures cannot be viewed using this technique, and that interpretation of the scans requires experience because of inherent measurement variability, ultrasound investigation of the tongue is a noninvasive and inexpensive procedure and is a potentially useful instrumental method of assessing tongue function in patients following TBI (Thompson-Ward & Murdoch, 1998).

Cineradiography, a high-speed x-ray motion picture technique provides simultaneous representation and quantification of a number of articulatory parameters (tongue, lip, and jaw mobility) from a lateral view of the pharyngo-oro-nasal complex (Kent, Netsell, & Bauer, 1975). To assist in the interpretation of the images, researchers have enhanced this procedure by attaching small radioopaque markers (lead pellets) to specific articulatory surfaces such as the dorsal surface of the tongue, the upper and lower lips, and the lower incisor, to track the movements of the articulators (Kent & Netsell, 1975; Kent et al., 1975; Kiritani, Ito, & Fujimura, 1975). Parameters such as range, velocity, consistency, and coordination of articulatory movement have been measured using this technique (Hirose, Kiritani, Ushijima, & Sawashima, 1978). Clinically, the most serious limitation of this technique, however, is the exposure of the patient to radiation (Hirose et al., 1978). As a result, the duration of the procedure must be limited, and repeat examinations restricted, thus reducing the capacity of this procedure to monitor treatment efficacy (Kiritani, 1986; Tuller, Shao, & Scott Kelso, 1990). Due to an increase in the availability of radiation-free procedures to evaluate articulatory dynamics, radiological imaging techniques are less likely to be used to assess this aspect of speech production in individuals following TBI.

Electromagnetic Articulography

Recently, a safe, nonradiological imaging technique, known as electromagnetic articulography (EMA), has been developed to track articulatory movements during speech, using alternating electromagnetic fields (Schönle, Gräbe, & Wenig, 1987). This technique detects and records over time, and along the midsagittal plane, the movement of miniature receiver coils attached to the midline of the tongue, upper and lower lips, mandible, and velum. The system is available commercially as the Electromagnetic Articulograph AG-100® (Carstens Medizinelektronik GmbH, Germany) and comprises of three transmitter coils that are housed in a light-weight plastic helmet and positioned around the subject's head in the midsagittal plane, at points that form an equilateral triangle (i.e., in front of the chin, in front of the forehead, and behind the neck). The three transmitter coils generate alternating magnetic fields at different frequencies (range 10–20 kHz) which, in turn, induce alternating signals in five miniature receiver coils attached to the articulators (Goozée, Murdoch, Theodoros, & Stokes, 2000). The magnitude of the alternating electrical signal induced in a receiver coil reflects the distance between the single receiver coil and a transmitter coil. The signal induced in the receiver coil within the magnetic fields generated by the three transmitter coils consists of three signal components. The location (x-y coordinates) of the receiver coil within the two-dimensional, midsagittal measurement plane is determined by separating the three signal components at each receiver coil and determining the distance between the receiver coil and each transmitter, based on the magnitude of each signal component. The position of each receiver coil is sampled rapidly over time to provide a two-dimensional representation of articulator movements along the midsagittal plane (Goozée et al., 2000). From this data, a number of kinematic parameters, including the trajectory, velocity, duration, and acceleration of articulatory movements are computed. While EMA has considerable potential for evaluating abnormal articulatory dynamics, research involving the use of this technique with dysarthric speakers has been limited, with only one study being reported in the literature to date (Goozée et al., 2000). This latter study used EMA to investigate articulatory dynamics in a dysarthric speaker following TBI, and provided considerable insight into the individual's articulatory patterns. (See "Physiological Features of Articulatory Dysfunction Following TBI" later in this Chapter.)

Electropalatography

Electropalatography (EPG) is another instrumental technique with the capacity to assess articulatory dynamics. This technique records the location and timing of tongue-to-palate contacts during continuous speech in real time, and provides visual representation of tongue gestures that are not usually seen (Dagenais, 1995; Hardcastle, 1984; Hardcastle, Gibbon, & Jones, 1991; Hardcastle, Jones, Knight, Trudgeon, & Calder, 1989). In most settings, EPG is conducted using the Reading Electropalatograph® (EPG3) system. Each subject is fitted with his/her own individual artificial acrylic palate. The artificial palate contains an array of 62 miniature touch-sensitive disc electrodes (1.4 mm in diameter) arranged in eight rows and eight columns according to a predetermined scheme based on anatomical landmarks (Hardcastle et al., 1991). The electrodes are equally spaced along each row, with the spacing between the anterior four rows equal to half that of the posterior four rows. This arrangement of the electrodes allows for comparison of contact patterns across different subjects (Hardcastle & Gibbon, 1997). Each palate covers the area bounded by the central incisors anteriorly, the junction of the hard and soft palates posteriorly, and the side teeth laterally (Hardcastle et al., 1991). The electropalatograph samples tongue-to-palate contacts at 10 millisecond intervals, while acoustic data is simultaneously collected at a rate of 10,000 Hz from a microphone connected to the EPG main unit. Prior to the recording of tongue-to-palate contacts, each subject requires a desensitization period to become accustomed to speaking with the artificial palate in position. The length of time for subjects to adapt to their EPG palates has been reported to vary from 20 minutes to up to 4 hours (Byrd, 1996; Fletcher, 1989; Hardcastle & Gibbon, 1997; Hardcastle et al., 1989). Following the desensitization period, tongue-to-palate contacts and acoustic data are recorded as the subject reads or repeats a series of single words, phrases, and/or sentences. While there have been only two studies reported in the literature to date that have used EPG to investigate dynamic tongue movements during speech in persons with dysarthria following TBI (Goozée, Murdoch, & Theodoros, 1999; Goozée, Murdoch, & Theodoros, In press, b), this instrumental technique would appear to have considerable potential in identifying and quantifying tongue dynamics in the speech disordered head-injured population. (See "Physiological Features of Articulatory Dysfunction Following TBI" later in this Chapter.)

Electromyography

Investigations of the status of the electrical activity of articulatory muscles during speech and nonspeech activities may be conducted using electromyography (EMG). The changes in muscle electrical activity are recorded using either surface, needle, or hook-wire electrodes, which are positioned either over or in the muscle under investigation (Thompson-Ward & Murdoch, 1998). EMG evaluations of muscle activity have identified degrees of hypertonicity and hypotonicity in articulatory muscles and abnormal variations in the activation and inhibition of muscle activity (Folkins, Linville, Garrett, & Brown, 1988; Leanderson, Meyerson, & Persson, 1972; McClean, 1991; Moore, Smith, & Ringel, 1988; Neilson & O'Dwyer, 1984; Shaiman, 1989; Sussman, MacNeilage, & Hanson, 1973). Although limitations of EMG exist with respect to the ability to isolate specific oral muscles anatomically and to access muscles for electrode placement, this technique has been used successfully to assess articulatory muscle activity in persons following TBI. Barlow and Burton (1988) utilized this technique to record the muscle activity of the orbicularis oris in 15 TBI subjects, using surface electrodes.

Physiological Features of Articulatory Dysfunction Following TBI

To date, a number of studies have investigated the physiological bases of articulatory disturbance in individuals following TBI (Barlow & Burton, 1988, 1990; Barlow & Netsell, 1989; Coelho, Gracco, Fourakis, Rossetti, & Oshima, 1994; Goozée et al., 1999; Goozée, Murdoch, & Theodoros, in press a; Goozée et al., 2000; Kent et al., 1975; McHenry, Minton & Wilson, 1994a; McHenry, Minton, Wilson, & Post, 1994b; Robin et al., 1991; Theodoros et al., 1995). The majority of these studies have focused on lip and tongue function during nonspeech tasks, with studies examining the dynamics of articulatory movement during speech in TBI individuals beginning to emerge in the literature. As yet, evaluation of jaw function in dysarthric speakers following TBI has not been specifically addressed.

Lip Dysfunction Following TBI

Labial force generation and control has been investigated in dysarthric speakers following TBI in a number of studies using specially designed instrumentation and assessment protocols. To date, however, the dynamics of lip function during speech have rarely been reported in the literature.

Strength, Endurance, Fine Force Control, and Rate

In a series of studies, Barlow and colleagues (Barlow & Burton, 1988, 1990; Barlow & Netsell, 1989) used strain-gauge instrumentation to examine the fine force control characteristics of the upper and lower lips in groups of individuals with dysarthria following TBI. During these assessments, a ramp-and-hold force paradigm was employed to investigate the subject's ability to generate lip force as rapidly and as accurately as possible to a submaximal target and then to maintain the target force during a hold phase (Barlow & Burton, 1990). In a preliminary study of 15 TBI dysarthric speakers, Barlow and Burton (1988) identified several aspects of impaired lip force control, including impairment in the rate of force recruitment, peak force overshoot, and instability during the hold phase. Similarly, Barlow and Netsell (1989) found that all 20 TBI subjects in their study exhibited lip force control impairments, with several subjects also demonstrating lip weakness. These latter subjects were, in fact, unable to generate a one Newton (N) force, which is within the presumed force operating range for speech (i.e., up to two N; Barlow & Burton, 1990). Furthermore, Barlow and Netsell (1989) identified greater impairment of force in the lower lips of these subjects as compared to their upper lips. A case study analysis of four adult TBI subjects by Barlow and Burton (1990) revealed a heterogeneous pattern of lip force control impairments. Three of the subjects demonstrated force overshoot during the ramp phase of lip contraction, while the remaining subject failed to reach the target force and exhibited a reduced speed of force generation. During the hold phase of the assessment paradigm, near-normal force stability and accuracy levels were achieved by two of the subjects, while one subject was noted to demonstrate excessive levels of force instability and lip weakness.

In similar studies by McHenry and colleagues (McHenry et al., 1994a; McHenry et al., 1994b) the dynamic and sustained lip-force-generating capacities of individuals following TBI were investigated. In a study involving groups of TBI dysarthric speakers with "more" (> 70%) or "less" (< 70%) speech intelligibility, McHenry et al. (1994b) sought to identify the relationship between speech intelligibility and orofacial strength and force control. The results revealed that the "more" and "less" intelligible subjects did not differ significantly in dynamic and sustained lip force generation.

Using a different type of strain-gauge instrument, Theodoros et al., (1995) investigated lip function in a group of 18 severely closed-head-injured (CHI) subjects with dysarthria. Four nonspeech tasks (maximum lip force, sustained maximum force, repetition of maximum lip force compressions, and maximum rate of maximum force compressions) were used to assess lip strength, endurance, and rate of repetitive lip movements in the group of head-injured subjects as compared to a group of matched control subjects. The CHI subjects were found to demonstrate significantly reduced lip strength and endurance as compared to the control subjects on all tasks, except for the maximum repetitive rate task. Although the CHI subjects failed to exhibit a reduction in mean lip force and endurance during rapid repetition of maximum lip compressions, these subjects did demonstrate a significantly slower rate of repetitive lip compressions as compared to the control group. This reduction in rate of repetitive lip compressions may have enabled the CHI subjects to maintain a lip strength within the normal range during this activity.

While previously mentioned studies have documented lip function in TBI dysarthric speakers using rather cumbersome instrumentation designed for nonspeech tasks only, the use of a miniature pressure transducer capable of measuring interlabial contact pressures during both nonspeech and speech activities in persons following TBI has been reported in the literature. Thompson et al. (1996) used an Entran flatline pressure transducer to investigate the interlabial contact pressures in a male adult with dysarthria following TBI. A range of nonspeech tasks, similar to those described in Theodoros et al. (1995) were employed in the study, in addition to a fine pressure control task (subject was required to sustain a target pressure of either 50%, 20%, or 10% of his maximum lip pressure for 5 seconds), a sustained submaximal pressure task (subject was required to sustain 50% of his maximal lip pressure for as long as possible), and a speech task involving the production of /p/ within a context of syllable, word, and sentence repetition.

The subject was found to produce normal lip pressure during the maximum effort task as well as a normal mean pressure across 10 repetitions of maximum lip compressions. Fine lip pressure control was also found to be comparable to normative data at each level. Mean lip pressure across the maximum rate repetition task, however, was reduced compared to normal, while the subject's rate of repetitive lip movements was markedly increased. The results indicated that the subject was using a strategy of reducing lip pressure to increase the rate of repetitive lip movements. Endurance of lip strength at a 50% submaximal pressure was found to be slightly reduced, compared to normal, indicating the potential for fatigue in lip function. In contrast, interlabial pressures during speech were found to be increased, compared to normal data. As a result, the percentage of maximum lip pressure produced during speech production was greater than that recorded for a normal control group. The authors suggested that high interlabial pressures during speech identified in this subject may reflect his slow and deliberate manner of articulation, which may have been partly due to the ataxic characteristics of his dysarthric speech disturbance, and/or to a compensatory technique adopted by him to increase speech intelligibility. Thompson et al. (1996) concluded that the use of the miniature lip pressure transducer was effective and time efficient in evaluating both the maximal effort components of lip function as well as lip pressures during speech.

Further development of the use of the Entran flatline transducer for assessing lip function in persons following TBI has been conducted in our laboratory with a study involving 19 TBI dysarthric speakers (mean age 30.6 years) and a matched control group. The assessment protocol used in this study was based on that used by Thompson et al. (1996) and included six nonspeech tasks (maximum interlabial contact pressure, sustained maximum pressure, sustained submaximal pressure, 10 repetitions of maximum lip-closing pressure, maximum rate of repetition of maximum lip-closing pressure, fine lip pressure control at 50%, 20%, and 10% levels of maximum pressure), and a speech task that incorporated repetition of syllables, words, phrases, and sentences containing bilabial stops /p/ and /m/ in the initial position. The results of this study revealed that the TBI subjects as a group demonstrated significantly reduced maximum interlabial contact pressure and mean pressure across 10 repetitions of maximum lip closing, as well as reductions in the mean pressure produced during the maximum rate of repetition of maximum lip closing, compared to the control group. For the TBI subjects, the rate of repetitive lip closure was also found to be significantly reduced, to a level that was slightly more than half that of the control group. The reduced rate of lip movement may be associated with the inherent physiological features of this muscle group. As lip muscles are composed of a large quantity of noncontractile tissue imposing a considerable viscous load (Luschei, 1991), substantial forces would be required for high rates of muscle fiber shortening to effect rapid lip movement. In the case of the TBI subjects in this study, their muscle weakness would be associated with low shortening velocities (Luschei, 1991), and, therefore, it is possible that the reduced lip strength identified in this group may have contributed to their reduced rate of repetitive lip movement.

With respect to lip strength endurance, the TBI subjects were found to be significantly impaired as compared to the control group when sustaining maximum lip pressure, but comparable to the control subjects when sustaining lip pressures at submaximal levels. In relation to their fine control of lip pressure, the TBI subjects were found to be significantly less accurate than the control subjects in producing target lip pressures at each of the 50%, 20%, and 10% levels of maximum pressure. The actual mean pressures generated by the TBI subjects were, on average, within 9.8%, 27%, 41% of the target pressure levels (50%, 20%, and 10% of maximum pressure), respectively, while the control subjects recorded actual mean pressures within 2.6%, 4.5%, and 5.7% of the respective target pressure levels. Interestingly, the greatest degree of inaccuracy demonstrated by the TBI subjects was during their attempts to match the 10% level of maximum pressure. Since this submaximal level corresponds to the pressures typically exhibited in normal speech production (10.5%, Hinton & Arokiasamy, 1997; less than 12%, Thompson et al., 1996), impairment in the accuracy of fine lip control at this level could have a negative effect on speech production. In contrast, the TBI subjects and their control counterparts demonstrated similar degrees of pressure stability at each of the three pressure levels. This latter result was inconsistent with the findings of Barlow and Burton (1988), who identified significant impairment in lip force stability in their group of 15 TBI adults. The inconsistency in results may be explained, however, in relation to the different instrumentation and tasks used in each study, and the inherent variability of TBI individuals with respect to lesion site and the severity and type of dysarthria.

During the speech tasks, the TBI subjects were found to generate similar interlabial contact pressures to those of the controls. However, when the mean pressures obtained for /p/ and /m/ were expressed as percentages of the individuals' maximum pressures, the TBI subjects were found to be using significantly greater percentages of their maximum lip pressures, compared to the control subjects, during the production of these phonemes. Indeed, the TBI subjects were utilizing higher percentages of their maximum lip pressures during speech than were required for normal speech production (i.e., approximately 10% of maximum lip pressure). This finding may partly explain why the TBI subjects demonstrated the greatest degree of inaccuracy when matching the 10% target level on the fine lip pressure control task, in that they may have experienced difficulty controlling the generation of small increments in pressure from their resting baseline levels. In that maximum lip pressure is considered to demarcate the extent of physiological capacity, the results obtained for the speech tasks indicated that the TBI subjects were actually producing pressures that were in the higher portion of their operating range (McHenry et al., 1994b). In doing so, the TBI subjects were utilizing increased physiological effort (McHenry et al., 1994b), which may result in fatigue during longer utterances and periods of speech, and subsequently may manifest as articulatory imprecision.

Lip Dynamics During Speech

In a single case study, Coelho et al. (1994) examined lip movements during speech in a closed-head-injured female with moderate-to-severe hypokinetic dysarthria. Her speech disturbance was characterized by breathiness, monotony of pitch, reduced loudness and stress, short, rapid bursts of speech, and inconsistent articulatory undershooting and spirantization. The dynamics of lip function were assessed during repetitive speech and nonspeech tasks, using a standard optoelectronic technique in which small light-emitting diodes (LEDS) were placed on the upper and lower lip vermillion borders in the midsagittal plane. Overall, the subject's repetitive movement was reduced for both speech and nonspeech tasks. Furthermore, the subject demonstrated reductions in displacement and velocity of upper and lower lip movements, with impairments in lip movements being exacerbated with increases in rate. Coelho et al. (1994) also found that the upper and lower lips of this subject were more impaired than her jaw in relation to movement displacements and velocities. Although this case study has provided some preliminary data, further instrumental studies of lip dynamics in this population are urgently required, to achieve a more complete understanding of the effects of TBI on lip function during speech.

Tongue Dysfunction Following TBI

Despite the fact that impaired tongue function is a common clinical feature of persons following TBI, and that integrity of tongue function is essential for the precise and rapid production of most speech sounds, comparatively little research investigating this aspect of articulatory function following TBI has been conducted to date. Studies that have investigated tongue function in this population have identified impairments in tongue strength, endurance, fine force control, and rate of repetitive movements during nonspeech activities as well as abnormalities in tongue placement and timing of lingual movements during speech.

Strength, Endurance, Fine Pressure Control, and Rate

Using the IOPI system, Robin et al. (1991) investigated the tongue strength and endurance of a 26-year-old female patient who exhibited a mild spastic-flaccid dysarthria following TBI. Tongue strength (maximum tongue pressure exerted) was found to be reduced, compared to a normal speaker, while endurance (sustained submaximal pressure at 50% of maximum tongue pressure) was recorded as comparable to that of normal speakers. A similar study by Stierwalt, Robin, Solomon,

Weiss, and Max (1996), involving 23 children and adolescents who had sustained a mild or severe TBI, revealed that tongue endurance was significantly reduced as compared to control subjects, while the maximal tongue strength of the TBI subjects was comparable to that of the control group. The results of this study, however, must be viewed in light of the fact that, within the TBI subject group, only seven of the subjects exhibited a mild or moderate dysarthria.

In a large group study investigating tongue function specifically in dysarthric speakers following TBI, Theodoros et al. (1995) identified significant impairments in tongue strength, endurance, and rate of repetitive movements in these subjects, compared to a matched control group. Significant reductions in tongue strength were identified during maximal effort tasks such as: production of maximum tongue pressure, sustained maximum tongue pressure, and 10 repetitions of maximum tongue pressure, and during maximum rate of repetition of maximum tongue pressures. Impaired tongue strength endurance was identified in the TBI subjects during 10 repetitions of maximum tongue pressure at a specific rate of one per second, with significantly lower pressures being produced at the end as compared to the beginning of this task. The rate of repetitive maximum tongue pressures was also found to be significantly reduced in the TBI subjects, compared to the controls. Interestingly, the TBI subjects did not demonstrate a decrease in tongue endurance during this task. This finding, however, may have been due to both the reduction in overall mean pressure and rate recorded for this activity, which together may have facilitated the maintenance of pressure across the task. Similarly, nonneurologically impaired subjects have demonstrated longer tongue endurance times at lower levels of maximum strength (Robin et al., 1992). In comparison to the results obtained during the assessment of lip function in the same subjects as previously outlined above, it was evident that tongue function was more severely compromised in this particular group of TBI subjects. Theodoros et al. (1995) proposed that both the lip and tongue dysfunction identified in this group of TBI subjects could conceivably account, at least in part, for the dysarthric speech disturbances observed.

To further investigate the relationship between physiological measures and articulatory proficiency, Goozée et al. (In press, a), using a more extensive physiological assessment battery and a computerized analysis procedure, examined the tongue strength, endurance, rate of repetitive movement, and fine tongue pressure control of a group of 20 TBI subjects, and correlated these findings with their group's perceived articulatory features (consonant and vowel imprecision and prolongation of phonemes). The physiological assessment of tongue function in the TBI subjects revealed that tongue strength was significantly impaired, compared to the control group, during both repetition tasks (10 repetitions of maximum tongue pressure and maximum rate of repetition of maximum pressure), although maximal tongue pressure exerted during the isolated maximum effort task was not found to differ significantly from the control group. The rate of repetitive tongue movements and endurance (duration for which tongue pressure could be maintained at 50% of maximum pressure) in this group of TBI subjects were also found to be significantly reduced as compared to the controls. With respect to fine control of tongue pressure, the TBI subjects were significantly less accurate than the control subjects in matching the targeted pressure levels of 50% and 20% of maximum tongue pressure, although their degree of tongue pressure stability was comparable to that of the control group. In an examination of the relationship between physiological measures and perceptual articulatory features, significant, but weak, correlations were obtained between consonant imprecision and maximum tongue pressure, sustained submaximal pressure, and degree of accuracy in matching a tongue pressure level of 10% of maximum pressure. The prolongation of phonemes feature was found to be weakly correlated with the pressure stability measure for fine pressure control at 20% of maximum pressure. A closer examination of each TBI subject's physiological tongue impairments and deviant perceptual articulatory features, however, revealed no obvious relationships between the physiological and perceptual parameters. Goozée et al. (In press, a) proposed that the high degree of inconsistency between the physiological and perceptual characteristics of the TBI subjects suggested that the subjects were compensating in different ways for the physiological impairments, with differing degrees of success.

Tongue Dynamics During Speech

While measurement of tongue strength, endurance, fine pressure control, and rate of repetitive movements during nonspeech activities is essential in determining the basic physiological status of lingual function, examination of tongue dynamics during speech provides the researcher and clinician with greater insight into the positioning, timing, and control of movement of this articulator. In the very limited number of studies to date, cineradiography, electropalatography, and electromagnetic articulography have been used to investigate dynamic parameters of tongue function.

Kent et al. (1975), investigating articulatory dynamics in dysarthric speakers using cineradiography, identified a restricted range of lingual mobility, limited flexibility in the directions of tongue movement, and slow rates of articulatory motion in one TBI subject. Another TBI individual was found to exhibit nonuniform and generally slower rates of articulatory motion, with tongue movements confined to within a narrow path of motion.

Recently, the use of electropalatography to examine the location and timing of tongue-to-palate contacts during speech in persons with dysarthria following TBI has been reported in the literature. The first of these studies, by Goozée et al. (1999), investigated the lingual timing characteristics of three subjects with dysarthria following TBI. For this study, the Reading Electropalatograph (See "Physiological Assessment of Articulatory Function Following TBI" in this Chapter.) was used to record tongue-to-palate contacts during the production of single-syllable words with the initial consonants /t/, /d/, /s/, /z/, /k/, and /g/. The duration of the approach, closure/stable constriction, and release phases of tongue movement that are important in the production of lingual consonants were measured for each subject and compared to those of a single control subject. Analyses of the EPG recordings revealed differential disturbances in the timing of tongue movements for the three subjects during the production of alveolar stops and fricatives, and velar stops.

Specifically, Case One, with mild spastic dysarthria, exhibited longer approach and release phase durations and shorter closure phases, compared to the control subject, for alveolar stop production. The shorter closure phase for alveolar stop production was considered to possibly reflect articulatory undershooting. For fricatives, the stable constriction and release phases were found to be similar to the control subject and the approach phase longer than normal. Closure for velar stops was not consistently recorded for this subject. Case Two who was also mildly spastic-dysarthric, demonstrated longer approach and closure/stable constriction phases and normal release phases for the production of alveolar stops and fricatives, while for velar stops, all phases were found to be longer than those of the control subject. The authors suggested that these findings were consistent with the perception of a moderately slow rate of speech in this case. Case Three was a moderately spastic-ataxic dysarthric male speaker, for whom the approach and closure phases were found to be longer than the normal control subject during the production of alveolar and velar stops. The release phases were found to be comparable to those of the normal subject. The longer phase durations evident in this case were considered to be consistent with the perception of phoneme prolongation in this subject's speech. Due to the deviant fricative closure pattern, it was not possible for valid durational data to be collected from this case. Where closure was identified, the contact patterns appeared to be a result of the overshooting of tongue placement, with the tongue extending anteriorly into the interdental position, as suggested by the phonetic transcriptions. Since overshooting is likely to be the result of incoordination in the force, accuracy, speed, and range of tongue movements frequently associated with involvement of the cerebellum, this pattern was thought to be consistent with the subject's diagnosis of spastic-ataxic dysarthria, in which both the upper motor neurons and the cerebellum are presumed to be impaired.

The second study by Goozée et al. (In press, b) sought to investigate the spatial characteristics of the tongue-to-palate contacts in the three TBI dysarthric speakers previously discussed, to determine if inaccurate tongue placement during consonant articulation was another factor contributing to the articulatory imprecision in these individuals. Five non-neurologically impaired adults served as the control subjects for this study. Spatial characteristics were analyzed in terms of the location, pattern, and amount of tongue-to-palate contact at the frame of maximum contact during the production of alveolar (/t/, /d/), fricative (/s/, /z/), and velar stop (/k/, /g/) initial consonants in single-syllable words. The TBI subjects were found to produce patterns and locations of contacts for the majority of consonants that were consistent with the contacts generated by the control subjects. One TBI subject, however, was noted to produce a very different pattern of tongue contact from that of the controls during the production of alveolar fricatives in that complete closure across the palate was evident for these phonemes, rather than the typical groove configuration. In addition, discrepancies were evident in the amount of tongue-to-palate contact exhibited, with two TBI subjects consistently demonstrating increased contacts compared to the control subjects. The investigators suggested that future studies examining tongue-to-palate contacts in dysarthric speakers following TBI should record consonants in the final word position and in consonant clusters to determine the possible presence of spatial disturbances in these phonetic environments.

To provide more detailed information regarding other aspects of tongue dynamics during speech, such as range and speed of tongue movements in the midsagittal plane, Goozée et al. (2000) conducted a kinematic analysis of tongue movements in a dysarthric speaker following TBI, using electromagnetic articulography (See "Physiological Assessment of Articulatory Function Following TBI" in this

Chapter.). Three receiver coils were attached to the tongue, and movements were recorded during the production of three single-syllable words with lingual consonants /t/, /s/, and /k/ in the initial position. The kinematic parameters investigated included movement trajectories, velocity, acceleration/deceleration, distance, and duration of tongue movements. Analyses of the results in comparison to a normal control subject revealed a disturbance in the *control* of tongue speed rather than a disturbance in the speed *per se*. Specifically, the subject with TBI demonstrated difficulty in decelerating his tongue movements appropriately when approaching the palate during consonant production. This difficulty resulted in inaccurate tongue movements that overshot the targeted articulatory position (as in production of /t/) and may have been instrumental in reducing the time that the tongue remained at the palate during the production of /s/ and /k/ in comparison to the control subject. The authors stressed the importance of examining a range of kinematic parameters, and the interactions among these when determining the nature of articulatory disturbances in dysarthric speakers following TBI and highlighted the value of electromagnetic articulography in achieving this aim.

Summary

Articulatory dysfunction in dysarthric speakers following TBI has been identified perceptually, acoustically, and physiologically using a range of techniques (see Table 3-1). Specifically, these subjects have been found to demonstrate a reduction in speech intelligibility, compared to normal speakers, with their speech output characterized by consonant and vowel imprecision, phoneme prolongation, and a reduced rate of speech. Acoustically, the dysarthric speakers with TBI demonstrated abnormal acoustic features consistent with articulatory undershooting and a slowed rate of speech. Physiological impairments in lip and tongue strength, endurance, fine force control, and rate of repetitive movements during nonspeech activities have been elucidated, while impairments in the dynamics of lip movement (displacement, velocity, and repetition rate) and tongue movement (placement, timing, displacement, velocity, and control of speed of movement) have been identified during speech production. Consistent with previous findings in dysarthric speakers and the variability inherent in this population, the TBI subjects were found to demonstrate differential articulatory subsystem impairment within individuals and between subjects. Clinically, the perceptual, acoustic, and physiological findings suggest that management of articulatory dysfunction in dysarthric speakers following TBI warrants an individualized approach to treatment, with an emphasis on enhancing the physiological status of the articulators, together with the use of compensatory techniques, to facilitate recovery of articulatory function and speech intelligibility in this population.

Table 3-1. Summary of the perceptual, acoustic, and physiological features of articulatory dysfunction identified in dysarthric speakers following TBI.

Perceptual	Acoustic	Physiological	
		Lip	Tongue
• Consonant imprecision • Vowel imprecision • Phoneme prolongation • Mild-moderate impairment in nonspeech tongue movements • Moderate tongue dysfunction during speech • Mild impairment in nonspeech lip movements • Mild-moderate lip dysfunction during speech (EPG) • ↑ or ↓ rate of speech • ↓ speech intelligibility	• ↑ syllable & word durations • Centralization of vowel formants (vowel reduction and distortion) • Spirantization • Large, slow amplitude cycles in formant trajectories associated with slow, exaggerated tongue protrusions and retractions • ↓ diadochokinetic rate	• ↓ rate of force recruitment • Peak force overshoot • Force instability during hold phase • ↓ lip strength • ↓ endurance • ↓ rate of repetitive lip movements (nonspeech) • ↓ accuracy fine force control • ↑ % maximum interlabial contact pressure used during speech • ↓ displacement upper and lower lips • ↓ velocities upper and lower lips	• ↓ tongue strength • ↓ endurance • ↑ rate of repetitive tongue movements (nonspeech) • ↓ accuracy fine force control • ↓ range lingual mobility (speech) • ↓ flexibility in direction of tongue movements (speech) • ↓ rate of movement (speech) • Abnormalities in lingual timing during consonant production • Deviations in amount of tongue-to-palate contact during consonant production (EPG) • Impaired control of speed of tongue movement (EMA)

↑or↓ = increased or reduced

References

Abbs, J.H. & Gilbert, B.N. (1973). A strain-gauge transduction system for lip and jaw motion in two dimensions: design criteria and calibration data. *Journal of Speech and Hearing Research, 16,* 248–256.

Abbs, J.H., Hartman, D.E., & Vishwanat, B. (1987). Orofacial motor control impairment in Parkinson's disease. *Neurology, 37,* 394–398.

Abbs, J.H., Hunker, C.J., & Barlow, S.M. (1983). Differential speech motor subsystem impairments with suprabulbar lesions: neurophysiological framework and supporting data. In W.R. Berry (Ed.), *Clinical Dysarthria* (pp. 21–56). San Diego: College Hill Press.

Abbs, J.H. & Netsell, R. (1973). An interpretation of jaw acceleration during speech. *Journal of Speech and Hearing Research, 16,* 421–425.

Amerman, J.D. (1993). A maximum-force-dependent protocol for assessing labial force control. *Journal of Speech and Hearing Research, 36,* 460–465.

Barlow, S.M. & Abbs, J.H. (1983). Force transducers for the evaluation of labial, lingual, and mandibular motor impairments. *Journal of Speech and Hearing Research, 26,* 616–621.

Barlow, S.M. & Abbs, J.H. (1984). Orofacial fine motor control impairments in congenital spasticity: evidence against hypertonus-related performance deficits. *Neurology, 34,* 145–150.

Barlow, S.M. & Abbs, J.H. (1986). Fine force and position control of select orofacial structures in the upper motor neuron syndrome. *Experimental Neurology, 94,* 699–713.

Barlow, S.M. & Burton, M. (1988). Orofacial force control impairments in brain injured adults. *Association for Research in Otolaryngology Abstracts,* 218.

Barlow, S.M & Burton, M.K. (1990). Ramp-and-hold force control in the upper and lower lips: Developing new neuromotor assessment applications in traumatically injured adults. *Journal of Speech and Hearing Research, 33,* 660–675.

Barlow, S.M., Cole, K.J., & Abbs, J.H. (1983). A new head-mounted lip-jaw movement transduction system for the study of motor speech disorders. *Journal of Speech and Hearing Disorders, 26,* 283–288.

Barlow, S.M. & Netsell, R. (1986). Differential fine force control of the upper and lower lips. *Journal of Speech and Hearing Research, 29,* 163–169.

Barlow, S.M. & Netsell, R. (1989). Clinical neurophysiology for individuals with dysarthria. In K.M. Yorkston & D.R. Beukelamn (Eds.), *Recent Advances in Clinical Dysarthria* (pp. 53–82). Boston: College Hill Press.

Barlow, S.M. & Rath, E.M. (1985). Maximum voluntary closing forces in the upper and lower lips of humans. *Journal of Speech and Hearing Research, 28,* 373–376.

Blumberger, J., Sullivan, S. J., & Clément, N. (1995). Diadochokinetic rate in persons with traumatic brain injury. *Brain Injury, 9,* 797–804.

Byrd, D. (1996). Influences on articulatory timing in consonant sequences. *Journal of Phonetics, 24,* 209–244.

Coelho, C.A., Gracco, V.L., Fourakis, M., Rossetti, M., & Oshima, K. (1994). Application of instrumental techniques in the assessment of dysarthria. A case study. In J.A. Till, K.M. Yorkston, & D.R. Beukelman (Eds.), *Motor Speech Disorders. Advances in Assessment and Treatment* (pp. 103–117). Baltimore: Paul Brookes Publishing Co.

Dagenais, P.A. (1995). Electropalatography in the treatment of articulation/phonological disorders. *Journal of Communication Disorders, 28,* 303–329.

DePaul, R., Abbs, J.H., Caligiuri, M.P., Gracco, V.L., & Brooks, B.R. (1988). Hypoglossal, trigeminal, and facial motor neuron involvement in amyotrophic lateral sclerosis. *Neurology, 38,* 281–283.

Dworkin, J.P. & Aronson, A.E. (1986). Tongue strength and alternate motion rates in normal and dysarthric speakers. *Journal of Communication Disorders, 19,* 115–132.

Dworkin, J.P., Aronson, A., & Mulder, D.W. (1980). Tongue strength in normals and in dysarthric patients with amyotrophic lateral sclerosis. *Journal of Speech and Hearing Research, 23,* 828–837.

Enderby, P.M. (1983). *Frenchay Dysarthria Assessment.* San Diego: College Hill Press.

Fletcher, S.G. (1989). Palatometric specification of stop, affricate, and sibilant sounds. *Journal of Speech and Hearing Research, 32,* 736–748.

Folkins, J.W. & Abbs, J.H. (1975). Lip and jaw motor control during speech: response to resistive loading of the jaw. *Journal of Speech and Hearing Research, 18,* 207–222.

Folkins, J.W., Linville, R.N., Garrett, J.D., & Brown, C.K. (1988). Interactions in the labial musculature during speech. *Journal of Speech and Hearing Research, 31,* 253–264.

Goozée, J.V., Murdoch, B.E., & Theodoros, D.G. (1999). Electropalatographic assessment of articulatory timing characteristics in dysarthria following traumatic brain injury. *Journal of Medical Speech-Language Pathology, 7,* 209–222.

Goozée, J.V., Murdoch, B.E., & Theodoros, D.G. (In press, a). Physiological assessment of tongue function in dysarthria following traumatic brain injury. *Logopedics, Phoniatrics Vocology.*

Goozée, J.V., Murdoch, B.E., & Theodoros, D.G. (In press, b). Electropalatographic assessment of tongue-to-palate contacts exhibited in dysarthria following traumatic brain injury: Spatial characteristics. *Journal of Medical Speech-Language Pathology.*

Goozée, J.V., Murdoch, B.E., Theodoros, D.G., & Stokes, P.D. (2000). Kinematic analysis of tongue movements in dysarthria following traumatic brain injury using electromagnetic articulography. *Brain Injury, 14,* 153–174.

Hardcastle, W.J. (1984). New methods of profiling lingual-palatal contact patterns with electropalatography. *Phonetics Laboratory Work in Progress, University of Reading, 4,* 1–40.

Hardcastle, W.J. & Gibbon, F. (1997). Electropalatography and its clinical applications. In M.J. Ball & C. Code (Eds.), *Instrumental Clinical Phonetics* (pp. 149–193). London: Whurr Publishers Ltd.

Hardcastle, W.J., Gibbon, F.E., & Jones, W. (1991). Visual display of tongue-palate contact: electropalatography in the assessment and remediation of speech disorders. *British Journal of Disorders of Communication, 26,* 41–74.

Hardcastle, W., Jones, W., Knight, C., Trudgeon, A., & Calder, G. (1989). New developments in electropalatography: a state-of-the-art report. *Clinical Linguistics and Phonetics, 3,* 1–38.

Hinton, V.A. & Arokiasamy, W.M. (1997). Maximum interlabial pressures in normal speakers. *Journal of Speech and Hearing Research, 40,* 400–404.

Hinton, V.A. & Luschei, E.S. (1992). Validation of a modern miniature transducer for measurement of interlabial contact pressures during speech. *Journal of Speech and Hearing Research, 35,* 245–251.

Hirose, H., Kiritani, S., Ushijima, T., & Sawashima, M. (1978). Analysis of abnormal articulatory dynamics in two dysarthric patients. *Journal of Speech and Hearing Disorders, 43,* 96–105.

Hughes, O.M. & Abbs, J.H. (1976). Labial-mandibular co-ordination in the production of speech: implications for the operation of motor equivalence. *Phonetica, 33,* 199–221.

Hunker, C., Abbs, J.H., & Barlow, S. (1982). The relationship between parkinsonian rigidity and hypokinesia in the orofacial system: a quantitative analysis. *Neurology, 32,* 755–761.

Kent, R. & Netsell, R. (1975). A case study of an ataxic dysarthric: cineradiographic and spectrographic observations. *Journal of Speech and Hearing Disorders, 40,* 115–134.

Kent, R., Netsell, R., & Bauer, L.L. (1975). Cineradiographic assessment of articulatory mobility in the dysarthrias. *Journal of Speech and Hearing Disorders, 40,* 467–480.

Kiritani, S. (1986). X-ray microbeam method for measurement of articulatory dynamics-techniques and results. *Speech Communication, 5,* 119–139.

Kiritani, S., Ito, K., & Fujimura, O. (1975). Tongue pellet tracking by a computer-controlled x-ray microbeam system. *The Journal of the Acoustical Society of America, 57,* 1516–1520.

Leanderson, R., Meyerson, B. A., & Persson, A. (1972). Lip muscle function in Parkinsonian dysarthria. *Acta Otolaryngologica, 74,* 350–357.

Luschei, E.S. (1991). Development of objective standards of nonspeech oral strength and performance: An advocate's views. In C.A. Moore, K.M. Yorkston, & D.R. Beukelman (Eds.), *Dysarthria and Apraxia of Speech: Perspectives on Management* (pp. 3–14). Baltimore: Paul Brookes Publishing Co.

McClean, M. (1991). Lip muscle EMG responses to oral pressure stimulation. *Journal of Speech and Hearing Research, 34,* 248–251.

McHenry, M., Minton, J., & Wilson, R. (1994a). Increasing the efficiency of articulatory force testing in traumatic brain injury. In J. Till, K.M. Yorkston, & D.R. Beukelman (Eds.), *Motor Speech Disorders: Advances in Assessment and Treatment* (pp. 135–146). Baltimore: Paul Brookes Publishing Co.

McHenry, M.A., Minton, J.T., Wilson, R.L., & Post, Y.V. (1994b). Intelligibility and nonspeech orofacial strength and force control following traumatic brain injury. *Journal of Speech and Hearing Research, 37,* 1271–1283.

McNeil, M.R., Weismer, G., Adams, S., & Mulligan, M. (1990). Oral structure nonspeech motor control in normal, dysarthric, aphasic, and apraxic speakers: isometric force and static position control. *Journal of Speech and Hearing Research, 33,* 255–268.

Moore, C.A., Smith, A., & Ringel, R.L. (1988). Task specific organization of activity in human jaw muscles. *Journal of Speech and Hearing Research, 31,* 670–680.

Muller, E.M. & Abbs, J.H. (1979). Strain gauge transduction of lip and jaw motion in the mid-sagittal plane: refinement of a prototype system. *The Journal of the Acoustical Society of America, 65,* 481–486.

Murdoch, B.E., Spencer, J., Theodoros, D.G., & Thompson, E.C. (1998). Lip and tongue function in multiple sclerosis: a physiological analysis. *Motor Control, 2,* 148–160.

Neilson, P.D. & O'Dwyer, N.J. (1984). Reproducibility and variability of speech muscle activity in athetoid dysarthria of cerebral palsy. *Journal of Speech and Hearing Research, 27,* 502–517.

Robin, D.A., Goel, A., Somodi, L.B., & Luschei, E.S. (1992). Tongue strength and endurance: relation to highly skilled movements. *Journal of Speech and Hearing Research, 35,* 1239–1245.

Robin, D.A., Somodi, L.B., & Luschei, E.S. (1991). Measurement of strength and endurance in normal and articulation disordered subjects. In C.A. Moore, K.M. Yorkston, & D.R. Beukelman (Eds.), *Dysarthria and Apraxia of Speech: Perspectives on Management* (pp. 173–184). Baltimore: Paul Brookes Publishing Co.

Schönle, P.W., Gräbe, K., & Wenig, P. (1987). Electromagnetic articulography: use of alternating magnetic fields for tracking movements of multiple points inside and outside the vocal tract. *Brain and Language, 31,* 26–35.

Shaiman, S. (1989). Kinematic and electromyographic responses to perturbation of the jaw. *The Journal of the Acoustical Society of America, 86,* 78–88.

Stierwalt, J.A.G., Robin, D.M., Solomon, N.P., Weiss, A.L., & Max, J.E. (1996). Tongue strength and endurance: Relation to the speaking ability of children and adolescents following traumatic brain injury. In D.A. Robin, K.M. Yorkston, & D.R. Beukelman (Eds.), *Disorders of Motor Speech: Assessment, Treatment, and Clinical Characterization* (pp. 241–256). Baltimore: Paul Brookes Publishing Co.

Stone, M. (1991). Imaging the tongue and vocal tract. *British Journal of Disorders of Communication, 26,* 11–23.

Sussman, H.M., MacNeilage, P.F., & Hanson, R.J. (1973). Labial and mandibular dynamics during the production of bilabial consonants: preliminary observations. *Journal of Speech and Hearing Research, 16,* 385–396.

Theodoros, D.G., Murdoch, B.E., & Chenery, H.J. (1994). Perceptual speech characteristics of dysarthric speakers following severe closed head injury. *Brain Injury, 8,* 101–124.

Theodoros, D.G., Murdoch, B.E., & Horton, S. (1999). Assessment of dysarthric speech: a case for a combined perceptual and physiological approach. *Language Testing, 16,* 315–351.

Theodoros, D.G., Murdoch, B.E., & Stokes, P.D. (1995). A physiological analysis of articulatory dysfunction in dysarthric speakers following severe closed-head injury. *Brain Injury, 9,* 237–254.

Thompson, E.C., Murdoch, B.E., & Stokes, P.D. (1995). Tongue function in subjects with upper motor neuron type dysarthria following cerebrovascular accident. *Journal of Medical Speech-Language Pathology, 3,* 27–40.

Thompson, E.C., Murdoch, B.E., Theodoros, D.G., & Stokes, P. D. (1996). Physiological assessment of interlabial contact pressures in normal and neurologically impaired adults. In J. Ponsford, P. Snow, & V. Anderson (Eds.), *International Perspectives in Traumatic Brain Injury* (pp. 259–266). Brisbane: Academic Press.

Thompson-Ward, E.C. & Murdoch, B.E. (1998). Instrumental assessment of the speech mechanism. In B.E. Murdoch (Ed.), *Dysarthria: A Physiological Approach to Assessment and Treatment* (pp. 68–101). Cheltenham: Stanley Thornes (Publishers) Ltd.

Tuller, B., Shao, S., & Scott Kelso, J.A. (1990). An evaluation of an alternating magnetic field device for monitoring tongue movements. *The Journal of the Acoustical Society of America, 88,* 674–679.

Vogel, M. & von Cramon, D. (1983). Articulatory recovery after traumatic midbrain damage: a follow-up study. *Folia Phoniatrica, 35,* 294–309.

Ward, E.C., Theodoros, D.G., & Murdoch, B.E. (In press). Changes in maximum capacity tongue pressures in surgical and non-surgical patients with Parkinson's disease following the Lee Silverman Voice Treatment Program. *Journal of Medical Speech-Language Pathology.*

Yorkston, K.M. & Beukelman, D.R. (1981). *Assessment of Intelligibility of Dysarthric Speech.* Austin: Pro-Ed.

Ziegler, W. & von Cramon, D. (1983a). Vowel distortion in traumatic dysarthria: A formant study. *Phonetica, 40,* 63–78.

Ziegler, W. & von Cramon, D. (1983b). Vowel distortion in traumatic dysarthria: lip rounding versus tongue advancement. *Phonetica, 40,* 312–322.

Ziegler, W. & von Cramon, D. (1986). Spastic dysarthria after acquired brain injury: an acoustic study. *British Journal of Disorders of Communication, 21,* 173–187.

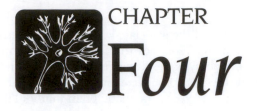

CHAPTER
Four

Velopharyngeal Dysfunction Following Traumatic Brain Injury

Deborah G. Theodoros and Bruce E. Murdoch

Introduction

The velopharyngeal valving mechanism is an essential functional component of the speech production process. Efficient opening and closing of the velopharyngeal port is required to produce the appropriate nasal and oral resonance in speech, as well as the intraoral pressures necessary for the articulation of various phonemes. The primary effect of velopharyngeal dysfunction on speech production in dysarthric speakers is the manifestation of hypernasal speech. Boone (1977) defined hypernasality as "an excessively undesirable amount of perceived nasal cavity resonance during the phonation of vowels." (p. 190). Similarly, Darley, Aronson, and Brown (1975) found that vowels were affected in dysarthric speakers with a mild degree of hypernasality, with the additional involvement of all consonants in the more severe cases. Although nasal resonance is appropriate for the three phonemes /m/, /n/, and /ŋ/, all other sounds in the English language primarily require oral resonance (Boone, 1977).

Velopharyngeal dysfunction, and the associated disturbance in resonance, is due to impairment of the basic motor processes that regulate the contraction of the muscles of the soft palate and pharynx, resulting in a reduction in the force of their contractions, limitations in the range of movements, and impaired coordination of muscle movement (Darley et al., 1975). Traumatic brain injury (TBI), which may result in diffuse damage to the central and peripheral nervous systems, has the potential to affect the motor control of the velopharyngeal valving mechanism, resulting in resonatory disturbances.

Clinically, TBI dysarthric speakers may demonstrate varying patterns and levels of severity of velopharyngeal dysfunction. Netsell (1969) described a range of different types of velopharyngeal dysfunction in a group of dysarthric speakers, including: gradual closing (velopharyngeal port opens at the beginning of an utterance, but gradually closes), anticipatory opening (velopharyngeal port opens in anticipation of a nasalized sound), retention opening (velopharynx slowly closes after production of a nasal sound, but not quickly enough to prevent nasal emission occurring during production of the next sound), and premature opening (velopharynx opens during the production of a "pressure" consonant, resulting in nasal emission of air).

In addition to causing hypernasality of speech, neurological impairment of the velopharyngeal valve may indirectly and adversely affect the articulation, prosody, and respiratory aspects of speech production in dysarthric speakers. Articulation may be affected by velopharyngeal dysfunction due to: the inability of the individual to generate sufficient intraoral pressure for the precise production of stops and fricatives; an inability to halt voicing during the articulation of voiceless plosive sounds because of an increase in glottal airflow associated with velopharyngeal incompetence (Kent & Rosenbek, 1982; Ziegler & von Cramon, 1986); slow closure of the velopharyngeal port during consonant formation, resulting in prolongation of these speech sounds (Netsell, 1969). As a result of the articulatory imprecision associated with velopharyngeal dysfunction, the prosody of speech may be adversely affected in relation to the equalization of emphasis and the disappearance of stress patterns (Darley et al., 1975). Furthermore, Kent and Rosenbek (1982) have demonstrated acoustically that nasalization of speech in dysarthric speakers is an important factor in the shaping of the syllable chain during speech, thus influencing the prosodic pattern. Respiratory support for speech may also be affected by velopharyngeal dysfunction in that wastage of expiratory air may occur as a result of inefficient valving of the breathstream at this level of the vocal tract.

Neuropathology of Velopharyngeal Dysfunction Following TBI

The neuropathological basis of the velopharyngeal dysfunction evident in dysarthric speakers following TBI is determined by the site(s) of lesion incurred at the time of injury. Impairment of the velopharyngeal valving mechanism may occur as a result of neurological damage to the upper motor neurons that supply the nuclei of the bulbar region of the brainstem, the lower motor neurons that supply the muscles of the soft palate and pharynx, subcortical structures, such as the basal ganglia, and/or the cerebellum and its connections.

Diffuse bilateral damage to the upper motor neurons supplying the bulbar nuclei of the cranial nerves results in hypertonicity, slowness of individual and repetitive movements, and a reduction in the range and force of movements of the muscles involved in speech production (Murdoch, 1990). The neurological damage involves both the direct and indirect corticobulbar pathways to the motor nuclei of the cranial nerves, causing impairment of movements and movement patterns. The spastic dysarthric speech disturbance that typically follows bilateral lesions of the upper motor neurons is frequently characterized by hypernasality. In a perceptual evaluation of the speech of 30 subjects with spastic dysarthria associated with pseudobulbar palsy, Darley et al. (1975) found that hypernasality was the eighth most frequently occurring deviant speech dimension in a series of 38 speech features. Similarly, hypernasality has been identified in other studies involving perceptual evaluations of persons with spastic dysarthria. Chenery, Murdoch, and Ingram (1992) found that 94% of their subjects with pseudobulbar palsy exhibited hypernasality of speech. In addition, in a physiological study, Thompson and Murdoch (1995) identified significantly greater degrees of nasality in 19 dysarthric subjects with upper motor neuron damage following cerebrovascular accident, compared to a matched control group of nonneurologically impaired individuals.

Following TBI, it is also possible for damage to occur to the vagus nerve, either at its origin in the nucleus ambiguous in the brainstem or to the nerve itself, as it passes peripherally to innervate the levator muscles of the soft palate. Such damage results in an associated flaccid dysarthria, accompanied by hypernasality. Bilateral lesions of the vagus nerve cause significant impairment of the elevation of the soft palate and marked hypernasality. Less severe hypernasality of speech will be perceived with a unilateral lesion of the vagus nerve where the elevation of the soft palate is reduced only on the affected side (Murdoch, 1990). Darley et al. (1975) found hypernasality to be the most prominent deviant speech dimension observed in 30 subjects with bulbar palsy and flaccid dysarthria.

Neurological impairment of subcortical structures deep within the brain (e.g., basal ganglia) due to a TBI, may result in hypokinetic dysarthria. Velopharyngeal dysfunction and hypernasality have been identified both perceptually and physiologically in persons with this form of dysarthria (Hoodin & Gilbert, 1989 a, b; Ludlow & Bassich, 1983; Netsell, Daniel, & Celesia, 1975; Theodoros, Murdoch, & Thompson, 1995). Theodoros et al. (1995) found that a group of hypokinetic dysarthric speakers demonstrated significantly greater nasality of speech physiologically, compared to a control group, while 74% of the subjects were perceived to demonstrate increased nasality of speech.

Damage to the cerebellum and/or its connections is often a frequent outcome of TBI. Lesions to this component of the central nervous system may result in ataxic dysarthria due to muscle hypotonicity and impairment of the coordination of the muscular activity involved in speech production. In particular, movements of the muscles of the soft palate and pharynx may be slow, dysrhythmic, unpredictable, and inaccurate in force, range, direction, and timing (Murdoch, 1990). As a result, individuals with cerebellar damage may possibly exhibit either hypernasality, hyponasality, or mixed nasality of speech due to the impaired coordination of palatal and pharyngeal muscle activity. To date, findings concerning the frequency of occurrence of resonatory disorders in persons with cerebellar impairment and ataxic dysarthria are equivocal. In an early study using spectrographic analysis of the speech of a subject with Friedrich's ataxia, Lehiste (1965) identified the presence of sporadic nasalization of non-nasal consonants, and the omission of nasals with compensatory nasalization. While Darley et al. (1975) did not identify hypernasality as a prominent feature of ataxic dysarthria, Chenery, Ingram, and Murdoch (1990) found that 11 of their 16 subjects with ataxic dysarthria exhibited hypernasal speech. Because damage to the cerebellum and its connections affects the coordination of motor control, it is possible that mixed nasality may also occur due to poorly timed velopharyngeal movements.

In that dysarthric speakers, following TBI, have been found to demonstrate either spastic, flaccid, ataxic, hypokinetic or a combination of these types of dysarthria (see Chapter 2, "Type and Severity of Dysarthria Following TBI"), velopharyngeal dysfunction must be considered a highly probable sequelae of TBI. Clinically, resonatory disturbances post-TBI have been noted to present across a continuum of severity, ranging from mild degrees of hypernasal speech to severe hypernasality that has a profound effect on speech intelligibility and the integrity of the speech mechanism.

Perceptual Features Of Velopharyngeal Dysfunction Following TBI

Detailed investigations of the perceptual manifestations of velopharyngeal dysfunction post-TBI are limited. Studies conducted to date, however, have identified hypernasality as the predominant type of resonatory disturbance in TBI subjects (McHenry, 1998; McHenry, Wilson, & Minton, 1994; Netsell & Daniel, 1979; Theodoros, Murdoch, & Chenery, 1994; Workinger & Netsell, 1992).

In general, single case studies of dysarthric speakers following TBI have reported the presence of severe hypernasality in these individuals (McHenry et al., 1994; Netsell & Daniel, 1979; Workinger & Netsell, 1992). In each case, the severe degree of hypernasality contributed significantly to a reduction in overall speech intelligibility and required prosthetic management in the form of a palatal lift to improve the physiological foundation of the speech mechanism to allow speech rehabilitation procedures to proceed and be effective. Group studies, however, have identified variable degrees of hypernasality in dysarthric speakers following TBI. A group study of 20 closed-head-injured (CHI) subjects by Theodoros et al. (1994), identified hypernasality in 95% of the subjects, with more than half (63%) of this group demonstrating hypernasal speech to a moderate-to-severe degree and 37% of the subjects exhibiting a mild degree of hypernasality. Mixed nasality was perceived to be present, mainly to a mild-to-moderate degree, in 90% of the subjects. Based on perceptual ratings of nasality, the CHI subjects examined by Theodoros et al. (1994) were found to demonstrate significantly greater degrees of hypernasality and mixed nasality, compared to their control counterparts. A similar incidence of hypernasality (98%) was identified in the speech output of an expanded cohort of 43 TBI dysarthric speakers investigated in our laboratory. Indeed, hypernasality was found to be the most frequently occurring deviant speech dimension, with the majority of the subjects (57%) exhibiting this abnormal speech feature to a moderate-to-severe degree. In this larger group of subjects, however, mixed nasality was perceived to occur less frequently (44%) than in the Theodoros et al. (1994) study, with the majority of these subjects demonstrating a mild degree of mixed nasality. The high incidence of perceived hypernasality identified in the 43 TBI dysarthric speakers was supported by the findings of the

Frenchay Dysarthria Assessment (Enderby, 1983), which identified mild-to-moderate impairment in palatal maintenance and a moderate impairment of palatal function during speech in this group of subjects (see Chapter 2, "Perceptual Features of Dysarthria Following TBI").

McHenry (1998), in a study of 83 TBI patients (90% of whom were dysarthric), reported that hypernasality was perceived to be present in approximately 47% of the subjects. The majority of the hypernasal subjects (59%) exhibited hypernasality to a mild degree. The discrepancy between the frequency of occurrence of hypernasality in the study by McHenry (1998) and that reported for our cohort of 43 TBI subjects may be related to: the differences in sample size between the two studies, differences in severity of dysarthria between the two groups (moderate-to-severe dysarthria in 49% of the authors' cohort, and in 32% of McHenry's subject cohort), the inadequacies of perceptual evaluation of nasality, and the inherent variability of impairment in dysarthric TBI subjects (McHenry, 1999; Theodoros, Murdoch, & Stokes, 1995).

Although the previous studies have identified increased nasality in dysarthric speakers following TBI, there is evidence to suggest that, of all the speech characteristics, the perceptual evaluation of nasality is particularly difficult, and potentially inaccurate, due to the "halo effect" in which other deviant speech features (e.g., articulatory imprecision, and phonatory and rate disturbances) may influence the listener's perception of this resonatory speech dimension (Brancewicz & Reich, 1989; Bzoch, 1989; Sherman, 1954). McHenry (1999), in a study of measures of nasality that would most accurately identify this speech dimension, found that perceived nasality was associated with reduced intelligibility and reduced speaking rate. The findings suggested, however, that it was the rate disturbance that would cause the listener to erroneously perceive excessive nasality in the individual's speech rather than the reduction in intelligibility (McHenry, 1999). Furthermore, McHenry (1999) determined that breathiness, evident physiologically in 71% of the sample, did not contribute to the perception of nasality in the sample of TBI subjects. In view of the inadequacies in the perceptual evaluation of nasality in dysarthric speakers, this form of assessment must be supplemented by objective measures of nasality to determine the presence or absence of velopharyngeal dysfunction in individuals following TBI.

Physiological Assessment of Velopharyngeal Function Following TBI

Physiological assessment of velopharyngeal function may involve a number of direct and indirect techniques, which provide either visualization of the velopharyngeal port, including soft palate and pharyngeal movement; an estimate of the size of the velopharyngeal orifice; representation of velar movement patterns in relation to other articulators during speech; or measures of nasal air flow and air pressure, nasal vibration, and acoustic output from oral and nasal cavities (Thompson-Ward & Murdoch, 1998). Some of these techniques have been used successfully to evaluate velopharyngeal function in dysarthric speakers following TBI, while others have the potential to provide useful diagnostic information regarding velopharyngeal competence in this population.

Direct Assessment Techniques

Since adequate velopharyngeal closure for speech involves the coordination of the velopharyngeal sphincter in three dimensions (David, White, Sprod, & Bagnall, 1982; Karnell & Morris, 1985), the need to evaluate this three-dimensional movement has led to the development of a number of dynamic instrumental techniques. These assessment techniques include endoscopy and nasendoscopy, videofluoroscopy, photodetection, and electromagnetic articulography (EMA). In addition, electromyography (EMG) has been used to directly record the electrical activity of velar and pharyngeal wall muscles.

A common clinical assessment of velopharyngeal function involves the use of oral and nasal videoendoscopic procedures, which allow the examiner to observe the completion, timing and coordination of palatal and pharyngeal wall movement. The nasoendoscopic procedure, involving the insertion of a thin, flexible fiberoptic tube into the nasopharynx via the nasal passages, allows for direct viewing of the velopharyngeal region from above, and permits observation of velar movements during speech (David et al.,1982; Karnell, Linville, & Edwards, 1988; Niimi, Bell-Berti, & Harris, 1982). Oral videoendoscopy involves the insertion of a rigid scope into the oral cavity. The endoscope is positioned laterally to the uvula so that an optimal view of the velopharyngeal port is obtained (Karnell & Morris, 1985). Although providing similar detail, the oral endoscopic procedure is problematic in that it does not allow for normal speech activity during this procedure (Willis & Stutz, 1972). Karnell and Morris (1985), however, found that when used in tandem, oral and nasal videoendoscopic procedures provided a more useful assessment of velopharyngeal function than when either procedure was used in isolation.

Further detail of the dynamic function of the velopharyngeal sphincter during speech may be obtained through videofluoroscopy, a radiographic imaging technique. Earlier technological versions of this technique included cineradiography and cinefluorography (Lock & Seaver, 1984; Williams & Eisenbach, 1981). Videofluoroscopy allows for the visualization of velopharyngeal sphincter function in the sagittal, frontal, and transverse plans of reference (Karnell & Morris, 1985). During this procedure, the velopharynx is coated with a barium sulphate contrast medium, applied through the nose (Henningsson & Isberg, 1991). The superior surface of the velum, and the lateral and posterior pharyngeal walls are subsequently coated with the contrast medium. In addition, the tongue and the contours of the lips are coated with the barium to allow for observation of the movements of the tongue and lips in relation to velopharyngeal movement. Henningsson and Isberg (1991), in a comparison of multiview videofluoroscopy and nasendoscopy found that the former technique was superior to the latter in demonstrating movements of the lateral pharyngeal walls. These investigators concluded that videofluoroscopy was indispensable in assessing velopharyngeal function.

Another technique that may be used to provide additional information concerning the total velopharyngeal area involves the use of a photodetector system that measures the intensity of light transmitted through the velopharyngeal port or reflected from the velar surface (Dalston & Seaver, 1990; Keefe & Dalston, 1989). The photodetector system comprises a light source, transmitting and receiving optical fibers, and a light detector (Keefe & Dalston, 1989). The dual-fiber photodetector probe is inserted into the nasal cavity to a position approximately 5 mm below the resting level of the velum (Keefe & Dalston, 1989). Light is introduced to the area below the velopharyngeal port by the transmitting fiber, while the optical receiving fiber detects the presence of light as the velopharyngeal port opens and closes. The photodetector output represents the total velopharyngeal area and reflects velar elevation and pharyngeal wall movement (Keefe and Dalston, 1989). These authors advocated that the photodetector system overcomes the problem of interpreting radiographic recordings of asynchronous movements of the lateral pharyngeal walls and the velum. Furthermore, photodetection has been found to be reliable and effective when used in conjunction with videoendoscopy (Karnell, Seaver, & Dalston, 1988).

Electromagnetic articulography (EMA) has been demonstrated to be a valuable tool in assessing velopharyngeal function in normal speakers (Engelke, Hoch, Bruns, & Striebeck, 1996), and therefore, has the potential for use in the TBI population. Engelke et al. (1996) suggested that the velum is a particularly suitable component of the speech mechanism to analyze because it has limited movement in a sagittal-vertical direction. As previously described in "Physiological Assessment of Articulatory Function Following TBI" in Chapter 3, EMA can provide real-time representation of movements of the lips, tongue, jaw, and velum during speech. In assessing velar movement using this technique, a sensor is adhered or sutured to the anterior margin of the velum in a midsagittal position and recordings are made during speech activities. From these recordings, the velocity, trajectory, and acceleration of velar movements may be determined. Due to the complexity of data collection and analyses, and the cost of this apparatus, however, this technique remains largely within the confines of the research arena at present.

Electromyography (EMG) has been used extensively to identify the specific muscles involved in the velopharyngeal sphincteric action (Bell-Berti, 1976; Bell-Berti & Hirose, 1975; Lubker, 1968). While this technique provides direct and detailed information of muscle activity in this area, its clinical application for assessing velopharyngeal function is limited due to the invasive nature of the procedure when using hook-wire electrodes, the difficulty with surface electrode placement, and the interference with articulatory movements during speech (Baken, 1987).

Indirect Assessment Techniques

To overcome the invasiveness and restricted applicability of many of the direct assessment techniques, noninvasive assessment techniques have been developed from which inferences regarding the status of velopharyngeal function may be made. These techniques include physiological measurement of nasal air flow and pressure, nasal accelerometry, and measurement of the ratio of acoustic output from the nasal and oral cavities.

Simultaneous measurement of nasal air flow and pressure and oral pressure has been reported by a number of investigators (Andreassen, Smith, & Guyette, 1992; Dalston & Warren, 1986; Dalston, Warren, & Smith, 1990). A greater increase in nasal airflow and a decrease in oral pressure are considered to be consistent with velopharyngeal incompetence (Warren & Devereux, 1966). With this technique, a catheter is positioned in one nostril and sealed with a cork, and another placed in the mouth. Static nasal and oral air pressures are measured by pressure transducers, while nasal air flow is recorded via tubing placed in the other nostril and connected to a heated pneumotachograph. A similar technique, which is less invasive, involves the use of a tight-fitting mask positioned over the nose and attached to a pneumotachograph, and a differential pressure transducer, to record nasal air flow and intraoral pressure during speech (McHenry, 1999). Intraoral pressure is measured using a small catheter, positioned just inside the lips behind the incisors, and attached to the pressure transducer. From this technique, a measure of velopharyngeal airway resistance can be obtained by dividing the peak intraoral air pressure during /p/ production by the corresponding air flow, and then subtracting nasal cavity resistance at the same nasal airflow (Barlow, Suing, Grossman, Bodmer, & Colbert, 1989; McHenry, 1998). The velopharyngeal airway resistance value may then be used to determine the velopharyngeal orifice area using the hydrokinetic orifice equation originally reported by Warren and DuBois (1964). This technique and derived calculations have been used successfully by McHenry (1997, 1998) to identify velopharyngeal airway resistance disorders and an estimate of velopharyngeal orifice area in individuals with dysarthric speech following TBI.

Indirect assessment of velopharyngeal function may also be achieved using nasal accelerometry which is designed to measure vibrations of the nose and throat during speech (Horii, 1980, 1983; Horii & Lang, 1981; Stevens, Kalikow, & Willemain, 1975). With this technique, one miniature, vibration-sensitive accelerometer is positioned externally on the nose, and one on the throat (on the thyroid lamina of the larynx), to record vibration. During the production of nasal utterances, the output of the nasal accelerometer is greater than that of the throat accelerometer. Horii (1980) introduced the use of an index of nasal coupling, the Horii Oral-Nasal Coupling (HONC) index, to quantify nasality. This index is the ratio of nasal accelerometric amplitude to voice amplitude recorded from the two accelerometers positioned on the nose and throat. From this type of assessment, a measure of nasality in speech can be obtained, and the degree of velopharyngeal function is inferred from the HONC index. A high nasality index is indicative of velopharyngeal incompetence, while a low index is consistent with normal velopharyngeal function. This technique, which is even less invasive than the previously mentioned nasal air pressure and air flow measurement techniques, has now been used in a number of studies to evaluate velopharyngeal function in dysarthric speakers (Theodoros et al., 1995; Thompson & Murdoch, 1995), and in particular, those persons with a dysarthric speech disturbance following TBI (Theodoros, Murdoch, Stokes, & Chenery, 1993).

Another indirect assessment of velopharyngeal function involves determination of the degree of nasality during speech derived from the ratio of acoustic output recorded from the nasal and oral cavities (Dalston & Seaver, 1992; Dalston, Warren, & Dalston, 1991; Nellis, Neiman, & Lehman, 1992). The most commonly used instrumentation to record this acoustic output is the commercially available Nasometer® (Kay Elemetrics), which consists of two directional microphones (one positioned in front of the nose, and the other in front of the mouth), separated by a sound-separating plate. During speech, the ratio of nasal to oral acoustic output is calculated by the accompanying software and displayed in real-time graphic form on the computer screen, and as a "nasalance" score. A high nasalance score is consistent with velopharyngeal dysfunction, while a low score is indicative of a normal level of velopharyngeal competency. As reported by

McHenry (1999), the Nasometer has been used successfully to assess velopharyngeal function in individuals following TBI, with the nasalance scores obtained for these subjects most accurately reflecting listener perception of nasality in speech.

Physiological Features of Velopharyngeal Dysfunction Following TBI

Physiological studies of velopharyngeal function in persons following TBI have identified impairment of this component of the speech production mechanism, using nasal accelerometry and aerodynamic assessment of velopharyngeal airway resistance. Of particular importance is the finding that instrumental assessment of velopharyngeal function following TBI has been pivotal in determining the validity of perceptual impressions of nasality in these speakers.

In the first group study of velopharyngeal function in dysarthric speakers with TBI, Theodoros et al. (1993) determined the degree of nasality in the speech of 20 dysarthric speakers using nasal accelerometry. The TBI subjects were found to demonstrate significantly higher mean HONC indices, expressed as a percentage (mean = 41.95%; SD = 19.88), for nonnasal utterances compared to a matched control group (mean = 26.35%; SD = 13.64), indicating a greater degree of velopharyngeal dysfunction in the former group. Although the TBI subjects were perceived to exhibit significantly greater degrees of hypernasality compared to the control group, the study failed to show any significant correlation between the perceptual ratings and the mean nasality indices obtained across nonnasal utterances for these subjects. In determining the relationship between these perceptual and physiological parameters, the data pertaining to each TBI subject was evaluated, and four subgroups of post-TBI dysarthric speakers were identified: group one consisted of those subjects who were perceived to be hypernasal and recorded high nasality indices; group two comprised subjects who were considered to be hypernasal, but recorded low nasality indices; group three subjects achieved high nasality indices while being perceived to exhibit minimal hypernasality during physiological assessment; and group four consisted of subjects who did not exhibit any marked hypernasality, and recorded low nasality indices across nonnasal utterances. Theodoros et al. (1993) concluded that the variation in these findings were not unexpected considering the diffuse nature of the brain injury associated with TBI and the difficulties inherent in the perceptual assessment of nasality. Furthermore, the investigators stressed the importance of evaluating both the perceptual and instrumental data relating to nasality in the TBI population on an individual basis.

In a larger cohort of 43 TBI subjects (including those of Theodoros et al., 1993) investigated in our laboratory (see "Perceptual Features of Dysarthria Following TBI" in Chapter 2), nasal accelerometry confirmed the findings of Theodoros et al. (1993) in relation to the mean HONC indices recorded for these subjects. The TBI dysarthric speakers demonstrated significantly greater mean percentage HONC indices (mean = 43.81%; SD = 19.74) for non-nasal utterances, compared to a matched control group (mean = 35.56%; SD = 17.67). These results were consistent with impairment of velopharyngeal function in the TBI subjects and the perceptual finding of hypernasality in 98% of these subjects.

Abnormal aerodynamics and velopharyngeal orifice area estimates associated with velopharyngeal function have also been reported in the TBI population (McHenry, 1997, 1998). McHenry (1998) investigated velopharyngeal airway resistance in a group of 83 severely TBI adults to determine the incidence of impairment in this parameter in mild, moderate, and severe dysarthric speakers, and to ascertain the relationship between perceived hypernasality and deficits in velopharyngeal airway resistance. A velopharyngeal airway resistance value of 100 $cmH_2O/L/sec$ was considered to be within normal limits based on clinical experience, while values from 50 to 99 $cmH_2O/L/sec$ indicated a mild or inconsistent resistance deficit. McHenry (1998) reported that a moderate deficit in velopharyngeal airway resistance was consistent with values from 25 to 49 $cmH_2O/L/sec$, while values less than 25 $cmH_2O/L/sec$ indicated a severe deficit. Of the 83 subjects, 52% exhibited normal velopharyngeal airway resistance, with 48% of the subjects recording abnormal values. Twenty percent of the subjects were found to have a mild or inconsistent resistance deficit, 11% were identified as having a moderate deficit, and 17% of the subjects recorded values consistent with a severe deficit in velopharyngeal airway resistance. In relation to the severity of dysarthria evident in these TBI subjects, the results indicated that most of the subjects with mild or no dysarthria recorded velopharyngeal airway resistance values within normal limits, while the majority of the 15 TBI subjects with severe dysarthria recorded resistance values of less than 25 $cmH_2O/L/sec$. In general, the perceptual findings for these subjects correlated with those of the physiological assessment. The majority of subjects who were not perceived to be hypernasal recorded velopharyngeal airway resistance values within normal limits, while most of the subjects who were rated as severely hypernasal obtained resistance values of less than 25 $cmH_2O/L/sec$. Consistent with the findings of Theodoros et al. (1993), however, McHenry (1998) also noted that a number of subjects evidenced discrepancies between the perceptual and physiological findings. These inconsistencies were attributed to the fact that the perception of hypernasality was possibly adversely influenced by other speech parameters such as pitch, loudness, vocal quality, speaking rate, and intelligibility (McHenry, 1998).

In a study of the effect of increased vocal effort on estimates of velopharyngeal orifice area (derived from a measure of velopharyngeal airway resistance), McHenry (1997) identified estimated velopharyngeal orifice areas that were inadequate or possibly inadequate in 50% of a group of 28 TBI subjects with below normal velopharyngeal airway resistance values. Within this group, 21% of the subjects were identified as having orifice areas of greater than 20 mm^2, 29% recorded areas between 19 mm^2 and 5 mm^2, and 50% of the subjects demonstrated velopharyngeal orifice areas of less than 5 mm^2. Warren, Dalston, and Mayo (1994) considered a velopharyngeal orifice area of less than 5 mm^2 to be adequate for normal resonance, while Warren (1979) suggested that an area greater than 20 mm^2 was indicative of inadequate velopharyngeal function, resulting in hypernasality and/or nasal emission. Estimated velopharyngeal orifice area values between 19 mm^2 and 5mm^2 were considered to be less discriminate and may or may not result in hypernasality and nasal emission (McHenry, 1997).

While studies of velopharyngeal function following TBI are emerging in the literature, this component of the speech mechanism in TBI dysarthric speakers has not yet been fully investigated, particularly in relation to the dynamic aspects of the sphincteric action of the valving mechanism. Additional physiological studies of velopharyngeal function are required to provide a basis for ongoing development of efficacious treatment programs for use in the clinical management of resonatory disturbances in individuals with dysarthric speech following TBI.

Summary

Velopharyngeal dysfunction and the perceptual manifestation of hypernasality has been identified as a frequently occurring consequence of TBI. Speakers who are dysarthric following TBI have been perceived to be significantly more hypernasal than normal speakers and have demonstrated physiological evidence of velopharyngeal dysfunction in a large proportion of individuals. Mild-to-severe degrees of hypernasality and velopharyngeal dysfunction have been noted in this population, with some individuals demonstrating such severe impairment of the velopharyngeal valve that the speech mechanism is profoundly compromised and speech intelligibility markedly affected. Although there is both perceptual and physiological evidence of velopharyngeal dysfunction in TBI individuals with dysarthric speech, each person must be evaluated on an individual basis because of the variability of impairment evident in this population, and the inherent difficulties in the perceptual evaluation of this speech dimension. The failure to closely examine individual assessment results in relation to velopharyngeal function, and failure to consider other deficits in the speech production mechanism that may be affecting these findings, may lead to the initiation of inappropriate management of the dysarthric speech disturbance.

References

Andreassen, M.L., Smith, B.E., & Guyette, T.W. (1992). Pressure-flow measurements for selected oral and nasal sound segments produced by normal adults. *Cleft Palate-Craniofacial Journal, 29*, 1–9.

Baken, R.J. (1987). *Clinical Measurement of Speech and Voice*. Boston: College-Hill Press.

Barlow, S.M., Suing, G., Grossman, A., Bodmer, P., & Colbert, R. (1989). A high-speed data acquisition and protocol control system for vocal tract physiology. *Journal of Voice, 3*, 283–293.

Bell-Berti, F. (1976). An electromyographic study of velopharyngeal function. *Journal of Speech and Hearing Research, 19*, 225–240.

Bell-Berti, F. & Hirose, H. (1975). Palatal activity in voicing distinctions: A simultaneous fiberoptic and electromyographic study. *Journal of Phonetics, 3*, 69–74.

Boone, D.R. (1977). *The Voice and Voice Therapy*. (Second edition). Englewood Cliffs: Prentice-Hall.

Brancewicz, T.M. & Reich, A.R. (1989). Speech rate reduction and "nasality" in normal speakers. *Journal of Speech and Hearing Research, 32*, 837–848.

Bzoch, K.R. (1989). Measurement and assessment of categorical aspects of cleft palate language, voice, and speech disorders. In K.R. Bzoch (Ed.), *Communicative Disorders Related to Cleft Lip and Palate* (pp. 137–173). Boston: College-Hill Press.

Chenery, H.J., Ingram, J.C.L., & Murdoch, B.E. (1990). Perceptual analysis of the speech in ataxic dysarthria. *Australian Journal of Human Communication Disorders, 18*, 19–28.

Chenery, H.J., Murdoch, B.E., & Ingram, J.C.L. (1992). The perceptual speech characteristics of persons with pseudobulbar palsy. *Australian Journal of Human Communication Disorders, 20*, 21–30.

Dalston, R.M. & Seaver, E.J. (1990). Nasometric and phototransductive measurements of reaction times among normal adult speakers. *Cleft Palate Journal, 27,* 61–67.

Dalston, R.M. & Seaver, E.J. (1992). Relative values of various standardized passages in the nasometric assessment of patients with velopharyngeal impairment. *Cleft Palate-Craniofacial Journal, 29,* 17–21.

Dalston, R.M. & Warren, D.W. (1986). Comparisons of Tonar II, pressure flow, and listener judgements of hypernasality in the assessment of velopharyngeal function. *Cleft Palate Journal, 32,* 108–115.

Dalston, R.M., Warren, D.W., & Dalston, E.T. (1991). A preliminary investigation concerning the use of nasometry in identifying patients with hyponasality and/or nasal airway impairment. *Journal of Speech and Hearing Research, 34,* 11–18.

Dalston, R.M., Warren, D.W., & Smith, L.R. (1990). The aerodynamic characteristics of speech produced by normal speakers and cleft palate speakers with adequate velopharyngeal function. *Cleft Palate Journal, 27,* 393–401.

Darley, F.L., Aronson, A.E., & Brown, J.R. (1975). *Motor Speech Disorders.* Philadelphia: W.B. Saunders Company.

David, D.J., White, J., Sprod, R., & Bagnall, A. (1982). Nasendoscopy: Significant refinements of a direct-viewing technique of the velopharyngeal sphincter. *Plastic and Reconstructive Surgery, 70,* 423–428.

Enderby, P.M. (1983). *Frenchay Dysarthria Assessment.* San Diego: College-Hill Press.

Engelke, W., Hoch, G., Bruns, T., & Striebeck, M. (1996). Simultaneous evaluation of articulatory velopharyngeal function under different dynamic conditions with EMA and videoendoscopy. *Folia Phoniatrica et Logopaedica, 48,* 65–77.

Henningsson, G. & Isberg, A. (1991). Comparison between multiview videofluoroscopy and nasendoscopy of velopharyngeal movements. *Cleft Palate-Craniofacial Journal, 28,* 413–417.

Hoodin, R.B. & Gilbert, H.R. (1989a). Nasal airflows in Parkinsonian speakers. *Journal of Communication Disorders, 22,* 169–180.

Hoodin, R.B. & Gilbert, H.R. (1989b). Parkinsonian dysarthria: An aerodynamic and perceptual description of velopharyngeal closure for speech. *Folia Phoniatrica, 41,* 249–258.

Horii, Y. (1980). An accelerometric approach to nasality measurement: A preliminary report. *Cleft Palate Journal, 17,* 254–261.

Horii, Y. (1983). An accelerometric measure as a physical correlate of perceived hypernasality in speech. *Journal of Speech and Hearing Research, 26,* 476–480.

Horii, Y. & Lang, J.E. (1981). Distributional analyses of an index of nasal coupling (HONC) in simulated hypernasal speech. *Cleft Palate Journal, 18,* 279–285.

Karnell, M.P., Linville, R.N., & Edwards, B.A. (1988). Variations in velar position over time: A nasal videoendoscopic study. *Journal of Speech and Hearing Research, 31,* 417–424.

Karnell, M.P. & Morris, H.L. (1985). Multiview videoendoscopic evaluation of velopharyngeal physiology in 15 normal speakers. *Annals of Otology, Rhinology, and Laryngology, 94,* 361–365.

Karnell, M.P., Seaver, E.J., & Dalston, R.M. (1988). A comparison of photodetector and endoscopic evaluations of velopharyngeal function. *Journal of Speech and Hearing Research, 31,* 503–510.

Keefe, M.J. & Dalston, R.M. (1989). An analysis of velopharyngeal timing in normal adult speakers using a microcomputer based photodetector system. *Journal of Speech and Hearing Research, 32,* 195–202.

Kent, R.D. & Rosenbek, J.C. (1982). Prosodic disturbance and neurologic lesion. *Brain and Language, 15,* 259–291.

Lehiste, I. (1965). Some acoustic characteristics of dysarthric speech. *Bibliotheca Phonetica, 2,* 1–124.

Lock, R.B. & Seaver, E.J. (1984). Nasality and velopharyngeal function in five hearing impaired adults. *Journal of Communication Disorders, 17,* 47–64.

Lubker, J.F. (1968). An electromyographic-cineradiographic investigation of velar function during normal speech production. *Cleft Palate Journal, 5,* 1–8.

Ludlow, C.L. & Bassich, C.J. (1983). The results of acoustic and perceptual assessment of two types of dysarthria. In W.R. Berry (Ed.), *Clinical Dysarthria* (pp. 121–154). San Diego: College-Hill Press.

McHenry, M.A. (1997). The effect of increased vocal effort on estimated velopharyngeal orifice area. *American Journal of Speech-Language Pathology, 6*, 55–61.

McHenry, M.A. (1998). Velopharyngeal airway resistance disorders after traumatic brain injury. *Archives of Physical Medicine and Rehabilitation, 79*, 545–549.

McHenry, M.A. (1999). Aerodynamic, acoustic, and perceptual measures of nasality following traumatic brain injury. *Brain Injury, 13*, 281–290.

McHenry, M.A., Wilson, R.L., & Minton, J.T. (1994). Management of multiple physiologic system deficits following traumatic brain injury. *Journal of Medical Speech-Language Pathology, 2*, 59–74.

Murdoch, B.E. (1990). *Acquired Speech and Language Disorders: A Neuroanatomical and Functional Neurological Approach*. London: Chapman and Hall.

Nellis, J.L., Neiman, G.S., & Lehman, J.A. (1992). Comparison of nasometer and listener judgements of nasality in the assessment of velopharyngeal function after pharyngeal flap surgery. *Cleft Palate-Craniofacial Journal, 29*, 157–163.

Netsell, R. (1969). Evaluation of velopharyngeal function in dysarthria. *Journal of Speech and Hearing Disorders, 34*, 113–122.

Netsell, R. & Daniel, B. (1979). Dysarthria in adults: Physiologic approach in rehabilitation. *Archives of Physical Medicine and Rehabilitation, 60*, 502–508.

Netsell, R., Daniel, B., & Celesia, G.G. (1975). Acceleration and weakness in Parkinsonian dysarthria. *Journal of Speech and Hearing Disorders, 40*, 170–178.

Niimi, S., Bell-Berti, F., & Harris, K.S. (1982). Dynamic aspects of velopharyngeal closure. *Folia Phoniatrica, 34*, 246–257.

Sherman, D. (1954). The merits of backward playing of connected speech in the scaling of voice quality disorders. *Journal of Speech and Hearing Disorders, 19*, 312–321.

Stevens, K.N., Kalikow, D.N., & Willemain, T.R. (1975). A miniature accelerometer for detecting glottal waveforms and nasalization. *Journal of Speech and Hearing Research, 18*, 594–599.

Theodoros, D.G., Murdoch, B.E., & Chenery, H.J. (1994). Perceptual speech characteristics of dysarthric speakers following severe closed head injury. *Brain Injury, 8*, 101–124.

Theodoros, D.G., Murdoch, B.E., & Stokes, P.D. (1995). Variability in the perceptual and physiological features of dysarthria following severe closed head injury: An examination of five cases. *Brain Injury, 9*, 671–696.

Theodoros, D.G., Murdoch, B.E., Stokes, P.D., & Chenery, H.J. (1993). Hypernasality in dysarthric speakers following severe closed head injury: A perceptual and instrumental analysis. *Brain Injury, 7*, 59–69.

Theodoros, D.G., Murdoch, B.E., & Thompson, E.C. (1995). Hypernasality in Parkinson's disease: A perceptual and physiological analysis. *Journal of Medical Speech-Language Pathology, 3*, 73–84.

Thompson, E.C. & Murdoch, B.E. (1995). Disorders of nasality in subjects with upper motor neurone type dysarthria following cerebrovascular accident. *Journal of Communication Disorders, 28*, 261–276.

Thompson-Ward, E.C. & Murdoch, B.E. (1998). Instrumental assessment of the speech mechanism. In B.E. Murdoch (Ed.), *Dysarthria: A Physiological Approach to Assessment and Treatment* (pp. 68–101). Cheltenham: Stanley Thorne Publishers Ltd.

Warren, D.W. (1979). Perci: A method for rating palatal efficiency. *Cleft Palate Journal, 16*, 179–285.

Warren, D.W., Dalston, R.M., & Mayo, R. (1994). Hypernasality and velopharyngeal impairment. *Cleft Palate-Craniofacial Journal, 31*, 257–262.

Warren, D.W. & Devereux, J.L. (1966). An analog study of cleft palate speech. *Cleft Palate Journal, 3*, 103–114.

Warren, D.W. & DuBois, A.B. (1964). A pressure-flow technique for measuring velopharyngeal orifice area during continuous speech. *Cleft Palate Journal, 1*, 52–71.

Williams, W.N. & Eisenbach, C.R. (1981). Assessing VP function: The lateral still technique vs. cinefluorography. *Cleft Palate Journal, 18*, 45–50.

Willis, C.R. & Stutz, M.L. (1972). The clinical use of the Taub oral panendoscope in the observation of velopharyngeal function. *Journal of Speech and Hearing Disorders, 37*, 495–502.

Workinger, M. & Netsell, R. (1992). Restoration of intelligible speech 13 years post-head injury. *Brain Injury, 6*, 183–187.

Ziegler, W. & von Cramon, D. (1986). Spastic dysarthria after acquired brain injury: An acoustic study. *British Journal of Disorders of Communication, 21*, 173–187.

CHAPTER
Five

Laryngeal Dysfunction Following Traumatic Brain Injury

Deborah G. Theodoros and Bruce E. Murdoch

Introduction

The laryngeal subsystem of the speech production mechanism provides the medium through which speech is delivered and contributes to the suprasegmental and articulatory features of speech (Ramig, 1992). Phonatory disturbances resulting from laryngeal dysfunction are frequently observed following traumatic brain injury (TBI) and are usually seen as part of a specific dysarthric speech impairment involving respiratory, articulatory, and resonatory deficits. Disordered phonation has been shown to have considerable adverse effects on the intelligibility of speech (McGarr & Osberger, 1978; Monsen, 1983; Parkhurst & Levitt, 1978), and therefore, this aspect of speech production may play a significant role in defining speech outcome in persons following TBI.

The Effects of Laryngeal Dysfunction on Speech

In addition to adequate respiratory support, consistent and efficient vibration of the vocal folds is essential for ensuring effective valving of the expiratory airflow for the generation of voice. Dysfunction of this aspect of the laryngeal mechanism involving hyperadduction, hypoadduction, or incoordination of the vocal folds may result in reduced vocal intensity and abnormal vocal quality. In the various dysarthric populations, reduced vocal loudness has been recognized as contributing to the difficulties in oral communication experienced by these speakers (Aronson, 1985; Rosenbek & La Pointe, 1991; Simpson, Till, & Goff, 1988). While not confirmed experimentally, abnormal vocal qualities such as harshness, strained-strangled voice, hoarseness, glottal fry, tremor, and wetness observed in dysarthric speakers (Aronson, 1985; Boone & McFarlane, 1988; Darley, Aronson, & Brown, 1975), clinically appear to adversely affect the intelligibility of speech (Ramig, 1992).

The suprasegmental features of speech, such as pitch and prosody and the articulatory characteristic of voiced/voiceless phoneme distinction, are dependent upon precise coordination of laryngeal, respiratory, and articulatory subsystems of the speech mechanism. Dysfunction in the laryngeal subsystem may cause a reduction in the variation of pitch, loudness, and duration of phonation such that dysprosody presents as an obvious deviant speech feature. The primary articulatory function of the larynx is to contribute to the distinction between voiced and voiceless phonemes. For some dysarthric speakers, hypoadduction of the vocal folds may result in voiced phonemes being produced as voiceless, while for other speakers with hyperadduction of the vocal folds, continuous voicing of all consonants may occur (Farmer, 1980; Freeman, Cannito, & Finnitzo-Heiber, 1985; Weismer, 1984). A disruption of laryngeal function in dysarthric speakers, therefore, may have a considerable, adverse effect on articulatory aspects of speech production.

Neuropathology of Laryngeal Dysfunction Following TBI

Complex central nervous system connections are required for the coordination of laryngeal function involving the control of vocal fold movement, and coordination with the respiratory, velopharyngeal, and articulatory subsystems of speech and reflex activities (e.g., swallowing). In that phonation requires highly integrated neurophysiological coordination, it is likely that laryngeal dysfunction may result from impairment at a number of levels of the central nervous system (Hanson, 1991).

The biomechanics of a TBI are such that damage may result in impairment of components of the central nervous system associated with laryngeal function. Following this type of brain injury, a broad spectrum of laryngeal dysfunction involving hyperfunctional, hypofunctional, and incoordinated laryngeal activity can be expected to result from bilateral lesions of the upper motor neurons, damage to specific lower motor neurons that supply laryngeal musculature, lesions of the extrapyramidal system and its connections, lesions of the cerebellum and its connecting pathways, and lesions involving several locations within the central and/or peripheral nervous systems. As a result of these lesions, the individual with TBI may exhibit features of spastic, flaccid, hypokinetic, hyperkinetic, or ataxic dysphonia, or a combination of these phonatory disturbances (Aronson, 1985: Hartman, 1984).

Spastic dysphonia associated with bilateral damage to the upper motor neurons in the pyramidal and extrapyramidal neuronal pathways is characterized by a harsh, strained-strangled vocal quality, with a reduction in pitch and loudness variation (Aronson, 1985; Colton & Casper, 1996a; Darley et al., 1975). The perceptual features of spastic dysphonia are consistent with hypertonicity and hyperadduction of the true vocal folds and supraglottic musculature (Colton & Casper, 1996a; Darley et al., 1975; Hartman, 1984). In that a TBI has the potential to result in diffuse axonal injury involving these neuronal pathways, a spastic dysphonia may readily occur following this type of brain insult.

Flaccid dysphonia is characterized by a hoarse, breathy, and often wet vocal quality (Aronson, 1985; Darley et al., 1975). The presentation and severity of flaccid dysphonia following TBI is determined by the effects of the injury to the vagus nerve in the brainstem or to specific laryngeal nerves such as the recurrent laryngeal and superior laryngeal nerves. Bilateral damage to the recurrent laryngeal nerves results in either adductor or abductor vocal fold paralysis. In the case of bilateral adductor vocal fold paralysis, where neither vocal fold can adduct to the midline, phonation may be impossible if the vocal folds are positioned too far apart. If the superior laryngeal nerve remains intact, however, the cricothyroid muscle will contract and contribute to adduction to some degree (Colton & Casper, 1996a). A unilateral vocal fold paralysis results in one vocal fold failing to adduct to the midline, resulting in a weak, hoarse, and breathy voice. Abductor vocal fold paralysis results in the vocal folds remaining in an adducted position such that the airway is compromised. In the case of bilateral abductor paralysis, the patient will require a tracheostomy to maintain an adequate airway.

Hypokinetic dysphonia may be evident following TBI due to damage to subcortical structures such as the basal ganglia and substantia nigra. The perceptual features of this type of dysphonia, include reduced vocal volume and pitch level, breathiness, hoarseness, variable rate, and reduced pitch and loudness variation (Aronson, 1985; Colton & Casper, 1996a; Hanson, 1991). The voice characteristics of hypokinetic dysphonia are thought to be the result of laryngeal muscle rigidity and hypokinesia associated with impaired basal ganglia function (Colton & Casper, 1996a).

Hyperkinetic dysphonia may also be a consequence of damage to the basal ganglia, parts of the cerebellar control circuit, and/or indirect activation pathways following TBI (Duffy, 1995). Vocal characteristics of hyperkinetic dysphonia, including harshness, strained-strangled vocal quality, excessive pitch and loudness variation, transient breathiness, and voice stoppages are associated with abnormal and unpredictable involuntary movements of laryngeal and respiratory musculature (Aronson, 1985; Colton & Casper, 1996a; Duffy, 1995; Hanson, 1991; Hartman, 1984).

Damage to the cerebellum and its connecting pathways may readily occur following TBI, possibly due to acceleration-deceleration or to direct damage to the brainstem region. Consequently, the individual's laryngeal muscle coordination and tone may be reduced, resulting in slowness, variability, and inaccuracy in the force, range, and timing of vocal fold movements (Colton & Casper, 1996a). The ensuing ataxic dysphonia is characterized by harshness, reduced pitch level, excess and equal stress, irregular variations in pitch and loudness, and pitch breaks (Colton & Casper, 1996a).

Determining the type and extent of phonatory disturbances and the impact of laryngeal subsystem dysfunction on speech intelligibility in dysarthric speakers following TBI necessitates perceptual, acoustic, and physiological evaluation. A range of assessments available to the clinician for this purpose are described in the following sections.

Perceptual Assessment of Voice Following TBI

Perceptual evaluation of the voice in dysarthric speakers following TBI is the initial, and most common, form of voice assessment undertaken in the clinical setting. This type of assessment involves a perceptual analysis of voice from a speech sample, clinical evaluation of respiratory and vocal parameters, and observation and evaluation of body and laryngeal postures, vocal tract characteristics, and associated behaviors.

The perceptual analysis of the TBI patient's voice begins during the initial consultation when the clinician obtains an informal impression of the patient's vocal problem in relation to general volume, pitch, and quality of the voice during conversational speech. Following this encounter, the clinician should obtain a tape-recorded speech sample of the patient reading or repeating a standard passage such as "The Grandfather Passage" (Darley et al., 1975) or the "Rainbow Passage" (Fairbanks, 1960), as well as a sample of conversational speech. Perceptual analysis of the voice sample may be performed using a specific rating scale, such as that used by Fitzgerald, Murdoch, & Chenery (1987), which evaluates vocal quality, and pitch and loudness parameters according to descriptive four-point and seven-point scales. Other perceptual voice rating scales that may be adopted are the Buffalo Voice Profile (Wilson, 1987), the Voice Profile Analysis (Laver, 1980), and the Voice Evaluation Format (Oates, 1983). Alternately, as is commonly the practice, respiratory and laryngeal parameters may be rated on the basis of a rating scale devised by the clinician.

One of the most comprehensive voice assessment protocols is The Voice Evaluation Format (Oates, 1983) in which five categories of phonation and associated factors are evaluated according to deviation from normal (normal/abnormal), consistency (present or intermittent), degree of severity according to a five-point scale, and any other variations. Initially, respiratory-phonatory capacity is evaluated to determine the type and pattern (arhythmical, shallow) of breathing and the degree of breath control during phonation. For this part of the assessment, it is noted if the patient is speaking on reserve air, and/or has poor phrasing with a tendency to run out of breath at the end of a sentence. The maximum duration of sustained vowels (/a/, /i/, /u/) and consonants (/s/, /z/, /m/) may also be measured in seconds. Calculation of the s/z ratio based on phonation time (Boone, 1977) is an additional diagnostic tool to identify the specific locus of dysfunction in the respiratory-phonatory systems. In the case of normal laryngeal and respiratory function, the individual should be able to produce equal durations of /s/ and /z/, resulting in a ratio of one. If the respiratory system is compromised and the laryngeal mechanism remains intact, then the /s/ and /z/ durations should be similar, with a ratio approximating one. However, if the laryngeal mechanism is compromised, resulting in reduced phonation time for the voiced /z/ phoneme while the expiratory airflow remains adequate, the s/z ratio will be greater than one (Colton & Casper, 1996b; Eckel & Boone, 1981). Colton and Casper (1996b), however, consider that the calculation of the s/z ratio should be viewed with caution and only considered a screening test that must be supplemented by other evaluations.

Second, clinical examination of the pitch of the voice is conducted to determine the modal pitch (pitch occurring most frequently in conversational speech), the highest and lowest pitches attained, and the degree of pitch variability. Evaluations of similar intensity parameters are also conducted in this assessment. The patient's vocal quality or phonation type (according to descriptors such as breathy, harsh, whispery, glottal fry, and falsetto) and the type and degree of discontinuity of voice (tremor, diplophonia, phonation breaks, voice arrests, pitch breaks, loudness breaks) are determined and rated according to a five-point scale of severity. The perceptual analysis of vocal quality by the clinician may be facilitated through an interactive multimedia learning package, A *Sound Judgment*, developed by Oates and Russell (1998).

The voice evaluation format also requires the clinician to observe the position of the larynx in the neck and the degree of neck muscle and general body tension. Although not specifically laryngeal, clinical observations of tongue (fronted, backed, raised, lowered) and jaw (closed, opened, protruded) position should also be noted as these components of the speech mechanism transform the voice into speech and in doing so, may alter vocal output. The resonance of the voice is assessed to determine the presence or absence of hypernasality, nasal emission, or hyponasality. Finally, observations and documentation of associated behaviors such as throat-clearing, coughing, and loud talking is required. The Voice Evaluation Format (Oates, 1983) is easy to administer and, when completed, provides a comprehensive profile of voice production from which treatment goals can be readily identified.

Despite the ease of administration and the minimal costs involved in perceptual voice assessment, the need to pursue acoustic and physiological assessment of voice in TBI dysarthric speakers remains paramount because of the perceptual difficulties encountered in the evaluation of voice in neurologically impaired populations. The difficulty in correctly perceiving specific phonatory disturbances in dysarthric speakers with concomitant impairment in other aspects of speech production, such as resonance and articulation, supports the need for objective assessment of laryngeal function in TBI dysarthric speakers.

Acoustic Evaluation of Voice Following TBI

Acoustic analysis provides quantification of the physical components of voice and involves the measurement of a number of parameters pertaining to frequency, amplitude, perturbation, signal noise, and temporal aspects of the acoustic signal. The acoustic evaluation of voice in individuals, following TBI, may be used to support perceptual and physiological findings, identify and clarify treatment goals, and monitor treatment efficacy.

A large number of acoustic analysis programs have been developed and vary according to levels of complexity (Read, Buder, & Kent, 1990). Some of the systems commercially available for acoustic analysis include the Computerized Speech Lab® (CSL)

(Kay Elemetrics Corp.), CSpeech®, the Canadian Speech Research Environment® (CSRE), the VisiPitch® (Kay Elemetrics Corp.), the MacSpeech Lab II®, and Dr. Speech Science for Windows® (Tiger Electronics) (Colton & Casper, 1996b; Thompson-Ward & Theodoros, 1998). The most commonly used acoustic instruments are the CSL and the VisiPitch, which are user-friendly, and provide real-time graphic displays of acoustic parameters, storage and analysis of data, and in the case of the CSL, spectrographic display of the voice signal.

The acoustic analysis programs incorporated into the instrumentation have the capacity to rapidly analyze the acoustic signal to provide a range of measures. A standard acoustic measure is that of fundamental frequency (Fo), which reflects the vibrating rate of the vocal folds and involves the calculation of the number of vibratory cycles per second, expressed as hertz (Hz). Fundamental frequency may be measured during sustained vowel and running speech tasks to obtain values of mean fundamental frequency, standard deviation of frequency, and frequency range. As TBI may result in neurological impairment of the laryngeal musculature affecting the elasticity and length of the vocal folds, and subsequently Fo, these measures are useful for quantifying the degree of pitch variation during speech and any marked pitch alterations that may occur. Because many dysarthric speakers with TBI demonstrate prosodic impairment associated with reduced pitch variation, acoustic analysis of this parameter is particularly relevant to this population.

Another standard acoustic measure of voice relates to vocal intensity, or amplitude. Measures of the average and standard deviation of vocal intensity can be obtained from any of the acoustic instruments previously mentioned, during the production of sustained vowels and connected speech. In addition, the individual's intensity, or dynamic range, can be determined by having the person produce their softest and loudest prolongation of /ah/. This measure may identify a reduction in the range of vocal intensity, which is consistent with reduced laryngeal flexibility, associated with laryngeal muscle impairment. As for Fo, vocal intensity measures are important in the assessment of laryngeal function in dysarthric speakers with TBI as perceived impairments in loudness level and variation have been identified in this subject group (Theodoros, Murdoch, & Chenery, 1994).

Perturbation measures that reflect rapid cycle-to-cycle changes in frequency and amplitude are frequently used in acoustic analysis to determine the aperiodicity in voicing that results from laryngeal pathology (Thompson-Ward & Theodoros, 1998). These changes in frequency and amplitude are related to small differences in mass, tension, and neural control of the vocal folds (Baer, 1979). Perturbation measures are obtained using only a sustained vowel task. The perturbation of frequency is referred to as "jitter", while short-term cycle-to-cycle variability in amplitude is called "shimmer". The presence of high degrees of jitter and shimmer correlates with perceived roughness, hoarseness, and harshness in the voice (Orlikoff, 1992). Gould and Korovin (1994) proposed that the presence of jitter indicates variations in the vibratory patterns of the vocal folds, while shimmer is indicative of vocal fold instability. Changes in vocal quality, such as hoarseness and harshness, have been perceived to be present in approximately 50% of dysarthric speakers following TBI (Theodoros, et al., 1994) and therefore, may be confirmed through acoustic measures of perturbation.

An additional acoustic measure related to the frequency and amplitude of the voice signal is the signal-to-noise/harmonic-to-noise ratio, which determines the proportion of total energy in the voice signal, compared to the proportion of aperiodic turbulence in the signal. A low signal-to-noise/harmonic-to-noise ratio is consistent with increased noise in the signal and can be related to breathiness and aphonia (Orlikoff, 1992). In the dysarthric speakers with TBI, breathiness and aphonia may be apparent in those individuals with a flaccid type of dysphonia and may be quantified using the signal-to-noise/harmonic-to-noise ratio.

A number of acoustic measures that relate to the temporal aspects of the voice signal may also be useful diagnostically and therapeutically in the assessment of laryngeal function in TBI dysarthric speakers. The most frequently used measure is maximum phonation time, which is calculated by recording the individual's maximum duration of phonation in seconds during the production of a sustained vowel. Although this assessment may also be conducted using a stopwatch, measurement of this parameter within an acoustic analysis program allows for the data to be recorded with reference to other acoustic values. Since this measure reflects glottal and respiratory efficiency, any reduction in duration of phonation, compared to normative values, is indicative of laryngeal and respiratory dysfunction, which may be directly related to neurological impairment associated with TBI. Another acoustic measure that may be useful for documenting laryngeal dysfunction in dysarthric speakers with TBI is voice onset time (VOT), which is used to determine the duration between the onset of the articulatory stop burst on a spectrogram and the first glottal pulse of the following vowel (Thompson-Ward & Theodoros, 1998). Tyler and Watterson (1991) suggested that this acoustic measure is indicative of coordination of the laryngeal and supralaryngeal behaviors (i.e., articulation). Effective coordination of voice onset is important in achieving voiced/voiceless consonant distinctions. For voiced sounds, it is necessary for vocal fold vibration to be synchronous with the plosive burst, while for voiceless sounds, there is a time interval between the burst and the beginning of vibration of the vocal folds (Fry, 1984). For some dysarthric speakers with TBI, it is difficult to coordinate this aspect of their voice production, and as a result, they produce imprecise and indistinct consonants, which reduce the overall intelligibility of their speech.

Assessment of the acoustic parameters described above in dysarthric speakers with TBI should provide a greater insight into the more intricate aspects of laryngeal function in these individuals and serve as a baseline for monitoring treatment efficacy. In addition, many of the instruments available for acoustic analysis provide visual and auditory feedback of vocal parameters, which may be adapted for therapeutic purposes.

Examination and Physiological Assessment of Laryngeal Function Following TBI

Although a large number of instrumental techniques have been developed for the assessment of laryngeal function, those most commonly used in clinical situations to evaluate this aspect of speech production in persons following TBI are described below. While this instrumentation specifically pertains to the assessment of laryngeal function, an essential component of any voice and laryngeal assessment protocol is an evaluation of respiratory function. Instrumentation and procedures for respiratory assessment are outlined in Chapter 6.

Indirect Laryngoscopy

A commonly used clinical technique for examining the larynx is an indirect laryngoscopy. This procedure involves the use of a laryngeal mirror that is inserted into the oropharynx and positioned carefully, so that it reflects an image of the vocal folds. The patient's tongue is pulled forward so that the laryngeal area may be visualized. The person is then requested to produce a high-pitched /ee/, which enhances the view of the larynx because of superior and anterior movement of the tongue and epiglottis (Colton & Casper, 1996b). While this technique is usually the most routinely used method for assessing the status of the larynx, it is limited by a number of factors such as the inability of the patient to speak normally due to the tongue being pulled forward, and the activation of hyperactive gag reflexes. For those TBI patients who present with hyperactive gag reflexes due to upper motor neuron damage, this latter limitation of the technique may become readily apparent and negate the use of this technique. Despite these limitations, indirect laryngoscopy may be quickly and effectively used to evaluate the status of the larynx in TBI subjects within the acute and chronic stages of rehabilitation.

Direct Laryngoscopy

For some patients, following TBI, a direct laryngoscopy may be required to enable the physician to examine laryngeal structure in detail. This procedure is particularly invasive in that it requires hospitalization and anesthetization. Such a procedure is limited by the inability to observe laryngeal function and is usually restricted to those cases requiring biopsies or laryngeal structure manipulation. In cases of severe neck injuries following TBI, direct laryngoscopy may be used to differentially diagnose the presence of vocal fold paralysis or some form of laryngeal cartilage dislocation.

Videolaryngoscopy

In order to provide a more superior view of vocal fold movement and laryngeal structures, and to overcome the limitations of other procedures, videolaryngoscopy has become the technique of choice for most physicians experienced in laryngeal examination. This technique involves the use of either a rigid endoscope or a flexible fiberscope attached to a video recorder, which allows for real-time recording of vocal fold movement, and provides a permanent record of the examination for future reference. The rigid endoscope is inserted into the mouth and positioned in the oropharynx so that the vocal folds can be viewed. As in the indirect laryngoscopic procedure, the patient is unable to speak normally, apart from the prolongation of a vowel, due to the tongue being pulled forward. A more sophisticated videolaryngoscopic procedure involves the use of a flexible fiberscope that is inserted through the patient's nasal cavity, over the soft palate, and into the oropharynx, where it is positioned to allow for observation of the supraglottal structures as well as the larynx. As the oral cavity is not obstructed in any way by the use of the flexible fiberscope, laryngeal function may be observed while the patient is speaking or singing. The use of the flexible fiberscope is particularly useful in circumventing the problem of hyperactive gag reflex by avoiding this region of the oropharynx, and therefore is a more suitable technique for evaluating laryngeal function in the TBI population.

To enable the vibratory detail of the vocal folds to be closely examined, a stroboscopic light source is used in conjunction with either type of endoscope, although the rigid endoscope does provide the clearer image. The stroboscopic light emits rapid pulses at rates that may be set by the examiner or controlled by the frequency of vocalization (Colton & Casper, 1996b). When the frequency of the light pulse is equal to the vocal frequency, the image will appear to be at a standstill. In contrast, when the frequency of the light pulse is slightly greater or less than the frequency of vocal fold vibration, the movement of the vocal folds will appear to be in slow motion, allowing for more detailed observation of the vibratory pattern of the vocal folds (Colton & Casper, 1996b). The information obtained from the stroboscopic image includes: the symmetry of movement of the vocal folds, presence of any non-vibrating portions of the vocal folds, periodicity of vibrations, presence and adequacy of the mucosal wave, glottal closure, amplitude or horizontal excursion of the vocal folds; and phase (open/closed phase) closure (Colton & Casper, 1996b).

Electroglottography

Electroglottography (EGG) is an indirect, noninvasive physiological assessment technique used to analyze the vibratory patterns of the vocal folds by providing an estimate of vocal fold contact during the glottal cycle (Baken, 1987; Colton & Conture, 1990; Hanson, Gerratt, Karin, & Berke, 1988). The measurement of vocal fold contact is based on the principle that tissue conducts electrical current. A high-frequency, low-current signal is passed between the vocal folds by means of electrodes positioned over the thyroid cartilage. When the vocal folds adduct and contact is made, there is an increase in the flow of the current between the electrodes, while a decrease in the current occurs when the vocal folds abduct during the vibratory cycle. The recordings of the changes in the flow of current between the vocal folds during various stages of the glottal cycle are displayed in the form of a glotttal waveform. From this waveform, it is possible to identify the opening and closing phases of the glottal cycle and the speed at which the vocal folds are closing (Colton & Casper, 1996b). A number of instruments are commercially available for measuring vocal fold contact area (Baken, 1987). These include the Fourcin® laryngograph, the Voiscope®, the F-J Electroglottograph®, and the Synchrovoice Quantitative Electroglottograph® (Baken, 1987; Gilbert, Potter, & Hoodin, 1984). Numerous studies in the literature have attempted to relate the shape of the waveform to the underlying physiology of vocal fold vibration (Childers, Moore, Naik, Larar, & Krishnamurthy, 1983; Dromey, Stathopoulos, & Sapienza, 1992), while others have identified characteristic waveforms associated with specific vocal pathology (Berry, Epstein, Fourcin, Freeman, & MacCurtain, 1982; Motta, Cesari, Iengo, & Motta, 1990). Despite a number of limitations with respect to electrode placement and degree of possible vocal fold contact (the signal is markedly reduced or absent in the case of unilateral paralysis), EGG is frequently used in both clinical and research environments and is readily applicable to the

TBI population. Theodoros and Murdoch (1994) reported the use of this technique in effectively identifying differing vocal fold vibratory patterns in dysarthric speakers following TBI.

Assessment of Laryngeal Aerodynamics

While EGG provides an analysis of the vibratory pattern of the vocal folds, a comprehensive assessment of laryngeal function in persons following TBI should also include an evaluation of laryngeal aerodynamics. An understanding of the interplay among the various physiological parameters of laryngeal function and voice production such as subglottal pressure, phonatory air flow, sound pressure level, and laryngeal airway resistance is essential for identifying appropriate treatment techniques.

Over the last couple of decades, a variety of instruments have been developed to measure these parameters of laryngeal aerodynamics (Baken, 1987; Thompson-Ward, & Murdoch, 1998). A commercially available instrument, the Aerophone II® Model 6800 (Kay Elemetrics Corp.), a voice function analyzer, has been used in our laboratory to assess laryngeal aerodynamics in normal and disordered speakers, including dysarthric speakers following TBI (Theodoros & Murdoch, 1994). This instrument is comprised of a handheld transducer module that consists of miniaturized transducers capable of simultaneously recording airflow, air pressure, and sound pressure level. A disposable anesthetic mask is placed over the nose and mouth of the patient while a thin flexible silicon tube is positioned in the mouth to record intraoral pressure. Subglottal pressure is estimated from a recording of intraoral pressure during the pronunciation of /ipipip/. The point of maximum oral pressure during the production of the /p/ is used as an estimate of subglottal pressure. Laryngeal airway resistance is measured indirectly by calculating the ratio of subglottal pressure to phonatory air flow during speech. In addition to measurements of subglottal pressure, phonatory air flow, sound pressure level, and laryngeal airway resistance, the Aerophone II measures the ad/abduction rate of the vocal folds by having the patient initiate and terminate voicing as quickly as possible (Theodoros & Murdoch, 1994).

McHenry (1996), using a different laryngeal aerodynamic equipment determined the laryngeal airway resistance, translaryngeal flow, and intraoral pressure of a group of TBI patients. In this study, a tight-fitting mask attached to a pneumotachograph (Hans Rudolph 4719) and a differential pressure transducer (Honeywell 163PC01D36), and a catheter inserted inside the lips and attached to another pressure transducer (Honeywell 162PC016), were used to collect the data.

While measurement of laryngeal aerodynamic parameters is an integral part of the assessment of laryngeal function in persons following TBI, high individual variability in performance is inherent in this form of assessment. Hammen and Yorkston (1994) recommended that a representative sample of an individual's performance be obtained through an average of at least five repetitions of a task. The issue of patient fatigue during extensive physiological testing, however, needs to be monitored carefully in clinical populations such as the traumatically brain-injured, who frequently demonstrate significant physical disability.

Perceptual Features of Laryngeal Dysfunction Following TBI

Perceptually, a range of phonatory disturbances have been identified in dysarthric speakers following TBI, a finding consistent with the potential for diffuse and varied neurological impairment following this type of brain injury. Abnormal phonation associated with both hypofunctional and hyperfunctional patterns of laryngeal activity have been identified in this population, in both single case and group studies. Single case study reports have revealed the presence of weak, breathy phonation in some subjects (McHenry, Wilson, & Minton, 1994; Netsell & Daniel, 1979), while a hyperfunctional phonatory pattern associated with a strained-strangled vocal quality has been identified in other individuals (Workinger & Netsell, 1992).

In an early study of dysphonia after traumatic midbrain damage in eight subjects, Vogel and von Cramon (1982) identified a transition from laryngeal hypofunction to a hyperfunctional pattern of laryngeal behavior during the course of recovery. A number of distinct stages in the recovery of phonation post-TBI were identified. In the initial stage, all subjects were mute immediately post-TBI, and phonation occurred reflexively, but not voluntarily. During the next stage of recovery, nonverbal vocalizations such as groaning, singing, laughing, and crying occurred spontaneously, or following stimulation. The transition to verbal utterances was achieved in the next recovery stage in the form of whispery speech that lasted one to three weeks and was accompanied by an increase in loudness and length of expiration. Following this stage, voiced phonation occurred when stimulated, although the voice was extremely breathy, low in volume, and increased in pitch. After approximately three weeks, constant phonation was stabilized, with loudness level during conversational speech reaching normal limits and pitch level reducing to a more appropriate level. Negative changes in phonation, however, were evident in the development of a mild to a considerably strained voice in these subjects. Laryngealizations (perceptually slow irregularities of vocal cord vibration), abrupt voice onset, and irregularities in vocal function such as tremolo, pitch breaks, and diplophonia became evident. The most severe phonatory impairments in these subjects, however, were reductions in pitch range and variation, resulting in monotonous speech. Vogel and von Cramon (1982) concluded that during recovery of phonation following TBI, the individual will initially present with a phonatory pattern consistent with hypokinetic dysphonia (high invariable pitch, reduced pitch range, invariable loudness, low intensity level, breathy vocal quality, and shallow breathing) which evolves into a mild form of spastic dysphonia characterized by effortful voice production. The authors stressed that although the recovery of voice varied in duration, the course of recovery was the same for all cases. Furthermore, they concluded that dysphonia following TBI was a mixed type of phonatory disturbance with elements of both hypokinetic and spastic dysphonia, the predominance of a particular dysphonia being dependent on the stage of recovery.

A recent study of 20 subjects with severe TBI and dysarthric speech, conducted by Theodoros et al. (1994), revealed features of hypofunctioning and hyperfunctioning laryngeal activity and laryngeal incoordination in this group. Deviant phonatory features, such as hoarseness, harshness, and intermittent breathiness, were found to be significantly more apparent in the vocal output of the TBI subjects, compared to a matched control group. The degree of strained-strangled vocal quality and glottal fry, however, were not found to be significantly greater in the TBI subjects, compared to their control counterparts. Hoarseness, associated with a hypofunctioning larynx, was perceived to be present in 55% of the TBI subjects, while harshness, consistent with a hyperfunctioning larynx was evident in 45% of cases. Intermittent breathiness, suggestive of laryngeal incoordination was perceived to be present in half of the subject group. All of the deviant phonatory perceptual features were present to a mild-to-moderate degree in the majority of the TBI subjects. Strained-strangled vocal quality was found to be present in only 6 (30%) of the 20 TBI subjects, while glottal fry was evident in only 5 (25%) of the subjects.

A perceptual study of laryngeal features in another group of 24 severely TBI dysarthric speakers recently conducted in our laboratory revealed the presence of deviant laryngeal features in 23 (96%) of the subjects, with only 1 subject being perceived to exhibit normal phonation. The majority of the subjects (66%) were perceived to exhibit glottal fry (66%), with hoarseness (54%), harshness (46%), strained-strangled vocal quality (42%), and intermittent breathiness (17%) also apparent in the subjects' vocal output. In this group of 24 cases, the abnormal laryngeal features were mainly perceived to be present to a mild degree, although hoarseness was evident to a moderate degree in approximately half of the subjects exhibiting this feature. In comparison to the previous findings of Theodoros et al. (1994), the results of this most recent study in our laboratory were consistent in relation to the frequency of occurrence of harshness and hoarseness, while glottal fry and strained-strangled vocal quality were found to be more frequently perceived in the latter investigation.

Aphonia following TBI is a frequently reported perceptual feature (Sapir & Aronson, 1985; Scholefield, 1987; Vogel & von Cramon, 1982). The etiology of aphonia post-TBI would appear to be individually determined, and not necessarily a result of impairment of motor control. A number of plausible explanations have been suggested for the occurrence of this phonatory characteristic. Sapir and Aronson (1985) have suggested that aphonia following TBI may be a consequence of an affective disorder resulting from damage to the limbic system and its neocortical, subcortical connections, rather than to laryngeal muscle paralysis or apraxia of phonation. These neural systems are thought to function as a drive-controlling mechanism that determines readiness to phonate and the intensity of phonation as it relates to the degree of expressiveness of an emotional vocal utterance (Jürgens & von Cramon, 1982). Secondly, they suggested that the aphonia may be due to an acute emotional reaction to the brain trauma and associated physical and cognitive losses. Such reactions are common in persons experiencing head trauma (Binder, 1984; Dembo, Levitan, & Wright, 1975). Thirdly, Sapir and Aronson (1985) proposed that the aphonia may have originally been due to vocal fold paralysis or apraxia of phonation but then remained in the form of an "inertial" aphonia, after these organic causes resolved and motor ability was restored (Aronson, 1985). Similarly, Scholefield (1987) proposed that the presence of aphonia in some cases following TBI may have its basis in impairment of the frontal lobe-limbic system and the right hemisphere. Research has indicated that lesions in a variety of locations within the limbic system can compromise vocalization (Botez & Barbeau, 1971), while damage to the right hemisphere may affect the use of emotional phonation and facial expression.

In view of the fact that the phonatory disturbances identified in dysarthric speakers following TBI are diverse and that perceptual assessment of voice is difficult against a background of other speech subsystem impairment, detailed investigation and confirmation of these features through objective assessment is warranted to ensure that the appropriate treatment is determined. In the case of voice disorder, it is critical that the nature of the phonatory disturbance be correctly identified since some vocal disorders require diametrically different treatment methods.

Acoustic Features of Laryngeal Dysfunction Following TBI

To date, there have been few studies that have investigated the acoustic features of laryngeal dysfunction following TBI. Early acoustic studies involved investigation of the recovery pattern of phonation following injury, while the most recent study has dealt with the acoustic analysis of a large number of persons with severe TBI. Hartmann and von Cramon (1984) employed a battery of acoustic parameters to evaluate recovery of normal phonation in a group of 24 subjects, 18 of whom had suffered a severe closed head injury. "Rough" voice quality was measured by a pitch perturbation parameter, "tense" vocal quality by the amount of spectral energy in the 1 to 5 KHz range, and "breathy" vocal quality by the amount of spectral energy in the 5 to 10 KHz range. The duration of aspiration noise preceding voice onset was also determined, with an increase in this value being consistent with overall breathy vocal quality. Another acoustic measure, the variance of spectral energy function above 5 KHz was indicative of increased tension in the vocal tract. Using these acoustic measures, two subgroups of patients and their recovery patterns were identified. One subgroup of patients demonstrated a vocal quality combination of breathy and tense, which gradually normalized, while the other subgroup of patients exhibited a normal or lax, breathy voice initially, which subsequently became more tense. While "breathy" and "tense" vocal qualities were evident in patients following TBI, a "rough" vocal quality was not a prominent feature of dysphonia after severe head trauma. These findings were consistent with those of Vogel and von Cramon (1982), who identified an early stage of recovery of phonation following TBI in which patients demonstrated hypokinetic dysphonia with further development to a mild spastic dysphonia at a later stage of recovery (See "Perceptual Features of Laryngeal Dysfunction Following TBI" in this chapter.). Hartmann and von Cramon (1984) stressed that the findings of two subgroups, the initial difference in their degree of severity, and the different recovery patterns for the two groups may well reflect different stages of the same recovery process.

In a recent study of acoustic features of laryngeal dysfunction following TBI, McHenry (2000) investigated the characteristics of 100 individuals post-TBI. Acoustic parameters utilized in the study included: amplitude perturbation quotient (APQ), indicating short-term irregularities in the amplitude of vocal fold vibration; jitter percent (JITT), indicating short-term cycle-to-cycle irregularity of pitch; noise-to-harmonics ratio (NHR), which is the average ratio of the inharmonic spectral energy in the frequency range of 1500 to 4500 Hz to that in the 70 Hz to 4500 Hz range; voice turbulence ratio (VTR), which reflects the relative energy level of high-frequency noise associated with turbulence caused by incomplete vocal cord adduction; frequency tremor intensity (FTRI), indicating the strength of low frequency modulation of the voice; and amplitude tremor intensity (ATRI), which reflects the strength of amplitude modulation in the voice. The results indicated that none of the subjects demonstrated vocal parameters within normal limits. The most frequently occurring abnormal acoustic parameter was amplitude perturbation, followed by the voice turbulence index. A small cohort (23%) of subjects exhibited abnormalities in all five parameters measured. Perceptual ratings of breathiness were found to be significantly correlated with both the APQ and NHR. McHenry (2000) suggested that these findings were indicative of hypofunctional phonation in this group of TBI subjects.

Physiological Features of Laryngeal Dysfunction Following TBI

To date, the exact nature of laryngeal dysfunction in dysarthric speakers following TBI remains controversial, with studies documenting the presence of hypofunctioning and hyperfunctioning laryngeal activity, as well as normal laryngeal function, in this population. These results are not unexpected, however, considering the diffuse nature of TBI, the diversity in the responses of individuals to such injury (Theodoros, Murdoch, & Stokes, 1995), and the variability inherent in physiological assessment of laryngeal parameters (Holmberg, Hillman, & Perkell, 1988). Although not confirmed physiologically, a general pattern of progression of laryngeal dysfunction post-TBI along a continuum of hypofunction to hyperfunction has been identified perceptually by a number of investigators and would appear to be related to the time postinjury (McHenry et al., 1994; Najenson, Sazbon, Fiselzon, Becker, & Schecter, 1978; Vogel & von Cramon, 1982).

Single case studies of individuals with dysarthric speech following TBI have largely identified physiological features of hypofunctional laryngeal behaviour such as high glottal airflow, reduced subglottal pressure, and low laryngeal airway resistance (McHenry et al., 1994; Netsell & Daniel, 1979; Netsell, Lotz, and Barlow, 1989). A group study of 26 TBI subjects by McHenry (1996) provided further data to support the presence of hypofunctional laryngeal activity in this population. In this study, in which 20 (77%) subjects demonstrated a mild dysarthria, four (15%) exhibited a moderate dysarthria, and two (8%) subjects exhibited normal speech, McHenry identified low laryngeal airway resistance consistent with hypofunctional laryngeal activity in the majority of the group (16 subjects [62%]). Five (19%) of the subjects exhibited increased laryngeal airway resistance consistent with a hyperfunctional pattern of laryngeal behavior, while the remaining five (19%) subjects recorded laryngeal airway resistance values within normal limits. To determine if laryngeal function changed over time postinjury as previously suggested, McHenry (1996) examined each individual's laryngeal airway resistance values in relation to duration postinjury. McHenry (1996) concluded from this analysis that these subjects did not conform to the suggested pattern of progression from laryngeal hypofunction to hyperfunction over time.

In contrast to McHenry's (1996) findings, Theodoros and Murdoch (1994) identified hyperfunctional laryngeal activity as the predominate form of laryngeal function in a group of 19 subjects with severe TBI and dysarthric speech. The majority of the subjects in this group (10; 53%) demonstrated moderate to severe degrees of dysarthric speech disturbances, while the remaining nine (47%) subjects exhibited mild dysarthria. The mean duration post-TBI for this group of subjects was 7.72 (SD = 6.34), which was longer than that recorded for the subjects in the study by McHenry (1996). Five subgroups of subjects with differential patterns of hyperfunctional laryngeal features, as determined electroglottographically and aerodynamically, were identified. Hyperfunctional features, such as increased fundamental frequency, decreased duty cycle and closing time, increased glottal resistance (laryngeal airway resistance) and glottal (subglottal) pressure, and reduced phonatory air flow rate and ad/abduction rate of the vocal folds were evident in the physiological findings, but never altogether in the one subject. Subgroup 1 (n = 1) was identified on the basis of a high glottal pressure, an elevated sound pressure level, a very high phonatory flow rate, and a slow ad/abduction rate. In Subgroup 2, the three subjects were distinguished on the basis of a high mean glottal pressure, normal glottal resistance, a high phonatory flow rate, and a reduced ad/abduction rate. Subgroup 3 (n = 9) consisted of subjects for whom laryngeal hyperfunction was reflected in a high fundamental frequency, a short open phase (duty cycle), and a fast closing time in the vibratory cycle. The subjects in Subgroup 4 (n = 3) demonstrated the most severe degree of hyperfunctional laryngeal behavior and were identified by a high glottal resistance, a low phonatory flow rate, glottal pressure, and sound pressure level, a slow ad/abduction rate, a high fundamental frequency, a short duty cycle, and a fast closing time, compared to normal subjects. Subgroup 5 (n = 3) consisted of subjects with a high glottal resistance, and low phonatory flow rates and sound pressure levels. It was suggested by Theodoros and Murdoch (1994) that the hyperfunctional laryngeal behavior exhibited by the group of subjects could be accounted for by the diffuse nature of neurological impairment following TBI involving cortical and subcortical neuronal damage to the upper motor neurons and corticobulbar fiber tracts, resulting in spasticity of the laryngeal musculature. Furthermore, Theodoros and Murdoch (1994) proposed that the different expressions of hyperfunctional laryngeal activity were indicative of glottal and respiratory force adjustments utilized by the individual subjects in response to spasticity in the vocal folds. It was also suggested by these investigators that the laryngeal hyperfunction noted in these subjects was a reflection of their attempts to compensate for impairments in other subsystems in the speech mechanism (e.g., an increase in laryngeal airway resistance may be a compensatory attempt on the part of the subject to conserve expiratory air flow being wasted by inefficient valving at the velopharynx).

While it is quite conceivable that both hyperfunctional and hypofunctional patterns of laryngeal behavior occur in dysarthric speakers post-TBI, the differences in results obtained in the studies by Theodoros and Murdoch (1994) and McHenry (1996) may also be explained in relation to the severity of the dysarthria exhibited by the subjects in each study, and the time post-TBI recorded for these subjects. As previously mentioned, the majority of the subjects (77%) in the McHenry study presented with mild dysarthria, while just over half of those (53%) in the Theodoros and Murdoch study demonstrated moderate-to-severe dysarthric speech disturbances. These latter subjects, therefore, may have experienced a greater degree and diversity of neuronal damage affecting upper motor neurons (resulting in spasticity), as well as other components of the speech mechanism for which they may be compensating. In

104 Chapter Five

addition, the subjects in the Theodoros and Murdoch (1994) study recorded a longer mean duration post-TBI (mean = 7.72 years), compared to that of the subjects in the McHenry (1996) study (mean = 4.21 years). It has previously been reported by a number of investigators that laryngeal function post-TBI tends to progress to a more hyperfunctional pattern over time. It may be the case that the hyperfunctional laryngeal behavior evident in the subjects in the Theodoros and Murdoch (1994) study reflects a later stage of recovery.

In an attempt to further elucidate the nature of laryngeal function post-TBI, the physiological laryngeal data of a cohort of 43 dysarthric speakers following TBI, representing a range of severity of dysarthria and duration post-TBI, was examined in our laboratory. This group of subjects consisted of the 19 subjects investigated in the Theodoros and Murdoch (1994) study together with an additional 24 severely TBI individuals with dysarthric speech. Within this group, 26 (60%) of the subjects demonstrated mild to mild to moderate degrees of dysarthria, with 17 (40%) of the subjects exhibiting moderate to severe degrees of dysarthric speech disturbances. The mean duration post-TBI for this group was 5.12 years (SD = 5.29). The laryngeal aerodynamics of each subject was evaluated to determine phonatory flow rate, sound pressure level, subglottal pressure, laryngeal airway resistance, and ad/abduction rate. The vibratory pattern of the vocal folds was analyzed to determine the fundamental frequency, duty cycle, and closing time of the vibratory cycle. Due to the extensive variability evident in the physiological data, the results were examined on an individual basis to determine the type of laryngeal activity present in each subject. A particular pattern of laryngeal activity was considered to be present in a subject if at least two laryngeal parameters consistent with a specific laryngeal behavior were found to be more than one standard deviation above or below the control group mean. Hyperfunctional laryngeal activity was considered to be present if there was evidence of at least two of the following: decreased air flow, increased laryngeal airway resistance, increased subglottal pressure, decreased ad/abduction rate, increased fundamental frequency, decreased duty cycle, and decreased closing time. In contrast, hypofunctional laryngeal behavior was identified if at least two of the following parameters were recorded: increased air flow, decreased laryngeal airway resistance, decreased subglottal pressure, decreased ad/abduction rate, reduced fundamental frequency, increased duty cycle, and increased closing time.

The results of this data analysis revealed the presence of three types of laryngeal activity in the group of 43 subjects: normal, hyperfunctional, and hypofunctional laryngeal activity. Normal laryngeal function was identified in 14 (32%) of the subjects. Hyperfunctional laryngeal activity was found to be present in 18 (42%) of the subjects while 11 (26%) of the subjects demonstrated a hypofunctional pattern of laryngeal behavior. Interestingly, these patterns of laryngeal activity appeared to be associated with both the severity of the dysarthria present and the mean duration post-TBI for each group, although these relationships were not confirmed statistically. The majority of the subjects in the hyperfunctional subgroup (61%) were found to exhibit moderate to severe degrees of dysarthria and recorded the longest mean duration post-TBI (mean = 6.91 years). The hypofunctional subgroup of subjects exhibited a predominantly mild dysarthric speech disturbance (64%), and recorded a mean duration post-TBI of 4.39 years. In contrast, the majority of the subjects with normal laryngeal function (71%) demonstrated mild dysarthria and recorded the shortest mean duration post-TBI (mean = 3.40 years). These findings suggest that the pattern of abnormal laryngeal function in dysarthric speakers following TBI may change over time, with laryngeal function evolving from a hypofunctional to a hyperfunctional pattern. This pattern is consistent with the previous findings of Vogel and von Cramon (1982), who identified, in the early stages of recovery, a hypokinetic dysphonia, which developed into a more spastic-like dysphonia in the later stages. Further support for this hypothesis is evident in a comparison of the characteristics of the subject group investigated in the McHenry (1996) study and the hypofunctional laryngeal subgroup in our study. The subjects in both of these groups demonstrated predominantly mild forms of dysarthria and recorded similar mean durations post-TBI (McHenry (1996): 4.21 years; current study: 4.39 years), suggesting that this pattern of laryngeal function is more likely in the early years post-TBI. To confirm this hypothesis, however, physiological monitoring of the laryngeal function of each dysarthric speaker following TBI is required on a longitudinal basis to determine the nature of change in laryngeal function over time. Furthermore, the results of our investigation tended to indicate that individuals with the more severe forms of dysarthria may be more likely to demonstrate a hyperfunctional pattern of laryngeal impairment. This finding, however, should be substantiated with the investigation of greater numbers of subjects who demonstrate a wide range of severity and types of dysarthria. The possibility of a progressive physiological change in laryngeal function over time, potentially has important clinical implications in that it may be necessary for clinicians to adjust treatment strategies for TBI dysarthric speakers with laryngeal dysfunction according to the time postinjury. Further research, however, is required to confirm this suggestion.

Summary

Phonatory disturbances and associated laryngeal dysfunction are prominent components of the dysarthric speech disturbance evident in persons following TBI. Assessment of laryngeal dysfunction following TBI should involve a comprehensive approach, incorporating physical examination of the larynx, and perceptual, acoustic and physiological evaluation of vocal output and the laryngeal mechanism. The diversity in the range of perceptual, acoustic, and physiological features of laryngeal dysfunction in this population is consistent with the diffuse nature of TBI. Both hyperfunctional and hypofunctional laryngeal activity has been identified in all modes of assessment post-TBI, with some individuals demonstrating normal laryngeal activity despite the presence of a dysarthric speech disturbance. There is also perceptual, acoustic, and physiological evidence to suggest that laryngeal dysfunction post-TBI may progress along a continuum from a hypofunctional level of laryngeal activity to a more hyperfunctional pattern as the time post-TBI increases. Future research involving comprehensive monitoring of laryngeal dysfunction in a range of dysarthric speakers post-TBI is required to ascertain the status of laryngeal function at different stages of recovery. Such information is critical to treatment planning, which may require specific adjustments as recovery progresses.

References

Aronson, A.E. (1985). *Clinical voice disorders: An interdisciplinary approach.* Second edition. New York: Thieme Inc.

Baer, T. (1979). Vocal jitter: A neuromuscular explanation. In V. Lawrence (Ed.), *Transcripts of the 8th symposium: Care of the Professional Voice* (pp. 19–22). New York: Voice Foundation.

Baken, R.J. (1987). *Clinical measurement of Speech and Voice.* Boston: College-Hill Press.

Berry, R.J., Epstein, R., Fourcin, J., Freeman, M., & MacCurtain, F. (1982). An objective analysis of voice disorder: Part one. *British Journal of Disorders of Communication, 17,* 67–76.

Binder, L.M. (1984). Emotional problems after stroke. *Stroke, 15,* 174–177.

Boone, D.R. (1977). *The Voice and Voice Therapy.* Second edition. Englewood Cliffs, New Jersey: Prentice Hall.

Boone, D.R. & McFarlane, S.C. (1988). *The Voice and Voice Therapy.* Englewood Cliffs, New Jersey: Prentice-Hall.

Botez, M.I. & Barbeau, A. (1971). Role of subcortical structures and particularly of the thalamus in the mechanisms of speech and language. *International Journal of Neurology, 8,* 300–320.

Childers, D.G., Moore, G.P., Naik, J.M., Larar, J.N., & Krishnamurthy, A.K. (1983). Assessment of laryngeal function by simultaneous synchronized measurement of speech, electroglottography, and high-speed film. In V. Lawrence (Ed.), *Transcripts of the 11th Symposium: Care of the Professional Voice* (pp. 234–244). New York: Voice Foundation.

Colton, R. & Casper, J.K. (1996a). Voice problems associated with nervous system involvement. In R. Colton & J.K. Casper (Eds.), *Understanding Voice problems: A Physiological Perspective for Diagnosis and Treatment.* Second edition (pp. 112–163). Baltimore: Williams & Wilkins.

Colton, R. & Casper, J.K. (1996b). The voice history, examination, and testing. In R. Colton & J.K. Casper (Eds.), *Understanding Voice problems: A physiological perspective for Diagnosis and Treatment.* Second edition (pp. 186–240). Baltimore: Williams & Wilkins.

Colton, R.H. & Conture, E.G. (1990). Problems and pitfalls of electroglottography. *Journal of Voice, 4,* 10–24.

Darley, F.L., Aronson, A.E., & Brown, J.R. (1975). *Motor Speech Disorders.* Philadelphia: W.B. Saunders Company.

Dembo, T., Levitan, G., & Wright, B. (1975). Adjustment to misfortune—a problem of social psychological rehabilitation. *Rehabilitative Psychology, 22,* 1–100.

Dromey, C., Stathopoulos, E.T., & Sapienza, C.M. (1992). Glottal airflow and electroglottographic measures of vocal function at multiple intensities. *Journal of Voice, 6,* 44–54.

Duffy, J.R. (1995). Hyperkinetic dysarthria. In J.R. Duffy, *Motor Speech Disorders: Substrates, Differential Diagnosis, and Management* (pp. 189–221). St. Louis: Mosby.

Eckel, F.C. & Boone, D.R. (1981). The s/z ratio as an indicator of laryngeal pathology. *Journal of Speech and Hearing Disorders, 46,*147–149.

Fairbanks, G.F. (1960). *Voice and Articulation Drillbook.* New York: Harper & Row.

Farmer, A. (1980). Voice onset time production in cerebral palsied speakers. *Folia Phoniatrica, 32,* 267–273.

FitzGerald, F.J., Murdoch, B.E., & Chenery, (1987). Multiple sclerosis: Associated speech and language disorders. *Australian Journal of Human Communication Disorders, 15,* 15–33.

Freeman, F., Cannito, M.P., & Finnitzo-Heiber, T. (1985). Classification of spasmodic dysphonia by perceptual-acoustic-visual means. In G. Gates (Ed.), *Spasmodic Dysphonia: The State of the Art* (pp. 5–18). New York: The Voice Foundation.

Fry, D.B. (1984). *The Physics of Speech.* Cambridge: Cambridge University Press.

Gilbert, H.R., Potter, C.R., & Hoodin, R. (1984). Laryngograph as a measure of vocal fold contact area. *Journal of Speech and Hearing Research, 27,* 178–182.

Gould, W.J. & Korovin, G.S. (1994). Laboratory advances for voice measurements. *Journal of Voice, 8,* 8–17.

Hammen, V.L. & Yorkston, K.M. (1994). Effect of instruction on selected aerodynamic parameters in subjects with dysarthria and control subjects. In J.A. Till, K.M. Yorkston, & D.R. Beukelman (Eds.), *Motor Speech Disorders: Advances in Assessment and Treatment* (pp. 161–173). Baltimore: Paul H. Brookes Publishing Co.

Hanson, D.G. (1991). Neuromuscular disorders of the larynx. In D.G. Hanson, *Otolaryngologic Clinics of North America: Voice Disorders* (pp. 1035–1051). Philadelphia: W.B. Saunders Company.

Hanson, D.G., Gerratt, B.R., Karin, R.R., & Berke, G.S. (1988). Glottographic measures of vocal fold vibration: An examination of laryngeal paralysis. *Laryngoscope, 98,* 541–548.

Hartman, D.E. (1984). Neurogenic dysphonia. *Annals of Otology, Rhinology, and Laryngology, 93,* 57–64.

Hartmann, E. & von Cramon, D. (1984). Acoustic measurement of voice quality in dysphonia after severe closed head trauma: A follow-up study. *British Journal of Disorders of Communication, 19,* 253–261.

Holmberg, E.B., Hillman, R.E., & Perkell, J.S. (1988). Glottal airflow and transglottal air pressure measurements for male and female speakers in soft, normal, and loud voice. *Journal of the Acoustical Society of America, 84,* 511–529.

Jürgens, U. & von Cramon, D. (1982). On the role of the anterior cingulate cortex in phonation: A case report. *Brain and Language, 15,* 234–248.

Laver, J. (1980). *Phonetic Description of Voice Quality.* Cambridge: Cambridge University Press.

McGarr, N.S. & Osberger, M.J. (1978). Pitch deviancy and intelligibility of deaf speech. *Journal of Communication Disorders, 11,* 237–247.

McHenry, M.A. (1996). Laryngeal airway resistance following traumatic brain injury. In D.A. Robin, K.M. Yorkston, & D.R. Beukelman, (Eds.), *Disorders of Motor Speech: Assessment, Treatment, and Clinical Characterization* (pp. 229–240). Baltimore: Paul H. Brookes Publishing Co.

McHenry, M. (2000). Acoustic characteristics of voice after severe traumatic brain injury. *Laryngoscope, 110,* 1157–1161.

McHenry, M.A., Wilson, R.L., & Minton, J.T. (1994). Management of multiple physiologic system deficits following traumatic brain injury. *Journal of Medical Speech-Language Pathology, 2,* 59–74.

Monsen, R.B. (1983). The oral speech intelligibility of hearing-impaired talkers. *Journal of Speech and Hearing Disorders, 48,* 286–296.

Motta, G., Cesari, U., Iengo, M., & Motta, G. (1990). Clinical application of electroglottography. *Folia Phoniatrica, 42,* 111–117.

Najenson, T., Sazbon, L., Fiselzon, J., Becker, E., & Schecter, I. (1978). Recovery of communicative functions after prolonged traumatic coma. *Scandanavian Journal of Rehabilitation Medicine, 10,* 15–21.

Netsell, R. & Daniel, B. (1979). Dysarthria in adults: Physiologic approach in rehabilitation. *Archives of Physical Medicine and Rehabilitation, 60,* 502–508.

Netsell, R., Lotz, W.K., & Barlow, S.M. (1989). A speech physiology examination for individuals with dysarthria. In K.M. Yorkston & D.R. Beukelman (Eds.), *Recent Advances in Clinical Dysarthria* (pp. 4–37). Boston: College-Hill Press.

Oates, J. (1983). *Voice Evaluation Format.* Unpublished.

Oates, J. & Russell, A. (1998). Learning voice analysis using an interactive multi-media package: Development and preliminary evaluation. *Journal of Voice, 12,* 500–512.

Orlikoff, R.F. (1992). The use of instrumental measures in the assessment and treatment of motor speech disorders. *Seminars in Speech and Language, 13,* 25–37.

Parkhurst, B. & Levitt, H. (1978). The effect of selected prosodic errors on the intelligibility of deaf speech. *Journal of Communication Disorders, 11,* 249–256.

Ramig, L.O. (1992). The role of phonation in speech intelligibility: A review and preliminary data from patients with Parkinson's disease. In R.D. Kent (Ed.), *Intelligibility in Speech Disorders: Theory, Measurement, and Management* (pp. 119–155). Philadelphia: John Benjamins Company.

Read, C., Buder, E., & Kent, R.D. (1990). Speech analysis systems: A survey. *Journal of Speech and Hearing Research, 33,* 363–374.

Rosenbek, J.C. & LaPointe, L.L. (1991). The dysarthrias: Description, diagnosis, and treatment. In D. Johns (Ed.), *Clinical Management of Neurogenic Communication Disorders* (pp. 97–152). Boston: Little, Brown & Co.

Sapir, S. & Aronson, A.E. (1985). Aphonia after closed head injury: Aetiologic considerations. *British Journal of Disorders of Communication, 20,* 289–296.

Scholefield, J.A. (1987). Aetiologies of aphonia following closed head injury. *British Journal of Disorders of Communication, 22,* 167–172.

Simpson, M.B., Till, J.A., & Goff, A.M. (1988). Long-term treatment of severe dysarthria: A case study. *Journal of Speech and Hearing Disorders, 53,* 433–440.

Theodoros, D.G. & Murdoch, B.E. (1994). Laryngeal dysfunction in dysarthric speakers following severe closed head injury. *Brain Injury, 8,* 667–684.

Theodoros, D.G., Murdoch, B.E., & Chenery, H.J. (1994). Perceptual speech characteristics of dysarthric speakers following severe closed head injury. *Brain Injury, 8,* 101–124.

Theodoros, D.G., Murdoch, B.E., & Stokes, P.D. (1995). Variability in the perceptual and physiological features of dysarthria following severe closed head injury: An examination of five cases. *Brain Injury, 9,* 671–696.

Thompson-Ward, E.C. & Theodoros, D.G. (1998). Acoustic analysis of dysarthric speech. In B.E. Murdoch (Ed.), *Dysarthria: A Physiological Approach to Assessment and Treatment* (pp. 102–129). Cheltenham: Stanley Thornes (Publishers) Ltd.

Thompson-Ward, E.C. & Murdoch, B.E. (1998). Instrumental assessment of the speech mechanism. In B. E. Murdoch (Ed.), *Dysarthria: A physiological approach to asssessment and treatment* (pp. 68–101). Cheltenham: Stanley Thornes (Publishers) LTD.

Tyler, A.A. & Watterson, T.L. (1991). VOT as an indirect measure of laryngeal function. *Seminars in Speech and Language, 12,* 131–141.

Vogel, M. & von Cramon, D. (1982). Dysphonia after traumatic midbrain damage: A follow-up study. *Folia Phoniatrica, 34,* 150–159.

Weismer, G. (1984). Acoustic descriptions of dysarthric speech: Perceptual correlates and physiological inferences. *Seminars in Speech and Language, 5,* 293–314.

Wilson, D.K. (1987). *Voice problems of children.* Third edition. Baltimore: Williams & Wilkins.

Workinger, M. & Netsell, R. (1992). Restoration of intelligible speech 13 years post-head injury. *Brain Injury, 6,* 183–187.

CHAPTER

Six

Speech Breathing Impairments Following Traumatic Brain Injury

Bruce E. Murdoch and Deborah G. Theodoros

Introduction

Speech breathing has been described as "a complex process requiring precise coordination of the components of the chest wall, namely the rib cage and abdomen/diaphragm, to maintain the subglottal pressures necessary for normal speech production" (Murdoch, Theodoros, Stokes, & Chenery, 1993, p. 2). Given the complexities of this process, it is not surprising that the diffuse brain damage associated with severe head trauma, which may include damage to the cerebral cortex, subcortical structures, cerebellum and/or brainstem, may disrupt the normal speech breathing process. According to McHenry and Minton (1998), the speech breathing strategies of persons with traumatic brain injury (TBI) may be influenced by a number of physiological and cognitive problems arising from the traumatic event, including verbal expressive limitations, impairments in valving at the level of the larynx and/or velopharynx, impaired coordination between respiratory and laryngeal function, incoordination of rib cage and abdominal-diaphragm displacements, and reduced vital capacity.

Studies using either perceptual (Theodoros, Murdoch, & Chenery, 1994) or physiological techniques (Murdoch, et al., 1993) have reported a number of speech breathing anomalies in individuals with severe TBI, including impaired respiratory support for speech, reduced vital capacity and impaired coordination of the rib cage and abdomen-diaphragm during performance of various speech tasks. A number of authors have suggested that disorders of speech breathing following neurological damage may contribute to the impairment of several aspects of the speech production process, namely prosody (Bellaire, Yorkston, & Beukelman, 1986; Darley, Aronson, & Brown, 1975; Metter, 1985) and phonation (Hixon & Putnam, 1983). Murdoch et al. (1993) commented that the respiratory abilities of the individuals with TBI examined in their study were aberrant in ways that could conceivably contribute to their speech abnormality. Consequently, the need for clinicians to recognize and account for the presence of speech breathing impairments in their management of speech disordered clients with TBI is important if they are to achieve the maximal effectiveness in their attempts to rehabilitate the communication deficits evidenced by this group of individuals. The present chapter will review contemporary procedures available for assessing the speech breathing abilities of individuals with TBI and will provide a synthesis of our current understanding of the range and nature of speech breathing anomalies exhibited by survivors of TBI as well as their possible contribution to any concomitant speech disorders.

Assessment of Speech Breathing Following TBI

The respiratory system provides the basic energy source for all speech and voice production. Consequently, the production of good quality voice, correct phoneme production, and appropriate intonation, stress, rhythm and phrasing rely on an adequate supply of air and precise control of exhalation. For this reason, accurate assessment of the speech breathing abilities of individuals with dysarthria subsequent to TBI is vital in formulating an appropriate plan and strategy for the treatment of their speech disorder. Two main groups of assessments are available for determining the speech breathing abilities of persons with TBI—perceptual assessments and physiological assessments.

Perceptual Assessment of Speech Breathing Following TBI

A number of commonly used perceptual assessments involve a clinical evaluation of respiratory function, and analyses of those deviant speech dimensions that are considered by clinicians to be related to the adequacy of respiratory support for speech. These assessments include the Frenchay Dysarthria Assessment (FDA; Enderby, 1983), the perceptual analysis devised by Darley et al. (1975) and the procedure for perceptual analysis used by FitzGerald, Murdoch, and Chenery (1987). In the FDA, respiratory control at rest and during speech is evaluated on a nine-point scale. The authors of the present chapter have found the perceptual speech analysis devised by FitzGerald et al. (1987) useful for evaluating respiratory function following TBI. The speech dimensions relating to respiratory function included in this perceptual rating scale fall into the areas of breath support for speech, loudness, and phrasing and breath patterning. The speech dimension, breath support for speech, is evaluated based on listening to a recording of the client reading the "Grandfather Passage" (Darley et al., 1975); the clinician is required to note whether there is sufficient supply and control of expiratory airflow to enable correct phrasing and maintenance of pitch and volume control for connected speech. Further, the clinician is required to note the presence of any features of the client's speech related to respiratory deficits such as: the presence of any interruptions to speech caused by sudden forced inspiratory or expiratory sighs, the presence of audible breathy inspiration or inspiratory stridor, and the presence of audible grunts at the end of expiration.

According to Yorkston, Beukelman and Bell (1988), loudness level is closely related to the level of subglottal air pressure generated by the respiratory system, and hence to the adequacy of respiratory support. Aspects of the client's speech that need to be considered by clinicians when assessing speech dimensions associated with loudness include:

Loudness level—is the volume of speech adequate and appropriate for the situation?

Loudness variation (monoloudness)—is the client able to increase the loudness level to a point appropriate to the discourse context?

Loudness maintenance—does loudness diminish over the course of a single breath group or over the course of connected speech?

Abnormal loudness variation—does the speaker produce sudden uncontrollable variations in loudness level that are not consistent with the meaning to be conveyed in a given passage?

Another feature suggestive of the presence of inadequate respiratory support for speech is the presence of short phrases or pauses for breath at inappropriate phrasal boundaries. According to Chenery (1998), when conducting perceptual assessments of phrasing and breath patterning, clinicians should note the following: whether the client is able to follow a quick inspiratory phase by a prolonged and coordinated expiratory phase; whether the client pauses during speech without the need for an inhalation or whether every utterance pause contains an inhalation; whether some air wastage occurs before the client begins to speak on his or her expired air or whether utterance commencement occurs simultaneously to the initial outflow of air; whether the client appears to run out of air at the end of a phrase, perhaps signalled by an increased rate of speech at the end of a phrase boundary, accompanied by reduced volume.

Speech breathing can influence or, in turn, be influenced by other components of the speech production process such as laryngeal, velopharyngeal, and orofacial function. Consequently, deficiencies in speech breathing may manifest as perceptual deficits in other aspects of speech (e.g., phonation). This lack of a one-to-one correspondence between the occurrence of a specific deviant speech dimension and impairment in a particular component of the speech production mechanism represents a major limitation to reliance on perceptual analysis alone when assessing speech breathing in clients with TBI or other neurological conditions. In many cases there is a need, therefore, for the results of a perceptual assessment of speech breathing to be supported by the findings of an objective, physiological assessment of speech breathing.

Physiological Assessment of Speech Breathing Following TBI

A variety of instrumental procedures are available for assessment of respiratory function and speech breathing in individuals with TBI. In general, these techniques can be divided into those that involve direct measurement of various lung volumes and capacities (e.g., spirometers) and those that indirectly measure respiratory function by monitoring the movements of the chest wall during performance of various respiratory exercises and during speech production (e.g., magnetometers, respiratory inductance plethysmographs, strain-gauge belt pneumographs).

Spirometric Assessment of Respiration

A range of portable, dry spirometers are now available to clinicians and are capable of providing simple-to-administer, yet accurate assessment of the major clinically relevant lung volumes and capacities, including vital capacity, forced expiratory volume (one second), inspiratory capacity, expiratory and inspiratory reserve volumes, as well as volume/flow relationships, tidal volume and respiration rate. In addition, the values for each of the respiratory parameters obtained by way of spirometric assessment can be compared to predicted values, based on the client's age, height, and sex using formulae weighted for age and/or height (Boren, Kory, & Synder, 1966; Kory, Callahan, & Boren, 1961). Despite being valuable for providing objective measures of lung volumes and capacities, however, spirometers are not useful for monitoring respiratory function during speech production because of the requirement that clients breathe through either a mouthpiece or fitted face mask during the procedure. Rather, for the purpose of quantifying speech breathing, kinematic respiratory assessments are required.

Kinematic Assessment of Speech Breathing

Kinematic assessment of respiratory function involves the indirect determination of airflow volume changes from displacements of the two components of the chest wall, i.e., the rib cage and abdomen. In that kinematic techniques do not require the client to wear a mouthpiece or nose clip, these methods allow for the measurement of various respiratory parameters during speech production. Kinematic assessment is based on kinematic theory, which suggests that the chest wall is a two-part system consisting of the rib cage and abdomen-diaphragm, arranged in mechanical parallel (Hixon, Goldman, & Mead, 1973). As the rib cage and abdomen-diaphragm move, they each displace a volume, and their combined displacements equal that of the lungs. Essentially, therefore kinematic analysis involves simultaneous but independent recording of changes in the dimensions of the rib cage and abdomen during performance of a range of speech and nonspeech tasks.

Three main types of kinematic instrumentation have been used by researchers to monitor respiration in clients with a variety of neurological disorders. These include: magnetometers (Hoit & Hixon, 1986; Solomon & Hixon, 1993; Stathopoulos & Sapienza, 1993); strain-gauge belt pneumographs (Murdoch, Chenery, Bowler, & Ingram, 1989a; Murdoch, Noble, Chenery, & Ingram, 1989b; Murdoch et al., 1993); and inductance plethysomography (McHenry & Minton, 1998; Winkworth, Davis, Adams, & Ellis, 1995). In particular, the latter two transduction systems have been used in the assessment of speech breathing in persons with TBI.

The strain-gauge belt pneumograph transduction system utilizes two elasticized straps with strain-gauges attached, one wrapped around the rib cage and the other around the abdomen, to monitor circumferential changes in these two components of the chest wall during speech production. This system was used by Murdoch et al. (1993) to assess the speech breathing abilities of a group of 20 subjects with dysarthria occurring subsequent to TBI. Murdoch, Sterling, Theodoros and Stokes (1995) have also used strain-gauge belt pneumographs to provide real-time biofeedback for the treatment of speech breathing deficits following TBI.

A more recently introduced system for measuring chest wall movements is respiratory inductance plethysmography (or "Respitrace®"). Respitrace has also been used to monitor the speech breathing abilities of a variety of neurologically disordered populations, including those with TBI (McHenry & Minton, 1998), and is currently the system of choice used in the authors' own laboratory. With this system, movements of the rib cage and abdomen during speech breathing are detected through changes in the electrical inductance of a zig-zag arrangement of fine wires inserted into two elasticized straps, one positioned around the rib cage and the other around the abdomen. An oscillator produces a frequency-modulated signal, which is directed through the wires in the elastic bands. Changes in the size of the chest wall circumference alter the shape and, therefore, the conductance of the zig-zag wires in the straps, leading to changes in the signal. In addition to providing an effective means of assessing respiratory function, the visual display of the signal output of the Respitrace system can be utilized as a biofeedback facility for those persons with TBI with an impairment in their ability to coordinate the two components of the chest wall during speech breathing.

Perceptual and Physiological Features of Respiratory Dysfunction Following TBI

To date, few reported studies have examined in detail the perceptual and physiological features of TBI dysarthria attributable to deficits in speech breathing. The most comprehensive studies to have been reported are those completed by Theodoros, Murdoch and colleagues (Murdoch et al., 1993; Theodoros et al., 1994; Theodoros, Shrapnel, & Murdoch, 1998). Consequently, these studies will provide the focus for this section of the present chapter.

Perceptual Features of Respiratory Dysfunction Following TBI

Theodoros et al. (1994) examined the perceptual speech characteristics of a group of 20 speakers with dysarthria occurring subsequent to severe TBI. Each subject participating in their study was required to read aloud a standard passage ("The Grandfather Passage") to obtain a tape-recorded speech sample for perceptual analysis. Each speech sample was subsequently rated by two speech-language pathologists on the same series of speech dimensions used by FitzGerald et al. (1987). The series comprised 32 dimensions covering the five aspects of speech production (i.e., prosody, respiration, phonation, resonance, and articulation). In addition, each subject was also administered the Frenchay Dysarthria Assessment (Enderby, 1983).

Reduced respiratory support for speech was noted by Theodoros et al. (1994) to be present in 85% of their subjects with TBI, with more than half of these subjects exhibiting a moderate-to-severe degree of impaired respiratory function. In addition, two abnormal respiratory features, namely audible inspirations and forced respiration, were reported to be present in the speech of 60% and 35% of the subjects with TBI, respectively. The frequent occurrence of reduced phrase lengths, present in the speech of 88% of the subjects with TBI, was also considered by Theodoros et al. (1994) to be indicative of an inadequate respiratory basis for speech in these cases, as was the high incidences of phonatory disturbance (e.g., variation of loudness, loudness level, maintenance of loudness).

Theodoros et al. (1994) suggested that the perception of impaired respiratory support for speech in subjects with TBI may be a function of two different processes. First, reduced respiratory support for speech may reflect a dysfunction of the respiratory mechanism per se, owing to various neuropathological processes that may be present in this group. Second, they suggested that the perception of impaired speech breathing in dysarthric speakers may be the result of the confounding influence of other deviant speech dimensions arising from associated inefficiency of laryngeal, velopharyngeal or articulatory valving of the expiratory breath stream. A number of authors have suggested that the perception of impaired breath support for speech is not entirely a result of dysfunction of the respiratory apparatus, but may also be related to impaired functioning in the laryngeal, velopharyngeal, and articulatory subsystems of the speech production mechanism (Murdoch et al., 1989b; Yorkston et al., 1988).

The diffuse pattern of brain damage usually found in individuals with severe TBI is consistent with the suggestion of Theodoros et al. (1994) that the perception of impaired breath support for speech in subjects with TBI may be related to the effects of inefficient valving of the expiratory breath stream. According to Theodoros et al. (1994), the diffuse nature of the neurological impairment inflicted by severe head trauma implies that the cause of reduced breath support for speech in a population of subjects with TBI would not simply be a dysfunction of the respiratory mechanism alone, but more likely the result of additional involvement of a number of other impaired speech subsystems. Impairment of the laryngeal, velopharyngeal, and articulatory subsystems may occur subsequent to TBI as a result of lesions to the upper and/or lower motor neurons, the extrapyramidal system, the cerebellum, or a combination of two or more of these levels of the nervous system. As indicated by Theodoros et al. (1994), however, final determination of the basis of the reported perceived impaired respiratory support for speech in individuals with TBI requires an instrumental evaluation of their respiratory systems, involving both spirometric and kinematic assessments of respiratory function.

Theodoros et al. (1994) also drew attention to the possibility that the basis of the perception of deviant articulatory features in the speech of their subjects with TBI may be impaired respiratory function. Impaired respiratory support for speech resulting from reduced vital capacity and/or incoordination of the movements of the chest wall may result in a weak and poorly maintained expiratory breath stream (Darley et al., 1975). As a result of respiratory dysfunction, the expiratory airflow may be inadequate for creating the essential intraoral pressures necessary for plosive consonant production and the intensity of airflow required for fricative consonant production (Darley et al., 1975). As pointed out by Theodoros et al. (1994), however, determination of the relative contribution of the respiratory mechanism to articulatory dysfunction in subjects with TBI requires simultaneous physiological examination of both subsystems.

Physiological Features of Respiratory Dysfunction Following TBI

As outlined in the previous section, a number of the features of the speech disorder exhibited by persons with TBI are possibly the outcome of disturbances in speech breathing. Although very few studies of speech breathing based on physiological analyses have been reported to date (McHenry, Wilson, & Minton, 1994; Murdoch et al., 1993), those that do appear in the literature have confirmed the perceptual impression that individuals with dysarthria subsequent to severe TBI have problems with speech breathing. In addition, these studies have identified a number of abnormal features of the speech breathing of persons with TBI that have the potential to disrupt normal speech production, including reduced lung volumes, abnormal chest wall movements during speech breathing, and a reduction in the number of syllables produced per breath.

Murdoch et al. (1993) carried out a spirometric and kinematic analysis of the speech breathing abilities of a group of 20 individuals with severe TBI, together with a group of 20 non-neurologically impaired controls matched for age and sex. A spirometric assessment of respiration was conducted using a portable, dry spirometer (Mijnhardt Vicatest$^{®}$ – P1), which yielded values for vital capacity (VC) and forced expiratory volume 1 second (FEV_1). The results of the spirometric assessment indicated that, as a group, the subjects with TBI had significantly lower VC and FEV_1 values than the control subjects, with 70% of the subjects with TBI recording VCs below the normal range (i.e., more than 20% below their predicted value). Tidal volumes, however, did not differ significantly between the two groups.

A reduction in VC has been observed in patients with a variety of neuromuscular disorders that involve the chest wall (Murdoch et al., 1989a; Murdoch, Chenery, Stokes, & Hardcastle, 1991; Putnam & Hixon, 1984). In most instances, researchers have attributed this reduction in VC to factors such as the presence of wasting and weakness in the muscles of the chest wall or the presence of rigidity in the respiratory muscles. For example, Putnam and Hixon (1984) suggested that the reduction in VC observed in 50% of their subjects with motor neuron disease was the outcome of wasting and weakness in the respiratory muscles as a result of atrophy of the muscles of the chest wall. With regard to subjects with Parkinson's disease, Murdoch et al. (1989a) suggested that the basis for the reduction in VCs noted in this group was limitations to the excursions of the chest wall caused by rigidity of the respiratory musculature. Murdoch et al. (1993) commented that, although some reduction in the excursion of the chest wall, as a result of increased muscle tone in association with spasticity, may have contributed to the lowering of VC in their subjects with TBI, they did not observe any significant degree of atrophy in the muscles of the chest wall in any of the brain-injured subjects. Consequently, they concluded that wasting and weakness of the respiratory musculature was not a major contributor to the reduction in the excursion of the chest wall in their subjects with TBI.

Disruption to the two-part coordination of the chest wall, leading to a reduction in the excursion of the respiratory apparatus, has been postulated as the mechanism underlying reduced VCs in patients with cerebellar disease (Murdoch et al., 1991). In that the kinematic analysis conducted by Murdoch et al. (1993) also revealed problems with the two-part coordination of the chest wall in subjects with TBI, these authors suggested that a mechanism similar to that proposed for individuals with cerebellar disease may also have contributed to the reduction in VC observed in their subjects with TBI. In support of this concept, Murdoch et al. (1993) noted that 40% of their subjects with TBI also exhibited clinical signs indicative of cerebellar involvement, including cerebellar ataxia and ataxic dysarthria.

Murdoch et al. (1993) examined the kinematics of speech breathing in their group of subjects with TBI, using the strain-gauge belt pneumograph transduction system developed by Murdoch et al. (1989a). The results of the kinematic analysis showed that although as an outcome of their lower VCs, the group with TBI expired smaller volumes of air during speech production than the control subjects, their pattern of speech breathing in terms of the relative volumes expired and relative contributions of the two components of the chest wall to the overall expiratory effort during speech was the same. One major difference in the patterns of speech breathing observed in the subjects with TBI and the control subjects, however, was that the relative motion charts recorded from the subjects with TBI consistently displayed a much higher incidence of slope changes and paradoxical movements of the chest wall than the controls. Unfortunately, as pointed out by Murdoch et al. (1993), the clinical significance of these abnormal breathing patterns is at present unclear. Although both gradual and abrupt changes in the relative contribution of the rib cage and abdomen to volume displacement do occur relatively frequently in normal speakers during speech production (Hodge & Rochet, 1989), the frequency of slope changes observed in the subjects with TBI examined by Murdoch et al. (1993) was approximately twice that observed in their control group. Paradoxical movements of the chest wall were also infrequently exhibited by the control subjects included in the study reported by Murdoch et al. (1993), leading the authors to conclude that the high incidence of slope changes and paradoxical movements observed in their subjects with TBI was in some way related to the brain damage caused by the severe head trauma experienced by these individuals, rather than being general features of speech breathing per se.

A high incidence of slope changes and paradoxical movements of the chest wall has also been reported in other neurologically disordered groups (Murdoch et al., 1989a; Murdoch et al., 1991; Putnam & Hixon, 1984), leading to a variety of explanations for their occurrence. Putnam and Hixon (1984) proposed that the abrupt slope changes in the relative motion diagrams recorded from individuals with motor neuron disease may be the outcome of rib cage/abdominal groping as a result of reduced afferent feedback for fine motor control of the chest wall caused by a loss of proprioception in atrophic muscles. As an alternate explanation, these authors suggested that the "trade-off" between the efforts of the rib cage and abdomen during speech observed in speakers with motor neuron disease may represent a strategy to counteract the effect of fatigue. Murdoch et al. (1993) concluded that, given that their subjects with TBI did not present with atrophy in the muscles of the chest wall, the explanation proposed for subjects with motor neuron disease was not appropriate for explaining the presence of slope changes and paradoxical movements of the chest wall in their subjects with TBI.

Aberrant coordination of the chest wall has been proposed as the basis for presence of bizarre movements of the rib cage and abdomen during speech production in individuals with cerebellar disorders (Abb, Hunker, & Barlow, 1983; Murdoch et al. 1991). Given the possible involvement of the cerebellum and/or its connections in at least 40% of their subjects with TBI, Murdoch et al. (1993) suggested that the high incidence of slope changes and paradoxical movements in these cases reflects problems, as the result of brain damage, with the temporal coordination of the two components of the chest wall as they act to maintain the subglottal pressures necessary for speech production.

Based on the work of Murdoch et al. (1993), therefore, it would appear that the majority of respiratory anomalies demonstrated by individuals with dysarthria subsequent to TBI most likely manifest as a consequence of a breakdown in the two-part coordination of the chest wall. Unfortunately, to date, no further group studies based on physiological analysis of the respiratory abilities of survivors of TBI have been reported. Consequently, there is a need for replication of the work of Murdoch et al. (1993) in order to verify and validate their findings. In a study recently completed in our laboratory, the authors of the present chapter have examined the speech breathing abilities of a further 15 subjects with dysarthria subsequent to severe TBI and 15 controls, using spirometric and kinematic procedures similar to those employed by Murdoch et al. (1993). One important change to the methodology, however, was that in the more recent study inductance plethysomography was used to monitor changes in the circumference of the chest wall during speech instead of the strain-gauge belt pneumograph transduction system utilized by Murdoch et al. (1993). The results of our latest study confirmed those of the earlier report, with the group of subjects with TBI recording significantly lower VC and FEV_1 values than the controls. As in the study reported by Murdoch et al. (1993), the overall pattern of speech breathing in terms of the relative volumes expired and relative contributions of the rib cage and abdomen to the expiratory effort during speech production was the same for both the TBI and control subjects. Also consistent with the findings of Murdoch et al. (1993) was the presence of frequent changes in the relative contribution of the rib cage and abdomen to the expiratory effort as well as a high number of paradoxical movements of the chest wall during speech production. Overall the findings of our more recent study based on inductance plethysmography support the proposal that respiratory anomalies evidenced in speakers with severe TBI are largely the outcomes of a breakdown in the two-part coordination of the chest wall. Collectively the findings of our recent study together with those of Murdoch et al. (1993) indicate that treatment for individuals with dysarthria subsequent to TBI should include a component directed at improving the coordinated action of the rib cage and abdomen during speech production. The treatment of dysarthria associated with TBI is covered in detail in Chapter 8.

Summary

Individuals with severe TBI exhibit a range of deficits in speech breathing that have the potential to interfere with normal speech production. Perceptually people with TBI demonstrate a high incidence of impaired respiratory support for speech and a range of other deviant speech dimensions that may, at least in part, be attributable to impaired respiratory function. Physiological analyses involving both spirometric and kinematic procedures have shown that people with TBI have reduced lung capacities (e.g., vital capacity), compared to non-neurologically impaired controls, as well as abnormal chest wall movements during speech production, possibly resulting from a breakdown in the two-part coordination of the chest wall. It is recommended that treatment aimed at improving the speech production abilities of individuals with TBI include a component aimed at improving coordination of the rib cage and abdomen during speech.

References

Abbs, J., Hunker, C., & Barlow, S. (1983). Differential speech motor subsystem impairments with supra bulbar lesions: Neurophysiological framework and supporting data. In W. Berry (Ed.), *Clinical Dysarthria* (pp.21–56). San Diego: College-Hill Press.

Bellaire, K., Yorkston, K.M., & Beukelman, D.R. (1986). Modification of breath patterning to increase naturalness of a mildly dysarthric speaker. *Journal of Communication Disorders, 19,* 271–280.

Boren, H.G., Kory, R.C., & Synder, J.C. (1966). The Veterans Administration-Army cooperative study of pulmonary function II. The lung volume and its subdivisions in normal men. *American Journal of Medicine, 41,* 96–114.

Chenery, H.J. (1998). Perceptual analysis of dysarthric speech. In B.E. Murdoch (Ed.), *Dysarthria: A Physiological Approach to Assessment and Treatment.* Cheltenham: Stanley Thornes Publishers Ltd.

Darley, F.L., Aronson, A.E., & Brown, J.R. (1975). *Motor Speech Disorders.* Philadephia: W.B. Saunders.

Enderby, P. (1983). *Frenchay Dysarthria Assessment.* San Diego: College-Hill Press.

FitzGerald, F.J., Murdoch, B.E., & Chenery, H.J. (1987). Multiple sclerosis: Associated speech and language disorders. *Australian Journal of Human Communication Disorders, 15,* 15–33.

Hixon, T.J., Goldman, M.D., & Mead, J. (1973). Kinematics of the chest wall during speech production: Volume displacements of the rib cage, abdomen and lung. *Journal of Speech and Hearing Research, 16,* 78–115.

Hixon, T.J. & Putnam, A.H. (1983). Voice disorders in relation to respiratory kinematics. *Seminars in Speech, Language and Hearing, 4,* 217–231.

Hodge, M.M. & Rochet, A. (1989). Characteristics of speech breathing in young women. *Journal of Speech and Hearing Research, 32.* 466–480.

Hoit, J.D. & Hixon, T.J. (1986). Body type and speech breathing. *Journal of Speech and Hearing Research, 29,* 313–324.

Kory, R.C., Callahan, R., & Boren, H.G. (1961). The Veterans Administration-Army cooperative study of pulmonary function I. Clinical spirometry in normal men. *American Journal of Medicine, 30,* 243–258.

McHenry, M.A. & Minton, J.T. (1998). Speech-breathing analysis procedures for speakers who are difficult to assess. In M.P. Cannito, K.M. Yorkston, & Beukelman, D.R., (Eds.), *Neuromotor Speech Disorders: Nature, Assessment and Management* (pp.167–180). Baltimore: Paul Brookes Publishing Company.

McHenry, M.A., Wilson, R.L., & Minton, J.T. (1994). Management of multiple physiologic system deficits following traumatic brain injury. *Journal of Medical Speech-Language Pathology, 2,* 59–74.

Metter, E.J. (1985). Motor speech production and assessment: Neurologic perspective. In J.K. Darby (Ed.), *Speech and Language Evaluation in Neurology: Adult Disorders* (pp. 343–362). New York: Grune and Stratton.

Murdoch, B.E., Chenery, H.J., Bowler, S., & Ingram, J. (1989a). Respiratory function in Parkinson's subjects exhibiting a perceptible speech deficit: A kinematic and spirometric analysis. *Journal of Speech and Hearing Disorders, 54,* 610–626.

Murdoch, B.E., Chenery, H.J., Stokes, P., & Hardcastle, W. (1991). Respiratory kinematics in speakers with cerebellar disease. *Journal of Speech and Hearing Research, 34,* 768–780.

Murdoch, B.E., Noble, J., Chenery, H.J. & Ingram J. (1989b). A spirometric and kinematic analysis of respiratory function in pseudobulbar palsy. *Australian Journal of Human Communication Disorders, 17,* 21–35.

Murdoch, B.E., Sterling, D.K., Theodoros, D.G., & Stokes, P.D. (1995). Physiological rehabilitation of disordered speech breathing in dysarthric speakers following severe closed head injury. In J. Fourez and N. Page (Eds.), *Treatment Issues and Long-Term Outcomes.* Brisbane: Australian Academic Press.

Murdoch, B.E., Theodoros, D.G., Stokes, P., & Chenery, H.J. (1993). Abnormal patterns of speech breathing in dysarthric speakers following severe closed head injury. *Brain Injury, 7,* 295–308.

Putnam, A. & Hixon, T.J. (1984). Respiratory kinematics in speakers with motor neuron disease. In M.R. McNeil, J.C. Rosenbek & A.E. Aronson (Eds.), *The Dysarthrias: Physiology, Acoustics, Perception, Management* (pp. 37–67). San Diego: College-Hill Press.

Solomon, N. & Hixon, T.J. (1993). Speech breathing in Parkinson's disease. *Journal of Speech Hearing Research, 36,* 294–310.

Stathopoulos, E.T. & Sapienza, C. (1993). Respiratory and laryngeal function of women and men during vocal intensity variation. *Journal of Speech and Hearing Research, 36,* 64–75.

Theodoros, D.G., Murdoch, B.E., & Chenery, H.J. (1994). Perceptual speech characteristics of dysarthric speakers following severe closed head injury. *Brain Injury, 8,* 101–124.

Theodoros, D.G., Schrapnel, N., & Murdoch, B.E. (1998). Motor speech impairment following traumatic brain injury: A physiological and perceptual analysis of one case. *Pediatric Rehabilitation, 2,* 107–122.

Winkworth, A.L., Davis, P.J., Adams, R.D., & Ellis, E. (1995). Breathing patterns during spontaneous speech. *Journal of Speech and Hearing Research, 38,*124–144.

Yorkston, K.M., Beukelman, D.R., & Bell, K.R. (1988). *Clinical Management of Dysarthric Speakers.* Philadelphia: Taylor & Francis.

CHAPTER

Seven

Dysarthria Following Traumatic Brain Injury in Childhood

Louise M. Cahill, Bruce E. Murdoch, and Deborah G. Theodoros

Introduction

Traumatic brain injury (TBI) is a leading cause of death and disability in the Western world, resulting in substantial social and economic costs to society (Sosin, Sniezek & Thurman, 1996). Epidemiological studies indicate that the incidence of TBI in child-hood is approximately 200 per 100,000 per year (Annegers, 1983; Kraus, 1995). Advances in medical treatment have increased the chances of surviving TBI, thereby increasing the need for rehabilitation and long-term services. Most children surviving TBI have a normal life expectancy, and many with moderate-to-severe injuries may require long term support to achieve a maximal level of independence and quality of life. Emanuelson, von Wendt, Lundälv, and Larsson (1996), in a study of the outcome of 25 children with severe TBI, found that almost all children were left with major impairments.

Dysarthria, a motor speech disorder resulting from damage to the neuromotor control mechanism, is a commonly reported sequela of severe TBI in children

(Bak, van Dongen, & Arts, 1983; Costeff, Groswasser, Landman, & Brenner, 1985; Costeff, Groswasser, & Goldstein, 1990). Ylviskaker (1986), reporting on a long-term follow-up study of children who had suffered severe TBI, found that 10% of children and 8% of adolescents were unintelligible. Several authors have reported on the persistent nature of dysarthria following TBI (Costeff et al., 1985; Thomsen, 1984; Rusk, Block, & Lowman, 1969). Costeff and colleagues (1985) found that 14 out of 36 children with a severe closed head injury (CHI) presented with dysarthria 2 years postinjury, while only one child remained aphasic. Hécaen (1976) reported that, second to writing disorders, articulatory disorders were the most prevalent and persistent communication deficit in a group of 15 children with severe CHI.

Dysarthria can have a negative impact on the child's quality of life, including withdrawal from family, social, and academic activities. Communication disorders are also recognized as having a negative influence on long-term vocational outcome (Brooks, McKinlay, Symington, Beattie, & Campsie, 1987) and social reintegration (Oddy, 1984; Malkmus, 1989). Some authors have even gone as far as to suggest that communication abilities may play the pivotal role in determining the quality of survival after head trauma (Najenson, Sazbon, Fiselzon, Becker, & Schechter, 1978).

Despite the persistent nature of dysarthria in TBI and its potential negative impact on the quality of life of many children, very little research into the nature and severity of the disorder has been reported. One reason for the dearth of research into childhood dysarthria is the presumption that the underlying physiological impairment in children and adults is similar. Therefore, in the past, data from the adult population has been used to describe childhood dysarthria. However, there are several reasons why the physiological manifestation of dysarthria in children subsequent to TBI may differ from that in adults subsequent to TBI: children may still be developing speech, there may be differences in recovery potential for children and adults, and there may be different mechanisms of neurological damage in children and adults. Consequently, there is a need for greater understanding of the nature of the physiological functioning of the motor speech impairment in children with dysarthria subsequent to TBI, so that more satisfactory strategies for the treatment of acquired childhood dysarthria can be developed.

The aim of this chapter, then, is to outline the characteristic features of dysarthria in children following TBI. The various procedures recommended by the authors for assessing the perceptual, acoustic and physiological features of dysarthria following TBI in childhood will be discussed. In addition to this, the physiological functioning of the major subsystems of the speech production apparatus in a group of children who have suffered TBI will be detailed. Furthermore, the speech outcome of three of these children will be discussed, to highlight the variable nature of the speech disturbance that can result following TBI.

Epidemiology of TBI in Childhood

Inconsistencies in the literature concerning the definitional issues related to TBI have led to difficulties in obtaining accurate estimates of the incidence of TBI in children and adolescents. Medical records often do not clearly define an injury as being a TBI, but rather as a "head injury," which may constitute injuries such as lacerations, but not brain damage. In addition, the cause of the injury (e.g., motor vehicle accident) may be stated, but not the actual result of that accident (e.g., TBI). Despite these methodological inconsistencies, however, it has been estimated that TBI is one of the most frequent neurological conditions that results in hospitalization of children under 19 years of age (Field, 1976) and that TBI is the leading cause of death or permanent disability in children and adolescents (Guyer & Ellers, 1990).

Incidence

Approximately 1 in 500 children will be hospitalized with TBI each year, and 1 in 30 children will sustain a TBI by the time they reach 18 years of age (Annegers, 1983). Each year in the U.S. more than 200,000 children are hospitalized as a result of TBI, with about 15,000 of these children experiencing a severe TBI (Di Scala, Osberg, Gans, Chin, & Grant, 1991). Incidence figures of 230 per 100,000 (Kalsbeek, McLaurin, Harris, & Miller, 1980) and 185 per 100,000, or 1 in every 550 school-aged children under 15 years of age (Kraus, Fife, Cox, Ramstein, & Conroy, 1986) have been reported. Several Australian studies have produced similar findings (Bogan, Hartley, & Ryan, 1991; Sakzewski, Ziviani, & Swanson, 1996). A recent study (Emanuelson & von Wendt, 1997) documented the incidence of children and adolescents (aged 0–17 years) who were admitted to a hospital for TBI in a particular region of Sweden in a 5-year period. The study looked solely at TBI, and excluded concussion and other mild injuries. They found a mean incidence rate for TBI in children and adolescents of 12 per 100,000, with 6 in every 100,000 cases being left with permanent functional impairment. They concluded that serious brain injury is a significant cause of permanent neurological disability in the pediatric age group in Sweden.

Age

Many studies have documented the incidence of TBI in various groups. The peak incidence for TBI has been reported to be between the ages of 15 and 24 years (Kraus, Rock & Hemyari, 1990; Mira, Tucker & Tyler, 1992). Sterling (1994), in a study across two Australian states, found that 17.8% of injuries occurred between the ages of 5 and 7 years, 35.6% between 8 and 11 years, 34.4% between 12 and 15 years, and 12% between 16 and 18 years. When age and cause of injury are examined, a consistent pattern emerges from the literature. Abuse and falls tend to be the most common cause of TBI in infants, toddlers, and preschoolers. In children aged 5 to 14 years the predominant cause of TBI appears to be motor vehicle accidents involving pedestrians or bicycles, and sporting injuries. In high school and late adolescence high-speed motor vehicle accidents have been found to be the major cause of severe TBI (Annegers, 1983; Craft, Shaw, & Cartlidge, 1972; Di Scala et al, 1991; Emanuelson & von Wendt, 1997; Goldstein & Levin, 1987; Kraus et al, 1986).

Gender

It is well established that boys are more at risk of TBI than girls, with ratios between 2:1 and 3:1 being reported (Goldstein & Levin, 1987; Rimel & Jane, 1983). This ratio is maintained throughout all age groups, and studies have found that males differ in both the degree of risk for TBI and in the type of risk (Frankowski, Annegers, & Whitman, 1985; Naugle, 1990). Males are more likely to be involved in motor vehicle accidents (MVA) and sustain sporting-related injuries. As well as this increased risk of injury, males are more likely to sustain fatal injuries because of their involvement in risk-taking activities and more aggressive sporting activities (Klauber, Barrett-Connor, Hofsetter, & Micik, 1986).

Predisposition to TBI

Klonoff and Paris (1974) reported a sex-related finding of premorbid learning difficulties and developmental delay in boys, but not in girls, with TBI. Mahoney et al, (1983) studied children who had suffered a severe TBI and found that 61% had pre-existing language and learning difficulties. Craft et al, (1972) reported that there was a higher incidence of teacher-reported premorbid behavioral difficulties in children with head injuries. It is thought that children with behavioral problems are more likely to take risks and enter into dangerous situations, thus predisposing them to head injuries (Goldstein & Levin, 1987).

Factors Influencing Outcome in Childhood TBI

The specific nature of impairment following TBI varies for each child, depending on the type of injury, the specific area of the brain affected, and the severity of the injury (Bigler, Clark, & Farmer, 1996). Furthermore, factors such as age, developmental level, academic achievement, and behavioral adjustment interact with the brain injury itself to determine the child's presentation and long-term outcome (Rivara et al., 1994). Typical long-term consequences of TBI in children and adolescents are functional limitations in the areas of sensory processing (vision, hearing), motor skills (including speech), cognition, language, self-care abilities and behavior. It has been suggested (Mira et al., 1992) that approximately 15% of children who are hospitalized will have long-term deficits in these areas. Cattelani, Lombardi, Brianti, and Mazzucchi (1998) studied the intellectual, behavioral, and social outcome of patients with a history of childhood TBI. They found that these patients displayed social maladjustment and poor quality of life, which were still present several years postinjury.

Variation in Recovery Potential for Children and Adults with TBI

Factors influencing the outcome of TBI in children vary from those that affect adults. Craft (1972) noted that children have a far better prognosis for recovery from severe head injuries than adults because of the plasticity of a child's brain. However, several authors have challenged this theory of cerebral plasticity (Costeff et al., 1985;

Mira et al., 1992). In a long-term study of 36 children who had suffered a severe TBI, Costeff et al, (1985) concluded that the overall degree of recovery for children was no better than in the adult population. Mira and colleagues (1992) postulated that TBI disrupts the learning process and hinders ongoing development and the ability to build on previously learned skills.

The most obvious difference in the recovery potential between children and adults is that a child's brain is still developing, and therefore the pathophysiological response to brain trauma will vary, depending on the age at the time of injury. As well as this, the skull reacts differently to trauma when the bone is thin and the sutures and fontanelle are open than after they have closed and fused. It has been suggested that because of its elasticity and greater degree of deformation, the skull of an infant absorbs the energy of the physical impact and thereby protects the brain better than the skull of an adult (Craft et al., 1972; Gurdjian & Webster, 1958; Menkes & Till, 1995). Therefore, the same traumatic event is likely to produce a different array of injuries at differing ages (Bruce, 1995).

There has been a widely held belief that children recover better than adults after a severe head injury, in relation to mortality rate and physiological effects of TBI. However, several authors have disputed this assumption. Carlsson, Von Essen, & Lofgren (1968) and Becker et al. (1977) found that although the mortality rate for children under 19 years was lower than that for adults, this could be accounted for by a lower secondary mortality, with the primary mortality being similar in adults and children. Bruce and colleagues (1979), in a study of the nature of brain injury subsequent to severe CHI in 85 children and adolescents, identified general cerebral swelling, but infrequent focal mass lesions. The authors attributed the cerebral swelling to vascular congestion produced by increased blood volume and flow. These findings contrast with studies in adults, where swelling is often associated with edema and decreased cerebral blood flow (Zimmerman et al., 1978). Bruce et al (1979) inferred that, because of this difference, the pathophysiological response of the child's brain to injury differs from that in adults.

Variation in the Type and Severity of Injury

Children are more prone to particular types of injuries at certain ages. While about half of adult TBI cases involve high-speed motor vehicle accidents, falls are responsible for half of the pediatric injuries (Levin, Benton, & Grossman, 1982). Even though motor vehicle accidents account for almost one-third of pediatric head injury cases, many of these are motor vehicle/pedestrian accidents occurring at low speeds (Levin et al., 1982). Since children are more likely to be injured as a result of low-speed accidents or falls, the rotational acceleration of the brain may be lower and briefer than that in high-speed motor vehicle accidents. Therefore, since high-speed vehicular accidents predominate in severely injured adolescents and adults, more diffuse brain injury would be expected in these cases (Levin et al., 1982). In fact, it was noted by Jamison and Kaye (1974) that persistent neurological deficits were only present in children injured in traffic accidents. Indeed, Moyes (1980) found traffic accidents to be the most common cause of long-term morbidity following head injury in childhood.

Type and severity of injury have commonly been linked to outcome following TBI. Although there is no consensus in the literature on the classification of severity of injury following TBI, it has commonly been measured by length and depth of coma, using the Glasgow Coma Scale (GCS; Teasdale & Jennett, 1974—see Chapter 1), and the length of post-traumatic amnesia (PTA). Although use of the GCS is widespread, its predictive value when used with children has been questioned (Lieh-Lai et al., 1992). In their study of 79 children with varying degrees of TBI, Lieh-Lai et al. found that 28% had initial GCS scores from 3 to 5, 36% had scores between 6 and 10, and 35.3% had scores between 11 and 13. Follow-up of these children found that those children with GCS scores of 3 to 5 frequently had favorable outcomes, but they required more aggressive therapy and their recovery period was longer than those children with higher GCS scores. Levin, Eisenberg, Wigg, and Kobayashi (1982) noted that head injuries in different age groups may not be strictly comparable in severity, even when they receive equal ratings on the GCS, and that the duration of impaired consciousness, rather than the initial GCS had the strongest relationship to cognitive outcome.

It is clear from the literature that many factors associated with TBI (mechanism of injury, cause of injury, pathophysiological response of the brain to the injury) vary with development, so care must be taken when comparing the outcome of children and adults following TBI. It is possible that functioning of the major components of the speech apparatus will be affected differently in children and adults following TBI. Further, it cannot be assumed that children will recover from TBI or respond to rehabilitative measures in the same manner as adults, as has been accepted in the past.

Dysarthria in Childhood TBI

As indicated earlier, childhood dysarthria has traditionally been described and classified using criteria pertaining to the adult dysarthric population. However, children with TBI may still be developing speech, and therefore the resultant motor speech disorder may well be an interaction of developmental and acquired components of the disorder (Murdoch & Hudson-Tennent, 1994). In particular, communication disorders, such as dysarthria, have not been comprehensively studied in childhood TBI. Until recently, there has been little information regarding the nature of dysarthria in children subsequent to TBI available in the literature. In the absence of a model of motor speech disorders for children most investigators have used the adult model of dysarthria, which correlates the type of dysarthria with the pathophysiology of the motor subsystems. This model is not totally satisfactory, particularly for younger children, whose speech and language skills are still developing. Therefore, there is an obvious need to investigate the specific nature of the speech disturbance following TBI as it relates to the pediatric population. The few studies to date that have attempted to relate features of pediatric dysarthria to a lesion site have been inconclusive (Bak et al., 1983; Stark, 1985), and few studies describe the nature and course of acquired childhood dysarthria (Bak et al., 1983; Murdoch & Hudson-Tennent, 1994; van Mourik, Catsman-Berrevoets, Paquier, Yosef-Bak, & van Dongen, 1997). Van Mourik et al. (1997) reviewed the literature relating to the analysis of speech features in acquired childhood dysarthria published since 1980, and observed that information on dysarthria in acquired childhood disorders was based on only a limited number of single case studies, most of which related to cases of cerebellar tumor resection. They noted that although acquired childhood dysarthria is not a rare disorder, the overall incidence and specific nature of the perceptual and physiological characteristics of dysarthria following TBI have not been fully investigated.

Hécaen (1976) studied 15 children with severe TBI and found that articulatory deficits were the second most prevalent and persistent communication deficit after writing disorders. Costeff and colleagues (1985) found that 14 of the 36 children with severe TBI in their study presented with dysarthria 4 years postinjury, while only one child remained aphasic. Ylvisaker (1986), in a long-term study of severe TBI, found that 10% of children and 8% of adolescents lacked intelligible speech. More recently, Boyer and Edwards (1991) studied 220 children and adolescents with severe TBI who were admitted consecutively to a rehabilitation program. They found that dysarthria was present in 33% of cases, while 25% were nonspeaking 1 to 3 years postinjury.

Assessment of Dysarthria in Childhood TBI

In the past, perceptual analysis has been the preferred method of assessing dysarthric speech. However, traditional perceptual assessments do not provide any direct information on the functioning of the speech subsystems (i.e., articulation, velopharyngeal, laryngeal, and respiration). It is now recognised that knowledge of the nature of the underlying pathophysiology of the speech production mechanism is necessary for the optimal treatment of motor speech disorders (Abbs & DePaul, 1989).

In recent years an extensive range of instrumentation has been developed for use in the assessment of the various components of the speech production mechanism. Instrumental assessment of the speech production mechanism provides an objective means of measuring the physiological nature of malfunctions at various stages of the speech production process. Peterson and Marquardt (1981) stated that including instrumental procedures in the process of diagnosing speech disorders enables clinicians to extend their senses and objectify their perceptual observations. Recently the emphasis in the management of motor speech disorders has been placed on improved objective measures of speech motor subsystem performance (Abbs & De Paul, 1989). Clinicians are increasingly considering the advantages of instrumental analysis, which provides quantitative, objective data on a wide range of different speech parameters that are beyond the scope of an auditory-based impressionistic judgment (Hardcastle, Morgan-Barry, & Clark, 1985).

Only a handful of studies, however, (Bak et al., 1983; Murdoch & Hudson-Tennent, 1993, 1994; Murdoch, Horton, Theodoros, & Thompson, 1997; Stierwalt, Robin, Solomon, Weiss, & Max, 1996; Theodoros, Shrapnel, & Murdoch, 1998; van Dongen, Catsman-Berrevoets, & van Mourik, 1994; Wit, Maassen, Gabreels, & Thoonen, 1993; Wit, Maassen, Gabreels, Thoonen, & de-Swart, 1994) have examined the physiological aspects of childhood dysarthria, and most of these studies have focused on children with dysarthria resulting from cerebral palsy, or dysarthria subsequent to resection of a posterior fossa tumor. The few studies that have looked at dysarthria following TBI in children have been single case studies (Murdoch et al., 1997; Theodoros et al., 1998; Wit et al., 1994) or have looked at only one aspect of the speech production mechanism (Stierwalt et al., 1996).

The authors of the current chapter recommend the integrated use of perceptual, acoustic, and instrumental measures when assessing children with dysarthria subsequent to TBI. The procedures for these assessments are briefly described in the following section. The reader is directed to Chapters 2, 3, 4, 5, and 6 of this book for a more detailed description of these procedures.

Perceptual Speech Assessment of Dysarthria in Childhood TBI

Various perceptual assessments have traditionally been used to characterize the disordered speech production of dysarthric speakers. A comprehensive perceptual assessment should evaluate the five major components of speech production: respiration, phonation, resonance, articulation, and prosody. It should provide information on specific deviant speech dimensions, an assessment of overall speech intelligibility, and a description of any motor speech subsystem dysfunction. The battery of perceptual assessments used in our research clinic has been designed to fully assess all of these categories. It includes:

• Assessment of Intelligibility of Dysarthric Speech (Yorkston & Beukleman, 1981)
• Frenchay Dysarthria Assessment (Enderby, 1983)
• Fisher-Logemann Test of Articulation Competence (Fisher & Logemann, 1971)
• Speech sample analysis (SSA)

The Assessment of Intelligibility of Dysarthric Speech (ASSIDS; Yorkston & Beukleman, 1981) provides an index of the severity of dysarthric speech by quantifying both single-word and sentence intelligibility as well as the speaking rate (words per minute), the rate of intelligible speech (i.e., the number of intelligible words per minute [IWPM]) and the communication efficiency ratio (CER) of dysarthric speakers. This test is designed for use with the adult population, but can be modified (by having the child repeat the words and sentences rather than read them) for children with reading difficulties or for those children who had not yet reached a reading level appropriate for administration of the test. The Frenchay Dysarthria Assessment (FDA; Enderby, 1983) provides a standardized assessment of speech neuromuscular activity, presented in a composite profile form and is easily administered to children. The Fisher-Logemann Test of Articulation Competence (Fisher & Logemann, 1971) provides an articulation profile and may be analyzed further to establish the presence of phonological processes, especially the presence of any developmental errors. Finally, a sample of the child's reading is analyzed perceptually (SSA). The children are asked to read aloud the standardized passage "The Grandfather Passage" (Darley, Aronson, & Brown, 1975) or, if the child cannot read, a picture description task is used. This sample is then rated by two experienced speech pathologists on a series of 33 different dimensions of speech, encompassing prosody, respiration, phonation, resonance, and articulation (FitzGerald, Murdoch, & Chenery, 1987). For full details of these assessments please see Chapter 2.

Instrumental Assessment of Dysarthria in Childhood TBI

The instrumental procedures used in our research clinic to assess the four major speech subsystems include:

- Respiratory Function
  - Spirometric assessment
  - Kinematic assessment (Respitrace®)
  - Aerodynamic assessment (Aerophone II®)
- Laryngeal Function
  - Electroglottographic assessment (Laryngograph®)
  - Aerodynamic assessment (Aerophone II®)
- Velopharngeal Function
  - Accelerometric assessment
  - Nasometer® (Kay Elemetrics)
  - Videofluroscopy (for special cases only)
- Articulatory Function
  - Lip and tongue pressure transduction systems
  - Electropalatography (EPG)
  - Electromagnetic articulography (EMA)

Respiratory Function

Respiratory function is assessed using both spirometric and kinematic techniques (as outlined in Chapter 6). The spirometric assessment yields measures such as vital capacity (VC) and forced expiratory volume per second (FEV_1). In addition to this, lung volume changes, percentage of relative contribution of the rib cage (%RC), mean syllables per breath, speaking rate, and the incidence of slope change and paradoxical chest wall movements are recorded using inductance plethysmography (Respitrace) during selected speech tasks (reading, conversation, vowel prolongation, syllable repetition and counting).

Laryngeal Function

Laryngeal function is assessed instrumentally using electroglottographic (EGG) and aerodynamic techniques. The EGG assessment is conducted using a Fourcin Laryngograph interfaced with a waveform display system (Kay Elemetrics Model 6091) running on an IBM-compatible computer. This system records the degree of vocal fold contact and the vocal fold vibratory patterns during phonation, and displays these features in the form of an Lx waveform. Three basic measures: fundamental frequency (Fo), duty cycle (DC), and closing time (CT) are obtained from this assessment. The fundamental frequency relates to the periodicity of the waveform, and is calculated as the length of time necessary for the vocal folds to complete one vibratory cycle. The duty cycle of the waveform is defined as the ratio of time that the vocal folds are open during the vocal period to the duration of the total vibratory cycle. The closing time is the duration of the closing phase, from totally open to totally closed.

Aerodynamic measures relating to air pressure, air flow, and sound pressure level are assessed via an Aerophone II airflow measurement system (Kay Elemetrics Model 6800). Several tasks are completed by each child to obtain measures of subglottic air pressure, sound pressure level, glottal resistance, phonatory flow, and ad/abduction rate (cycles/second). See Chapter 5 for full details of these assessments.

Velopharyngeal Function

Velopharyngeal function is assessed using two different systems. The first is a modified version of the nasal accelerometric technique proposed by Horii (1980), in which two miniature transducers are attached to the side of the nose and throat to detect the degree of vibration of air through these structures. A ratio of nasal to laryngeal vibrations is calculated, thereby providing a nasality index, which is referred to as the Horii Oral Nasal Coupling Index (HONC).

The second system is commercially marketed as the Nasometer (Kay Elemetrics), and consists of two directional microphones, one at the level of the nasal cavity and the other in front of the oral cavity. An efficient sound separator plate separates the two microphones. The ratio of acoustic output from the oral and nasal cavities is calculated in terms of percentage as a "nasalance" score.

In certain cases videofluoroscopy is also utilized in the assessment of velopharyngeal function. These procedures are outlined in more detail in Chapter 4 of this book.

Articulatory Function

The assessment of articulatory function involves measurement of lip and tongue strength, endurance, fine force control, and rate of repetitive movements, using two pressure transduction systems. Interlabial pressures are measured during speech and nonspeech tasks using a miniaturised pressure transducer (Entran Flatline® No. EPL 5081-7S) with factory calibration, similar to that described by Hinton and Luschei (1992). Tongue function is assessed during nonspeech tasks only, using a rubber-bulb pressure transduction system similar to that described by Murdoch, Attard, Ozanne, and Stokes (1995) and Robin, Somodi, and Luschei, (1991).

Electropalatography and electromagnetic articulography are instrumental assessments, used for the measurement of dynamic articulatory function, in some cases. Electropalatography is a technique that provides information on the location and timing of tongue contacts with the hard palate during speech. The subject is required to wear a thin acrylic plate fitted with miniature electrodes. When tongue contact with the hard palate occurs, a signal is conducted to an external processing unit, which stores the contact patterns and enables them to be displayed on a monitor.

The Electromagnetic Articulograph® AG-100 (Carstens Medizinelektronic, Germany) uses magnetic fields for tracking the movements of multiple points on supraglottic structures in the midsagittal plane. The system comprises of three transmitter coils arranged in an equilateral triangle and housed in a plastic helmet. This systems enables the study of displacements, timing, speed, and coordination of the articulators during speech.

For further details on these assessments, see Chapter 3 of this book.

Acoustic Assessment of Dysarthria in TBI

Acoustic analysis of vocal function has been used by many researchers to examine fundamental frequency, frequency range, laryngeal perturbation measures, voice amplitude, voice onset time, intonation contours, formant structure, and other aspects of phonation (Hartman & von Cramon, 1984; Hillenbrand, Cleveland, & Erickson, 1994; Kent et al, 1992). Acoustic analysis has been described as the least expensive and least intrusive instrumental approach to the evaluation of dysarthria, requiring minimal equipment, and providing detailed information on disordered behavior (Keller, Vigneux, & Laframboise, 1991). Many programs are commercially available for the acoustic analysis of speech, and a discussion of these systems is beyond the scope of this chapter. For a more detailed overview of acoustic assessment, see Thompson-Ward and Theodoros (1998).

There are only a limited number of acoustic studies of dysarthria following TBI in adults, and they have focused on the prosodic and articulatory aspects of spastic dysarthria (Morris, 1989; Weismer, 1984, Ziegler & von Cramon, 1986). There is, to our knowledge, no literature on the acoustic analysis of dysarthric speech following TBI in childhood. We are presently collecting acoustic data from a group of subjects who have acquired a TBI in childhood.

Perceptual and Physiological Functioning of the Speech Mechanism Following TBI in Childhood

Recently, the authors of the present chapter have assessed the perceptual and physiological features of speech functioning in a group of 22 individuals who sustained a TBI during childhood. All four functional components of the speech mechanism (respiratory, laryngeal, velopharyngeal, and articulatory function) were assessed using the various perceptual and instrumental procedures described previously. Of the 22 subjects assessed, 10 were classified as dysarthric, on the basis of a perceptual analysis, and 12 were nondysarthric. Fourteen (64%) of the total sample of TBI subjects were male ($M = 13.52$ years; $SD = 3.16$; range = 8–18 years), and eight were female ($M = 11.35$ years; $SD = 3.26$; range = 5–15 years). The mean age of the total sample of TBI subjects was 12.73 years ($SD = 3.29$), with ages ranging from 5 to 18 years. All subjects were at least 6 months postinjury. Subjects were excluded from the study if they had a prior history of a speech disturbance, or a prior or coexisting neurological disorder. Eighteen non-neurologically impaired individuals (mean age = 12.57 years; $SD = 3.33$; range = 5–17 years) served as controls. For biographical and clinical details of the 22 TBI subjects please see Table 7-1. The results of the perceptual and physiological assessment of this group of children with TBI are detailed below.

Perceptual Speech Features in Childhood TBI

The perceptual analysis of the speech of the 22 TBI subjects, when compared to the control group, revealed a significant disturbance in various aspects of prosody, resonance, phonation, and articulation. In addition to this, assessment on the ASSIDS revealed that the TBI group demonstrated a significant reduction in the rate of speech, intelligible words per minute, and communication efficiency, when compared to the control group, with the dysarthric TBI subjects also demonstrating a reduced sentence intelligibility. The TBI group also exhibited significant impairment in reflex, lip, palate, laryngeal, and tongue function, when the results of the FDA were compared to the control group.

Table 7-1. Biographical and clinical details of the TBI subjects.

Subject	Age at Assess. (years)	Sex	Months Postinjury	Nature of Accident	GCS	Site of Lesion(s) Confirmed by CT/MRI	Severity of Dysarthria
1	15.17	M	7	HBT	4	Depressed skull; diffuse cerebral edema	Mild
2	11.17	M	6	MV/B	3	Right parietal skull #	Absent
3	9.17	M	10	MV/B	8	Mild cerebral swelling	Absent
4	8.25	M	25	MV/B	8	Left upper hematoma, narrowing of ventricular system; linear fracture left frontal lobe	Absent
5	8.57	F	14	BA	4	Skull #; left frontal contusion; edema	Absent
6	15.00	F	31	MV/P	3	# right petrous temporal bone & left maxilla; small bleed in right basal ganglia	Absent
7	16.08	M	19	MV/B	9	Subdural hemorrhage temporoparietal region; edema left cerebral hemisphere	Absent
8	14.67	M	29	MV/P	3	# through occipital & basal regions with severe diffuse cerebral edema	Absent
9	14.33	M	21	MV/P	8	Left frontal petechial hemorrhages with diffuse cerebral swelling, left > right	Absent
10	11.00	F	36	MV/P	12	Deep white matter changes consistent with diffuse axonal injury	Absent
11	5.42	F	8	MVA	12	# right parietal bone; hematoma right temporoparietal area	Absent
12	12.08	F	40	Fall	3	Depressed compound # left parietooccipital region; edema	Absent
13	15.17	M	72	MV/B	3	Diffuse axonal injury	Mild-moderate

(continues)

Table 7-1. (*continued*)

Subject	Age at Assess. (years)	Sex	Months Postinjury	Nature of Accident	GCS	Site of Lesion(s) Confirmed by CT/MRI	Severity of Dysarthria
14	15.42	F	24	MV/P	3	Cerebral edema; subarachnoid & intraventricular hemorrhage	Mild
15	10.75	M	42	Fall	7	Diffuse axonal injury; right cerebral edema & hematoma	Absent
16	18.25	M	10	MV/B	3	Right temporoparietal, cerebral edema	Moderate-severe
17	9.83	M	18	MBA	5	Posterior interhemispheric hematoma extending over left tentorium; profuse edema; dilation of temporal horns	Moderate
18	16.00	M	78	MV/B	4	Edema and effacement of sulci & compression of ventricles; hematoma in left parietal lobe lateral to thalamus	Severe
19	17.17	M	40	MV/B	4	Intracranial petechial hemorrhages and contusion right basal ganglia	Moderate
20	11.08	F	13	MV/B	3	Brainstem/pontine hemorrhage; prominent lateral ventricles secondary to diffuse axonal injury	Moderate
21	13.25	M	6	MV/B	7	Brainstem hemorrhages; diffuse bilateral cerebral contusions and axonal injury	Moderate
22	12.25	F	78	MV/P	3	Pneumoencephaly, contrecoupe lesions parietal lobes; depressed right parietal #, pituitary fossa #; obliteration of basal cisterns, 3rd and 4th ventricle effacement; hemorrhage into right thalamus	Moderate

GCS = Glasgow Coma Score; HBT = hit by train; MV/B = motor vehicle/bicycle accident; BA = bicycle accident; MV/P = motor vehicle/pedestrian accident; MVA = motor vehicle accident; MBA = motor bike accident; # = fracture.

Speech Sample Analysis

A speech sample was collected from each individual with TBI, using the techniques described above, and then rated separately by two experienced speech pathologists on 33 dimensions, encompassing the five aspects of speech production: prosody (including features of pitch, loudness, rate, stress, and phrasing), respiration, phonation, resonance, and articulation. The ratings for the TBI group and the control group were compared by a Mann-Whitney U test for independent measures, using a stringent alpha level ($p < .01$) to allow for the multiplicity of tests. The TBI group displayed significant impairment on 5 of the 33 speech dimensions, compared to the matched control group. Specifically, the TBI group as a whole demonstrated: a lack of pitch variation, a decreased general rate of speech, hypernasality, glottal fry, and imprecision of consonants.

When the 10 dysarthric TBI subjects were compared to the control group, 9 of the 33 dimensions were noted to be significantly impaired. Three of these deviant speech dimensions related to prosody (lack of variation in pitch, decreased general rate of speech, and excess stress on usually unstressed parts of speech) and two related to articulation (imprecision of consonants, and increased length of phonemes). In addition, the dysarthric TBI subjects were noted to have significantly impaired breath support for speech, significant degrees of hypernasality and glottal fry, and a significant reduction in speech intelligibility, when compared to the control group.

The frequency of occurrence of each deviant speech dimension exhibited by the TBI group as a whole was also determined to provide a descriptive measure of the perceptual speech sample analysis. The most frequently occurring deviant speech dimension was that of imprecision of consonants, with 59% of all TBI subjects being rated with some degree of consonant imprecision, ranging from a mild to a severe degree. The speech dimensions of hypernasality, inappropriate pitch level, lack of variation in pitch, and glottal fry were present in 54% of the subjects. Excess stress for the context was the next most frequently occurring deviant speech dimension, being present in 41% of all TBI subjects. Impaired breath support for speech, a shortened phrase length, increased length of phonemes, and hoarseness were present in 36% of all subjects. Other frequently occurring deviant speech dimensions included maintenance of rate, prolonged intervals, and decreased overall intelligibility (27%). Maintenance of loudness, hyponasality, and imprecision of vowels were noted to be present in 22% of subjects. The speech dimensions of mixed nasality, harshness, strain-strangled phonation, intermittent breathiness, wetness, pitch breaks, excessive fluctuation of rate and pitch, excessive loudness variation, short rushes of speech, forced inspiration/expiration, and audible inspiration were noted in only one or two subjects. Table 7-2 contains a summary of the occurrence and severity of the TBI group's deviant speech features.

Table 7-2. Occurrence and severity of speech deviations found in the TBI group

Speech Dimension	Frequency of Deviation		Severity of Deviation					
			Just Noticeable Deviation		Moderate Deviation		Severe Deviation	
	n	%	n	%	n	%	n	%
Pitch Level	12	54.54	11	50.00	1	4.54	0	0.00
Variation of Pitch	12	54.54	6	27.27	6	27.27	0	0.00
Steadiness of Pitch	4	18.18	3	13.64	1	4.54	0	0.00
Loudness Level	4	18.18	4	18.18	0	0.00	0	0.00
Variation of Loudness	4	18.18	3	13.64	1	4.54	0	0.00
Maintenance of Loudness	5	22.73	3	13.64	2	9.09	0	0.00
Phrase Length	8	36.36	4	18.18	2	9.09	2	9.09
General Rate	12	54.54	7	31.82	3	13.64	2	9.09
Maintenance of Rate	6	27.27	5	22.73	1	4.54	0	0.00
General Stress Pattern	9	40.91	4	18.18	5	22.73	0	0.00
Breath Support for Speech	8	36.36	4	18.18	4	18.18	0	0.00
Hypernasality	12	54.54	5	22.73	7	31.82	0	0.00
Hyponasality	5	22.73	5	22.73	0	0.00	0	0.00
Mixed Nasality	2	9.09	2	9.09	0	0.00	0	0.00
Harshness	2	9.09	2	9.09	0	0.00	0	0.00
Strain-Strangled	2	9.09	2	9.09	0	0.00	0	0.00
Intermittent Breathiness	2	9.09	2	9.09	0	0.00	0	0.00
Hoarseness	8	36.36	6	27.27	2	9.09	0	0.00
Glottal Fry	12	54.54	11	50.00	1	4.54	0	0.00
Wetness	1	4.54	1	4.54	0	0.00	0	0.00
Precision of Consonants	13	59.09	9	40.91	3	13.64	1	4.54
Length of Phonemes	8	36.36	7	31.82	1	4.54	0	0.00
Precision of Vowels	5	22.73	4	18.18	1	4.54	0	0.00
Overall Intelligibility	6	27.27	4	18.18	1	4.54	1	4.54
Pitch Breaks	2	9.09	2	9.09	0	0.00	0	0.00
Ex. Fluctuation of Pitch	1	4.54	1	4.54	0	0.00	0	0.00
Ex. Loudness Variation	1	4.54	0	0.00	0	0.00	1	4.54
Rate Fluctuations	2	9.09	1	4.54	0	0.00	1	4.54
Prolonged Intervals	6	27.27	2	9.09	1	4.54	3	13.64
Short Rushes of Speech	3	13.64	2	9.09	0	0.00	1	4.54
Forced Insp./Expir.	1	4.54	0	0.00	0	0.00	1	4.54
Audible Inspiration	1	4.54	0	0.00	1	4.54	0	0.00
Grunt	0	0.00	0	0.00	0	0.00	0	0.00

Assessment of Intelligibility of Dysarthric Speech

Based on the results of the ASSIDS, the TBI group as a whole was found to exhibit significant reductions in rate of speech (WPM), intelligible words per minute (IWPM), and communication efficiency (CER), compared to the control subjects. Although the sentence intelligibility score was lower for the TBI group, it was not significantly different from that of the control group. However, when the dysarthric TBI subjects were compared to the control group, significant reductions were noted in sentence intelligibility as well as in WPM, CER, IWPM, and an increase was noted in unintelligible words per minute (UWPM). It was also noted that the nondysarthric TBI subjects demonstrated significantly reduced WPM, CER, and IWPM, when compared to the control group. Therefore, although not perceived to be dysarthric, certain elements of speech intelligibility, such as rate of speech, as measured on the ASSIDS, were found to be impaired in the nondysarthric group, compared to their control counterparts.

Frenchay Dysarthria Assessment

Evaluation on the FDA indicated that, when compared to the control group, the TBI subjects' performance was significantly impaired on 19 of the 25 subsystem components. The TBI group demonstrated impairments in all subsystems of the speech mechanism, except for jaw and respiratory function. Further, the 10 dysarthric speakers were found to demonstrate significantly impaired function on all measures of lip, tongue, and laryngeal function, with impairment also noted in respiration during speech and palatal function. Interestingly, the non-dysarthric TBI subjects also demonstrated significantly impaired function in many areas of lip, tongue, and laryngeal function, when compared to the control group. Therefore, some degree of subclinical impairment in speech neuromuscular activity was evident in the speech of these speakers, even though they had been rated perceptually as non-dysarthric. A profile of the mean scores and standard deviations for the TBI group's performance on the FDA can be found in Figure 7-1.

Physiological Functioning of the Speech Mechanism Following Childhood TBI

Physiological assessment of speech function identified varying degrees of impairment across all speech subsystems in the TBI subjects when compared to the control group. Velopharyngeal function was found to be the most impaired subsystem, with significantly increased nasality present in all the TBI group's non-nasal utterances, when compared to the control group. Articulatory function in the TBI group was also found to be significantly impaired, compared to the control group, with lip function being more impaired than tongue function. Spirometric assessment of respiratory function identified significantly reduced mean predicted values for VC and FEV_1 in the TBI group, with associated reduced syllables per breath and syllables per minute. Kinematic assessment revealed relatively normal respiratory values with the exception of a reduced lung volume initiation (LVI) and abdominal volume initiation (ABVI), when expressed as a percentage of VC, during conversation. Assessment of laryngeal function on aerodynamic and electroglottographic measures identified no areas of significant impairment in the TBI group, with the exception of a reduced ad/abduction rate, when compared to the control subjects. A summary of the deviant physiological speech features of the TBI group can be found in Table 7-3.

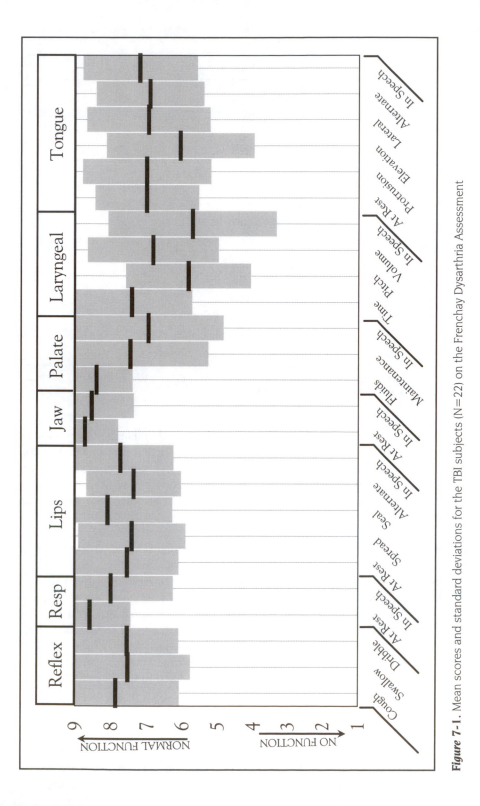

Figure 7-1. Mean scores and standard deviations for the TBI subjects (N=22) on the Frenchay Dysarthria Assessment

Table 7-3. Summary of the deviant physiological speech features identified in the childhood TBI group.

Speech Subsystem		Deviant Physiological Speech Features
Respiratory		↓ vital capacity
		↓ FEV_1
		↓ LVI in conversation
		↓ ABVI in conversation
		↓ syllables per breath
		↓ syllables per minute
Velopharyngeal		↑ nasality NN sounds
		↑ nasality NN words
		↑ nasality NN sentences
		↑ nasality NN utterances
Laryngeal		↓ ad/abduction rate
Articulatory	*Lip*	↓ maximum lip pressure
		↓ sustained maximum lip pressure
		↓ lip pressure in repetitive tasks
	Tongue	↓ rate in fast tongue repetition task

↓ = decreased; ↑ = increased; LVI = lung volume initiation; ABVI = abdominal volume initiation; FEV_1 = forced expiratory volume in first second; NN = non-nasal.

Respiratory Function

Respiratory function was assessed using both spirometric and kinematic techniques, as previously described. The TBI group was found to have a significant reduction in the mean predicted values for both VC (74%) and FEV_1 (69%), when compared to the control group (VC = 91%; FEV_1 = 83%). The 10 dysarthric TBI subjects were found to have a significantly reduced VC (68%), but not FEV_1 (70%), when compared to the control group.

Kinematic evaluation revealed essentially normal respiratory function in the TBI group, with the exception of a reduced lung volume initiation (LVI) when expressed as a percentage of VC, during conversational speech. This could largely be accounted for by a decrease in abdominal volume initiation (ABVI) in conversation. Even though the respiratory kinematics of the TBI group were relatively normal, significant impairments in breath control and speaking rate were noted, with significant reductions in syllables per breath (M = 6.52) and syllables per minute (M = 114.98), when compared to the control group (M = 10.51 syllables per breath; M = 174.31 syllables per minute). The dysarthric TBI speakers also demonstrated a significantly reduced number of syllables per breath (M = 4.55) and syllables per minute (M = 84.55), supporting the perceptual findings of significantly impaired breath support for speech on both the FDA and SSA.

Laryngeal Function

Laryngeal function was assessed using both electroglottographic (Laryngograph) and aerodynamic (Aerophone II) measures, as previously described. No significant differences were detected between the TBI group and the control group on electroglottographic measures. As well as this, no significant differences were found between the dysarthric speakers in the TBI group, the nondysarthric speakers, and the control group. The results of the aerodynamic assessment indicated that the ad/abduction rate was significantly reduced in the TBI group as a whole ($M = 2.56$ cps; $SD = 0.91$) and the 10 dysarthric TBI subjects ($M = 2.44$ cps; $SD = 0.63$), when compared to the control group ($M = 3.26$ cps; $SD = 1.05$). The lack of statistically significant differences on most physiological measures of laryngeal function between these groups is interesting, given that the presence of glottal fry was detected in 54% of the TBI subjects, and 36% were reported as being hoarse. Similarly, all measures of laryngeal function measured on the FDA were found to be significantly impaired, compared to the control group. Several factors may have contributed to these conflicting results. The wide age range of the TBI subjects meant that subjects with prepubertal and pubertal stages of laryngeal development were present in the group, and the effect of endocrinological changes on the vocal qualities of both male and female adolescents is well documented (Hollien & Malcik, 1967; Michel, Hollien, & Moore, 1966). Another reason may be that the FDA and the physiological assessments are assessing quite different measures of laryngeal function. Other factors that may have influenced the results include the relatively low number of dysarthric TBI speakers, and the intersubject variability present in the electroglottographic and aerodynamic data. Therefore it may be more appropriate that analysis of laryngeal function involves the identification of subgroupings of subjects with similar ages and/or similar vocal function to allow for these confounding influences.

Velopharyngeal Function

Results of accelerometric assessment indicated that the TBI group as a whole ($M = 39.82$, $SD = 26.50$), and the dysarthric TBI subjects ($M = 47.80$, $SD = 25.59$), exhibited a significant degree of increased nasality on all non-nasal utterances, when compared to the control group ($M = 20.44$, $SD = 8.95$). Similarly, assessment on the Nasometer revealed that the TBI group ($M = 17.76$, $SD = 14.86$) and the dysarthric TBI subjects ($M = 24.79$, $SD = 17.59$) demonstrated significantly higher nasalance levels than the control subjects ($M = 9.35$, $SD = 4.95$). These results support the results of the perceptual assessment, which identified hypernasality as the second most frequently occurring deviant speech dimension in the TBI speakers, with 54% perceived to have some degree of hypernasality in their speech.

Articulatory Function

Instrumental assessment of lip function revealed significant impairment in the TBI group as a whole, and in the dysarthric and nondysarthric TBI subjects, when compared to the control group, in the areas of maximum lip pressure, sustained maximum lip pressure, repetition of maximum lip pressure, and a reduced pressure in the fast lip repetition task. See Table 7-4 for a comparison of the means and standard deviations recorded for these tasks. These results support the perceptual findings of consonant imprecision and impaired lip function on the FDA. The presence of significantly impaired lip function in the nondysarthric TBI subjects indicated that, although speech was perceived to be normal in this group, there were in fact subclinical impairments present in lip function. This fact is supported by the presence of significantly impaired function on the FDA in the areas of lips at rest and alternating lip movements in the nondysarthric TBI subjects, when compared to the control group.

Table 7-4. Means and standard deviations for the whole TBI group (TBIG), dysarthric TBI group (DTBI), nondysarthric TBI group (NDTBI), and control group, for lip tasks where significant impairment was noted.

Parameter	TBIG (n = 22)		DTBI (n = 10)		NDTBI (n = 12)		CONTROL (n = 18)	
	Mean	SD	Mean	SD	Mean	SD	Mean	SD
MLP (kPa)	19.88	7.87	16.97	9.19	22.31	5.93	32.79	11.80
Sustained MLP (Units^2)	14150	6927	12115	7220	15847	6484	22817	9407
Repetition MLP (kPa)	13.52	7.40	11.47	8.58	15.06	6.33	24.74	10.86
Fast repetition press. (kPa)	12.51	6.64	11.76	6.02	13.00	7.24	21.18	8.07

MLP = maximum lip pressure; press. = pressure; SD = standard deviation.

Physiological assessment of tongue function identified a significantly reduced rate of tongue movement in the fast tongue repetition task in the TBI group, when compared to the control group. This finding supports the perceptual finding of a reduced general rate of speech in the TBI group. However, it is surprising that other elements of impaired tongue function were not identified on the instrumental assessment, given that significant impairment was noted in all areas of tongue function on the FDA. The most obvious reason for this discrepancy is that the FDA evaluates quite different measures of tongue function than the instrumental assessment of tongue function. The tongue pressure transduction system assesses static measures of tongue strength, endurance, fine force control, and rate of repetitive movements, while the FDA rates range and coordination of tongue movements. Stierwalt and colleagues (1996), in their study of children and adolescents with TBI, also found that the TBI group did not differ from the control group in terms of maximal tongue strength. They did, however, identify significant correlations between the nonspeech measures of tongue performance and the perceptual judgments of overall speech defectiveness and articulatory imprecision in their TBI subjects. This discrepancy in results highlights the need for more dynamic assessment of tongue function during speech, using procedures such as electropalatography and electromagnetic articulography.

Case Discussions

The comprehensive evaluation of the perceptual and physiological features of the speech of a group of children following TBI, which was discussed previously, identified a number of speech motor subsystem impairments in the TBI subjects with dysarthria. While this group information is valuable, it fails to illustrate the variability and the specific nature of the speech disturbances demonstrated by individual subjects. An extensive variation in the type and severity of speech impairment present in individual children was noted by the authors. This finding was not surprising given that the diffuse nature of the brain damage that may result from TBI leads to extreme variability in injury and the type of dysarthria, depending on the site(s) of lesion. Several studies of adults following TBI have noted an array of deficits in the neuromuscular control of the speech mechanism (Marquardt, Stoll, & Sussman, 1990; Theodoros, Murdoch, & Chenery, 1994; Theodoros, Murdoch, & Stokes, 1995; Ylvisaker, 1992). To demonstrate the variation in the nature and extent of the physiological and perceptual speech impairments that can occur in children following TBI, three cases will be discussed. The childrens' speech was comprehensively evaluated using both perceptual and physiological measures described earlier in this chapter. For each case, data from the assessment of respiratory, velopharyngeal, and articulatory systems were compared with that of the non-neurologically-impaired control group previously described ($n = 18$; mean age $= 12.57$ years; $SD = 3.33$; range $= 5$–17 years). Due to the large variation in age of the subjects, data for laryngeal function recorded from each child was compared to that of a matched control subject.

Case 1 - Neville

Neville is an 18-year-old male who sustained a severe TBI at the age of 9 years 10 months when his bicycle was hit by a motor vehicle. CT scan data indicated a fracture in the right frontoparietal region, some blood in the third ventricle and ethmoid sinuses, and mild cerebral edema on the right side with compression of the right antennae horn of the ventricle. Neville was mute for a period of at least 6 months postinjury. Results of the perceptual and instrumental assessments revealed that Neville displayed varying degrees of dysfunction at all levels of the speech production apparatus (respiratory, laryngeal, velopharyngeal, and articulatory subsystems). He was rated as having a moderate flaccid dysarthria. See Table 7-5 for a summary of the results of his perceptual and physiological assessments.

Table 7-5. Case 1 - results of perceptual and physiological assessments.

Case 1: 18-year-old male assessed 8.5 years post-MVA (hit from bike). GCS = 3. CT scan data indicated damage in the right parietal region and mild cerebral edema. He was rated as having a moderate flaccid dysarthria.

Speech Subsystem	Perceptual Assessment	Physiological Assessment
Respiratory	FDA - Very mild impairment at rest SSA - Mod.↓ breath support for speech - Mild intermittent breathiness	↓ vital capacity ↓ forced expiratory volume

Laryngeal	FDA - Mod/severe impairment
	SSA - Mild ↓ in pitch variation
	  - Mild ↓ in loudness level
	  - Mild intermittent breathiness
		↓ peak air pressure
		↓ phonatory resistance
		↓ adduction/abduction rate

Velopharyngeal	FDA - Mod.↓ in palatal function SSA - Severe hypernasality	Moderate ↑ nasality in non-nasal utterances

(continues)

Table 7-5. (continued)

Speech Subsystem	Perceptual Assessment	Physiological Assessment
Articulatory		
Lip	FDA - Mod/severe impairment SSA - Mod. consonant impreciseness	↓ maximum lip strength ↓ rate of repetitive lip movements ↓ lip endurance
Tongue	FDA - Mod/severe impairment SSA - Mod. consonant impreciseness - Mod. ↓ in general rate	↓ maximum tongue strength ↓ rate of repetitive movements ↓ tongue endurance ↓ fine force control

Intelligibility	ASSIDS - Sentence intelligibility 45% of normal
	   - ↓ rate of speech
	SSA - Moderate ↓ in speech intelligibility
	   - Moderate ↓ in general rate of speech	

FDA = Frenchay Dysarthria Assessment; SSA = speech sample analysis; ASSIDS = Assessment of Intelligibility of Dysarthric Speech; ↑↓ = greater than 1 standard deviation above or below the control group mean. (Laryngeal values are compared to a single matched control subject.)

Respiratory Function

Spirometric assessment of Neville's respiratory function revealed that both the vital capacity (VC = 45%) and forced expiratory volume (FEV_1 = 47%), when compared to their predicted values, were markedly reduced. Kinematic assessment indicated increased lung volume initiation (↑ 3.24 SD), lung volume termination (↑ 1.75 SD) and lung volume excursion (↑ 2.67 SD) during reading, when compared to the control group. This pattern of speech breathing indicated that Neville was using the higher end of lung volume during this task, which was inconsistent with a normal pattern.

Laryngeal Function

Perceptual assessment of Neville's laryngeal subsystem on the FDA indicated moderate-to-severe impairment of laryngeal characteristics. Electroglottographic measures (fundamental frequency, closing time, and duty cycle) were found to be comparable to a matched control subject. However, aerodynamic measures (Aerophone II) of laryngeal function revealed decreased phonatory resistance and adduction/abduction rate, when compared to a control subject matched for age and sex. These factors are consistent with hypofunctioning of the laryngeal valving mechanism, and with the diagnosis of flaccid dysarthria.

The discrepancies in the perceptual and physiological assessment results highlight the need to identify the underlying physiological impairment and not rely solely on the perceptual analysis of speech, especially when planning therapy. Theodoros and Murdoch (1994) stated that an understanding of the physiological nature of the laryngeal subsystem is very important, since this component of the speech mechanism not only provides the acoustic medium through which speech is delivered, but also contributes to the suprasegmental and articulatory features of speech.

Velopharyngeal Function

Accelerometric assessment of Neville's speech indicated an increased degree of nasality in the production of non-nasal utterances (↑ 2.07 SD), which confirmed the perceptual rating of moderate hypernasality. An inadequate velopharyngeal mechanism can place increased burdens on the respiratory system, which, in turn, may lead to shortened phrases and phonatory abnormalities involving pitch and loudness as well as articulatory disturbances (Johns & Salyer, 1978).

Articulatory Function

The perceptual analysis of Neville's speech sample (SSA) identified moderate impairment of articulation and prosody in the form of imprecision of consonants, decreased overall speech intelligibility, and a slowed rate of speech. Results of the FDA, in which moderate-to-severe impairment of the lips and tongue were observed, and a reduced sentence intelligibility score (45%) on the ASSIDS, support the perceptual finding of articulatory imprecision.

Lip and tongue pressure transducer analyses demonstrated impaired labial and lingual function, when compared to the control group. Significant impairments were noted in the areas of lip strength (↓ 1.82 SD) and sustained maximal lip pressure (↓ 1.83 SD) and in the repetitive movement tasks, where both the rate (↓1.38) and pressure (↓ 1.76) were reduced, when compared to the control group. Tongue function was also significantly impaired, most noticeably in the areas of tongue strength (↓ 3.04 SD), endurance (↓ 2.38 SD), repetition of maximum tongue pressure (↓ 2.91 SD), and rate in the fast repetition task (↓ 2.91 SD). On the basis of these assessments, it was noted that tongue function appeared to be more severely affected than lip function. This finding may account for the perception of articulatory imprecision, as well as a reduction in the general rate of speech and in the perception of prolonged intervals during speech production.

Summary and Implications for Treatment

Neville presented with a moderate flaccid dysarthria characterized by a decreased rate of speech, moderate hypernasality, moderate imprecision of consonants, and moderately decreased speech intelligibility. Physiological assessment revealed impairments across all speech subsystems. Based on both the perceptual and instrumental assessments, treatment would concentrate on the following areas:

1. *Articulatory function*
   Increase tongue strength and endurance
   Increase lip strength and endurance
   Increase rate and maintenance of pressure on repetitive lip and tongue tasks
2. *Velopharyngeal function*
   Decrease nasality in speech/increase oral resonance
3. *Laryngeal function*
   Increase phonatory effort to improve vocal fold adduction

4. *Respiratory function*

Increase vital capacity to improve breath support for speech

Neville would benefit from a multisystem approach to therapy, working on respiratory, laryngeal, and velopharyngeal function to facilitate adequate breath and voice to support articulation. Since the velopharyngeal system plays an important role in the maintenance of intraoral pressure for the production of plosive and fricative sounds, therapy should also be focused on increasing velopharyngeal valving. Treatment aimed at increasing laryngeal valving could also incorporate exercises aimed at increasing respiratory support, vocal fold adduction, and volume, pitch, and loudness variation. Both traditional and biofeedback techniques could be used to remediate lip and tongue deficits.

Case 2 - Troy

Troy sustained a severe TBI at age 10 years 7 months, after the bicycle he was riding was struck by a motor vehicle. He was assessed in our research clinic at age 11 years 2 months, 7 months postinjury. CT scan data revealed a fracture in the right parietal region. Perceptual and instrumental assessment of Troy's speech revealed minimal deficits. Troy was not considered to demonstrate any perceptible dysarthria. Table 7-6 summarizes the results of his perceptual and physiological assessments.

Table 7-6. Case 2 -results of perceptual and physiological assessments.

Case 2: 11-year-old male assessed 7 months post-MVA (hit from bike). GCS = 3. CT scan data indicated a right parietal fracture. He was rated as nondysarthric.

Speech Subsystem	Perceptual Assessment	Physiological Assessment
Respiratory	FDA - No impairment noted SSA - No features noted	↓ vital capacity ↓ forced expiratory volume ↓ syllables/breath
Laryngeal	FDA - No impairment noted SSA - No features noted	↑ phonatory flow rate ↓ phonatory resistance ↓ adduction/abduction rate
Velopharyngeal	FDA - Mild hyponasality noted SSA - Mild hyponasality noted	↑ nasality in non-nasal sounds & sentences
Articulatory Lip	FDA - Very mild ↓ in coordination SSA - No features noted	↓ lip pressure in fast repetition tasks
Tongue	FDA - Very mild ↓ in coordination SSA - No features noted	↓ maximum tongue strength ↓ tongue pressure in fast repetition tasks
Intelligibility	ASSIDS - Mild decrease in rate of speech SSA - No features noted	

FDA = Frenchay Dysarthria Assessment; SSA = speech sample analysis; ASSIDS = Assessment of Intelligibility of Dysarthric Speech; ↑↓ = greater than 1 standard deviation above or below the control group mean. (Laryngeal values are compared to a single matched control subject.)

Respiratory Function

Perceptual assessment of Troy's speech (FDA, SSA) identified no areas of impairment in respiratory function. Spirometric assessment, however, identified reduced vital capacity (VC = 67%) and forced expiratory volumes (FEV_1 = 45%), when compared with their predicted values. Kinematic assessment indicated that LVI and LVT during reading were reduced when compared to the control group, and that Troy produced a reduced number of syllables per breath during reading, which supports the notion that respiratory support for speech was not totally adequate.

Laryngeal Function

Aerodynamic assessment (Aerophone II) identified an increased phonatory flow rate, decreased phonatory resistance, and a decreased adduction/abduction rate, when compared to a matched control subject, consistent with mild hypofunctioning of the laryngeal valve. However, all measures taken from the electroglottographic assessment were found to be comparable to the control subject matched for age and sex. Perceptual analysis of Troy's speech found no evidence of laryngeal dysfunction.

Velopharyngeal Function

Perceptual assessment of Troy's speech identified mild hyponasality, which was in direct contrast to the findings of the accelerometric assessment, which identified moderately increased nasality in non-nasal utterances (↑ 2.86 SD).

Articulatory Function

Perceptual assessment on the FDA identified mild incoordination of the lips and tongue. No deviant features relating to articulatory function were noted on the SSA. Physiological assessment of lip and tongue function, using pressure transduction systems, identified mild subclinical deficits in articulatory function, especially apparent in tasks requiring rapid repetitive movements of the tongue. These results support the perceptual finding of mild incoordination of lip and tongue movements noted on the FDA.

Summary and Implications for Treatment

Perceptually Troy presented as nondysarthric, with only a mild degree of hyponasality noted in his speech. However, mild subclinical deficits in some speech subsystems were noted on instrumental assessment. The nature and degree of these deficits, however, would not be sufficient to recommend any intervention. The absence of dysarthria in this child is interesting, given that he sustained an injury of similar type and severity to Case 1. This disparity highlights the differential nature of speech outcome that can occur following TBI in childhood.

Case 3 - Connor

Connor presented to our research clinic for assessment at the age of 15 years. He had sustained a severe TBI 6 years earlier, when his bicycle was hit by a motor vehicle. CT scan data revealed diffuse axonal injury. Connor was reportedly mute for several weeks postinjury. Perceptual and instrumental assessment of Connor's speech revealed mild-to-moderate impairment in articulatory, laryngeal and velopharyngeal function, but essentially normal respiratory function. His speech was characterized by prosodic disturbances such as reduced pitch variation, decreased general rate of speech, and excess stress for context, resulting in an overall rating of mild-to-moderate ataxic dysarthria. See Table 7-7 for a summary of the results of his perceptual and physiological assessments.

Respiratory Function

Spirometric assessment of respiratory function revealed that Connor's vital capacity and forced expiratory volumes were within normal limits. Kinematic assessment indicated essentially normal respiration patterns when compared to the control group, with the exception of a reduced LVI during reading. These results confirm the perceptual rating on the FDA and SSA of normal respiratory function. The exception to this was the finding of a reduced number of syllables per breath. However, it is possible that the reduced syllables per breath were a result of Connor's slowed rate of speech rather than impaired respiratory function per se.

Table 7-7. Case 3 - results of perceptual and physiological assessments.

Case 3: 15-year-old male assessed 6 years post-MVA (hit from bike). GCS = 3. CT scan revealed evidence of diffuse axonal injury. He was rated as having a mild-to-moderate ataxic dysarthria.

Speech Subsystem	Perceptual Assessment	Physiological Assessment
Respiratory	FDA - No impairment noted SSA - No features noted	↓ syllables/breath
Laryngeal	FDA - Mod. impairment noted SSA - Mild ↓ in pitch variation	↓ peak air pressure ↓ phonatory resistance ↑ closing time
Velopharyngeal	FDA - Mild impairment noted SSA - Mild hypernasality noted	Mod. ↑ nasality in non-nasal utterances
Articulatory Lip	FDA - Mild impairment in lip function SSA - No features noted	↓ maximum lip strength ↓ pressure in fast repetition tasks ↓ fine force control of lips
Tongue	FDA - Mild/mod.↓ in tongue function SSA - Mild ↓ in general rate of speech	↑ maximum tongue pressure ↓ rate in fast repetition task
Intelligibility	ASSIDS - ↓ sentence intelligibility - ↓ rate of speech SSA - Intelligibility rated as within normal range	

Prosody	SSA - Mild decrease in general rate of speech
	  - Mild decrease in pitch variation
	  - Moderate excess of stress for context	

FDA = Frenchay Dysarthria Assessment; SSA = speech sample analysis; ASSIDS = Assessment of Intelligibility of Dysarthric Speech; ↑↓ = greater than 1 standard deviation above or below the control group mean. (Laryngeal values are compared to a single matched control subject.)

Laryngeal Function

Although perceptual analysis on the FDA identified moderate impairment in pitch, volume, and vocal quality, the only feature rated as deviant on the SSA was mildly impaired variation of pitch. Aerodynamic assessment (Aerophone II) of laryngeal function identified decreased peak air pressure and decreased phonatory resistance, while electroglottographic assessment (Laryngograph) revealed an increased closing time, when compared to a matched control subject. In general, these features are consistent with hypofunctioning of the laryngeal valve.

Velopharyngeal Function

Instrumental assessment of Connor's velopharyngeal function, when compared to the control group, revealed a moderate-to-severe degree of hypernasality on production of non-nasal utterances ($\uparrow$ 3.64 SD). This finding conflicts with the perceptual rating on both the FDA and SSA, which indicated only mildly increased nasality. This inconsistency highlights the need to confirm perceptual judgements with physiological information before commencing therapy. A finding of only mildly increased nasality may not warrant specific intervention, and the deficit may remain untreated. Hypernasality typically results from paralysis, paresis, or incoordination of the muscles involved in velopharyngeal closure (Johns & Salyer, 1978). However, it has also been suggested by Hoodin and Gilbert (1989) that a decreased rate of speech may affect velopharyngeal closure. In their study of subjects with Parkinson's disease, Hoodin and Gilbert (1989) found that these subjects demonstrated a break in the velopharyngeal seal at slower speaking rates. Therefore, it is conceivable that the increased nasality identified instrumentally in Connor's speech could be due to poor functioning of the velopharyngeal valve, or possibly could be a side effect of his reduced rate of speech.

Articulatory Function

Perceptual assessment of articulatory function using the FDA identified mild impairment in lip function and mild-to-moderate impairment in tongue function. A mild decrease in the general rate of speech was identified perceptually on the SSA, and a decreased number of words per minute (77 WPM, $\downarrow$ 3.13 SD) was identified on the ASSIDS. Physiological assessment of tongue function identified an increased maximum tongue pressure ($\uparrow$ 1.35 SD), but a reduction in the rate of rapid repetitive tongue movements ($\downarrow$ 1.29 SD), when compared to the control group. This finding of reduced rate of tongue movements would contribute directly to the perceptual finding of a reduction in the general rate of speech.

Instrumental assessment of lip function revealed decreased maximum lip strength ($\downarrow$ 1.30 SD) and decreased pressure in repetition of maximum lip pressure, when compared to the control group. It is surprising that, despite these impairments in lip function, Connor was perceived as having normal consonant precision. It has been suggested (Robin, Goel, Somodi, & Luschei, 1992) that there is a "critical level" of strength reduction (i.e., the degree of strength reduction that is sufficient to affect speech production). Although there was a considerable reduction in lip strength, the weakness appears not to be within the critical range that affects the accuracy of consonant production.

Prosodic Aspects of Speech

The most salient aspect of Connor's speech was a decreased general rate of speech, with reduced pitch variation and excess stress for context. With the absence of impairments in the area of breath support for speech, Connor's decreased rate of speech would most likely be explained by the reduced rate of tongue movements identified in repetitive tasks. The decreased pitch variation may be related to the presence of hypofunctioning of the laryngeal valve, which results in reduced laryngeal tone and a subsequent reduction in pitch range (because of the impaired ability of vocal folds to increase tone). It is also likely that Connor's slowed rate of speech contributes to the perception of decreased pitch variation and excess stress for context.

Summary and Implications for Treatment

Connor presented perceptually with a mild-to-moderate ataxic dysarthria, characterized by a slowed rate of speech, decreased pitch variation, excess stress for context, and mild-to-moderate hypernasality. Instrumental assessment of the speech mechanism identified mild-to-moderate impairment in all subsystems except respiration, when compared to the control group. Based on these findings, the following treatment regimen would be suggested to address the underlying pathophysiology of the dysarthric speech pattern exhibited by this subject.

1. *Prosody*

   Increase speech rate

2. *Velopharyngeal function*

   Decrease nasality in speech/increase oral resonance

3. *Articulatory function*

   Increase rate and maintenance of pressure on repetitive lip and tongue tasks

4. *Laryngeal function*

   Increase phonatory effort to improve vocal fold adduction

Since velopharyngeal functioning appears to be the most severely impaired aspect of speech production, based on instrumental assessment, treatment should initially commence in this area. However, therapy aimed at increasing articulatory function, especially rapid repetitive movements of the tongue, would be beneficial in increasing Connor's rate of speech, and hence improve prosody. Treatment aimed at increasing laryngeal valving may also benefit Connor by increasing air pressure essential for the production of bilabial sounds.

The differential nature of speech outcome following TBI in childhood was highlighted by these three cases. Despite the similar age at injury, and the comparable type and severity of injury, each case presented with a different profile of speech subsystem impairment. The diffuse, nonspecific nature of TBI means that damage may occur to many areas of the central nervous system, resulting in impairment in one or more of the motor speech subsystems. Using a combination of perceptual and instrumental investigations allows for a more accurate determination of the underlying pathophysiology of the speech disorder and, hence, enables more effective planning for therapy programs.

Summary

Until recently, there has been a dearth of physiological studies of the speech mechanism in children following TBI, despite the frequent occurrence of TBI in childhood and potential negative effects of this condition on the quality of life of these children. In the absence of information regarding the physiological nature of the speech impairment in children following TBI, data from the adult population has been used in the assessment and treatment of these children. This chapter has outlined the characteristic features of dysarthria in childhood TBI, and reported on the results of a recent study in our research clinic, in which 22 subjects with TBI acquired in childhood were assessed on the recommended perceptual and physiological battery of speech assessments.

Extreme variability in injury and type of dysarthria has been reported in the adult literature, due to the diffuse nature of the brain damage that can result from TBI. Marked variability in speech outcome was also evident in this study of children who had suffered a TBI. To demonstrate the differential speech outcome that may result following childhood TBI, three case studies were reported. These case discussions highlighted the need for a full perceptual and physiological assessment of the speech apparatus of children with dysarthria following TBI, to increase the accuracy of the clinical speech diagnosis, and to provide appropriate individually tailored treatment programs.

References

Abbs, J. & DePaul, R. (1989). Assessment of dysarthria: The critical prerequisite to treatment. In M.M. Leahy (Ed.) *Disorders of Communication: The Science of Intervention*, (pp. 206–227). London: Taylor and Francis.

Annegers, J.F. (1983). The epidemiology of head trauma in children. In K. Shapiro (Ed.), *Pediatric Head Trauma* (pp. 1–10). New York: Frutura Publishing Company.

Bak, E., van Dongen, H.R. & Arts, W.F.M. (1983) The analysis of acquired dysarthria in children. *Developmental Medicine and Child Neurology, 25*, 81–94.

Becker, D.P., Miller, J.D., Ward, J.D., Greenberg, R.P., Young, H.F., & Sakalas, R. (1977). The outcome from severe head injury with intensive management. *Journal of Neurosurgery, 47*, 491–502.

Bigler, E.D., Clark, E., & Farmer, J. (1996). Traumatic brain injury: 1990s update - Introduction to the special series. *Journal of Learning Disabilities, 29(5)*, 512–513.

Bogan, J., Hartley, P., & Ryan, L. (1991). *The Student with a Brain Injury: Reintegration, Assessment and Strategies for Mainstream Teachers*. Sydney: Department of School Education, Metropolitan West Region.

Boyer, M.G. & Edwards, P. (1991). Outcome 1 to 3 years after severe traumatic brain injury in children and adolescents. *Injury: The British Journal of Accident Surgery, 22(4)*, 315–320.

Brooks, N., McKinlay, W., Symington, C., Beattie, A., & Campsie, L. (1987). Return to work within the first seven years of severe head injury. *Brain Injury, 1*, 5–19.

Bruce, D.A. (1995). Pathophysiological responses of the child's brain following trauma. In S.H. Broman & M.E. Michel (Eds.) *Traumatic Head Injury in Children*. New York: Oxford University Press.

Bruce, D.A., Raphaely, R.C., Goldberg, A.I., Zimmerman, R.A., Bilaniuk, L.T. & Schut, L. (1979). Pathophysiology, treatment and outcome following severe head injury in children. *Child's Brain, 5*, 174–191.

Carlsson, C.A., Von Essen, A., & Lofgren, J. (1968). Factors affecting the clinical course of patients with severe head injury. *Journal of Neurosurgery, 29*, 242–251.

Cattelani, R., Lombardi, F., Brianti, R., & Mazzucchi, A. (1998). Traumatic brain injury in childhood: intellectual, behavioral and social outcome into adulthood. *Brain Injury, 12(4)*, 283–296.

Costeff, H., Groswasser, Z., & Goldstein, R. (1990). Long-term follow-up review of 31 children with severe closed head trauma. *Journal of Neurosurgery, 73*, 684–687.

Costeff, H., Groswasser, Z., Landman, Y., & Brenner, T. (1985). Survivors of severe traumatic brain injury in childhood. Late residual disability. *Scandinavian Journal of Rehabilitation Medicine, Supplement 12*, 10–15.

Craft, A.W., Shaw, D.A., & Cartlidge, N.E.F. (1972). Head injuries in children. *British Medical Journal, 4*, 200–203.

Darley, F.L., Aronson, A.E., & Brown, J.R. (1975). *Speech Motor Disorders*. Philadelphia: W.B. Saunders.

Di Scala, C., Osberg, S., Gans, B.M., Chin, L., & Grant, C. (1991). Children with traumatic brain injury: Morbidity and postacute treatment. *Archives of Physical Medicine and Rehabilitation, 72(August)*, 662–666.

Emanuelson, I. & von Wendt, L. (1997). Epidemiology of traumatic brain injury in children and adolescents in south-western Sweden. *Acta Paedratrica, 86*, 730–5.

Emanuelson, I., von Wendt, L., Lundälv, E., & Larsson, J. (1996). Rehabilitation and follow-up of children with severe traumatic brain injury. *Child's Nervous System, 12*, 460–465.

Enderby, P.M. (1983) *Frenchay Dysarthria Assessment*. San Diego: College-Hill Press.

Field, J.H. (1976). *Epidemiology of Head Injury in England and Wales: With Particular Application to Rehabilitation*. Leicester, UK: Willsons.

Fisher, H.B. & Logemann, J.A. (1971). *The Fisher-Logemann Test of Articulation Competence*. Boston, MA: Houghton Mifflin Co.

FitzGerald, F.J., Murdoch, B.E. & Chenery, H.J. (1987). Multiple sclerosis: Associated speech and language disorders. *Australian Journal of Human Communication Disorders, 15*, 15–33.

Frankowski, R.F., Annegers, J.F., & Whitman, S. (1985). *Epidemiological and Descriptive Studies Part 1: The Descriptive Epidemiology of Head Trauma in the United States*. Bethesda, MD: National Institute of Neurological and Communicative Disorders and Stroke, National Institutes of Health.

Goldstein, F.C. & Levin, H.S. (1987). Epidemiology of pediatric closed head injury: Incidence, clinical characteristics, and risk factors. *Journal of Learning Disabilities, 20*, 518–524.

Gurdjian, E.S. & Webster, J.E. (1958). *Head Injuries: Mechanisms, Diagnosis and Management*. Boston: Little Brown & Co.

Guyer, B. & Ellers, B. (1990). Childhood injuries in the United States. *American Journal of Diseases of Children, 144*, 649–652.

Hardcastle, W.J., Morgan-Barry, R.A. & Clark, C.J. (1985). Articulatory and voicing characteristics of adult dysarthric and verbal dyspraxic speakers: An instrumental study. *British Journal of Disorders of Communication, 20*, 249–270.

Hartman, E. & von Cramon, D. (1984). Acoustic measurement of voice quality in central dysphonia. *Journal of Communication Disorders, 17*, 425–440.

Hécaen, H. (1976). Acquired aphasia in children and the otogenesis of hemispheric functional specialization. *Brain and Language, 3*, 114–134.

Hillenbrand, J., Cleveland, R.A. & Erickson, R.L. (1994). Acoustic correlates of breathy voice quality. *Journal of Speech and Hearing Research, 37*, 769–778.

Hinton, V.A. & Luschei, E.S. (1992). Validation of a modern miniature transducer for measurement of interlabial contact pressure during speech. *Journal of Speech and Hearing Research, 35*, 245–251.

Hollien, H. & Malcik, E. (1967). Evaluation of cross-sectional studies of adolescent voice changes in males. *Speech Monographs, 34*, 80–84.

Hoodin, R.B. & Gilbert, H.R. (1989). Nasal airflows in Parkinsonian speakers. *Journal of Communication Disorders, 22*, 169–180.

Horii, Y. (1980). An accelerometric approach to nasality measurement: A preliminary report. *Cleft Palate Journal, 17*, 254–261.

Jamison, D.L & Kaye, H.H. (1974). Accidental head injury in children. *Archives of Disease of Childhood, 49*, 376–381.

Johns, D.F. & Salyer, K.E. (1978). Surgical and prosthetic management of neurogenic speech disorders. In: D. Johns (Ed.). *Clinical Management of Neurogenic Communication Disorders*, (pp 311–331), Boston, MA: Little-Brown.

Kalsbeek, W., McLaurin, R., Harris, B., & Miller, J. (1980). The national head and spinal cord survey: Major findings. *Journal of Neurosurgery, 53*, 519–531.

Keller, E., Vigneux, P., & Laframboise, M. (1991). Acoustic analysis of neurologically impaired speech. *British Journal of Disorders of Communication, 26*, 75–94.

Kent, J.F., Kent, R.D., Rosenbeck, J.C., Weismer, G., Martin, R., Sufit, R. & Brooks, B.R. (1992). Quantitative description of the dysarthria in women with amyotrophic lateral sclerosis. *Journal of Speech and Hearing Research, 35*, 723–733.

Klauber, M.R., Barrett-Connor, E., Hofsetter, C.R., & Micik, S.H. (1986). A population-based study of non-fatal childhood injuries. *Preventive Medicine, 15*, 139–149.

Klonoff, H. & Paris, R. (1974). Immediate, short-term, and residual effects of acute head injuries in children. In R.M. Reitan & L.A. Davison (Eds.), *Clinical Neuropsychology: Current Status and Applications* (pp. 179–210). New York: John Wiley.

Kraus, J.F. (1995). Epidemiological features of brain injury in children: Occurrence, children at risk, causes and manner of injury, severity, and outcomes. In S.H. Broman & M.E. Michel (Eds.), *Traumatic Head Injury in Children.* (pp. 22–39). New York: Oxford University Press.

Kraus, J.F., Fife, D., Cox, P., Ramstein, K., & Conroy, C. (1986). Incidence, severity, and causes of pediatric brain injury. *American Journal of Diseases in Children, 140*, 687–693.

Kraus, J.F., Rock, A., & Hemyari, P. (1990). Brain injuries among infants, children, adolescents, and young adults. *American Journal of Diseases in Children, 144*, 684–691.

Levin, H.S., Benton, A.L. & Grossman, R.G. (1982). *Neurobehavioral Consequences of Closed Head Injury*. New York: Oxford University Press.

Levin, H.S., Eisenberg, H.M., Wigg, N.R., & Kobayashi, K. (1982). Memory and intellectuaal ability after head injury in children and adolescents. *Neurosurgery, 11(5)*, 668–673.

Lieh-Lai, M.W., Theodorou, A.A., Sarnaik, A.P., Meert, K.L., Moylan, P.M., & Canady, A.I. (1992). Limitations of the Glasgow Coma Scale in predicting outcome in children with traumatic brain injury. *Journal of Pediatrics, 120*, 195–199.

Mahoney, W.J., D' Souza, B.J., Haller, J.A., Rogers, M.C., Epstein, M.H., & Freeman, J.M. (1983). Long-term outcome of children with severe head trauma and prolonged coma. *Paediatrics, 71*, 756–762.

Malkmus, D.D. (1989). Community re-entry: Cognitive-communication intervention within a social skill context. *Topics in Language Disorders, 9*, 50–66.

Marquardt, T.P., Stoll, J., & Sussman, H. (1990). Disorders of communication in traumatic brain injury. In E.D. Bigler (Ed.), *Traumatic Brain Injury: Mechanisms of Damage, Assessment, Intervention and Outcome* (pp. 181–205). Austin, TX: Pro-Ed.

Menkes, J.H. & Till, K. (1995). Postnatal trauma and injuries by physical agents. In J.H. Menkes (Ed.)., *Textbook of Child Neurology* (pp. 557–597). Baltimore: Williams and Wilkins.

Michel, J.F., Hollien, H., & Moore, P. (1966). Speaking fundamental frequency characteristics of 15, 16 and 17 year-old girls. *Language and Speech, 9*, 46–51.

Mira, M.P., Tucker, B.F., & Tyler, J.S. (1992). *Traumatic Brain Injury in Children and Adolescents: A Sourcebook for Teachers and Other School Personnel*. Austin, Texas: Pro-Ed.

Morris, R.J. (1989). VOT and dysarthria: A descriptive study. *Journal of Communication Disorders, 22*, 23–33.

Moyes, C.D. (1980). Epidemiology of serious head injuries in childhood. *Child, Care, Health and Development, 6*, 1–9.

Murdoch, B.E., Attard, M.D., Ozanne, A.E., & Stokes, P.D. (1995). Impaired tongue strength and endurance in developmental verbal dyspraxia: A physiological analysis. *European Journal of Disorders of Communication, 30*, 51–64.

Murdoch, B.E., Horton, S.K., Theodoros, D.G., & Thompson, E.C. (1997). Cinical application of speech science instrumentation in the determination of treatment priorities in acquired and congenital childhood dysarthria. In W. Hulstijn, H.F.M. Peters, & P.H.H.M. Van Lieshout (Eds.), *Speech Production: Motor Control, Brain Research and Fluency Disorders* (pp. 621–630). New York: Elsevier Science.

Murdoch, B.E. & Hudson-Tennent, L.J. (1993). Speech breathing anomalies in children with dysarthria following treatment for posterior fossa tumors. *Journal of Medical Speech-Language Pathology, 1(2)*, 107–119.

Murdoch, B.E. & Hudson-Tennent, L.J. (1994). Speech disorders in children treated for posterior fossa tumors: Ataxic and developmental features. *European Journal of Disorders of Communication, 29*, 379–397.

Najenson, T., Sazbon, L., Fiselzon, J., Becker, E., & Schechter, I. (1978). Recovery of communicative functions after prolonged traumatic coma. *Scandinavian Journal of Rehabilitative Medicine, 10*, 15–21.

Naugle, R.I. (1990). Epidemiology of traumatic brain injury in adults. In E.B. Bigler (Ed.), *Traumatic Brain Injury* (pp. 69–103). Austin, Texas: Pro-Ed.

Oddy, M. (1984). Head injury and social adjustment. In N. Brooks (Ed.) *Closed Head Injury: Psychological, Social and Family Consequences.* New York: Oxford University Press.

Orlikoff, R.F. (1992). The use of instrumental measures in the assessment and treatment of motor speech disorders. *Seminars in Speech and Language, 13*, 25–37.

Peterson, H.A. & Marquardt, T.P. (1981). *Appraisal and Diagnosis of Speech and Language Disorders*, Englewood Cliffs, NJ: Prentice Hall.

Rimel, R.W. & Jane, J.A. (1983). Characteristics of the head-injured patient. In M.R. Rosenthal, M.R. Bond, J.D. Miller, & E.R. Griffith (Eds.), *Rehabilitation of the Head Injured Adult* (pp. 9–12). Philadelphia: Davis.

Rivara, J.B., Jaffe, K.M., Polissar, N.L., Fay, N.L., Martin, G.C., Shurtleff, H.A., & Liao, S. (1994). Family functioning and children's academic performance and behavior problems in the year following traumatic brain injury. *Archives of Physical Medicine and Rehabilitation, 75*, 269–279.

Robin, D.A., Goel, A., Somodi, C.B. & Luschei, E.S. (1992). Tongue strength and endurance: relation to highly skilled movements. *Journal of Speech and Hearing Research, 35*, 1239–1245.

Robin, D.A., Somodi, C.B., & Luschei, E.S. (1991). Measurement of tongue strength and endurance in normal and articulation disordered subjects. In C.A. Moore, K.M. Yorkston, & D.R. Beukelman (Eds.), *Dysarthria and Apraxia of Speech: Perspectives on Management.* Baltimore, MD: Paul H. Brooks.

Rusk, H., Block, J., & Lowmann, E. (1969). Rehabilitation of the brain-injured patient: A report of 157 cases with long-term follow-up of 118. In E. Walker, W. Caveness, & M. Critchley (Eds.), *The Late Effects of Head Injury* (pp. 327–332). Springfield: Charles C. Thomas.

Sakzewski, L., Ziviani, J., & Swanson, C. (1996). Impact of early discharge planning and case management on length of hospital stay for children with acquired brain injury. *Australian Occupational Therapy Journal, 45*, 105–112.

Sosin, D.M., Sniezek, J.E., & Thurman, D.J. (1996). Incidence of mild and moderate brain injury in the United States, 1991. *Brain Injury, 10(1)*, 47–54.

Stark, R.E. (1985). Dysarthria in children. In J.K. Darby (Ed.), *Speech and Language Evaluation in Neurology: Childhood Disorders.* (pp. 185–217). Orlando, FL: Grune and Stratton Inc.

Sterling, L. (1994). *Students with Acquired Brain Injuries in Primary and Secondary Schools.* Canberra, Australia: Government Printing Service.

Stierwalt, J.A., Robin, D.A., Solomon, N.P., Weiss, A.L., & Max, J.E. (1996). Tongue strength and endurance. Relation to the speaking ability of children and adolescents following traumatic brain injury. In D.A. Robin, K.M. Yorkston, & D.R. Beukelman (Eds.), *Disorders of Motor Speech Assessment, Treatment and Clinical Characterization* (pp. 241–256). Baltimore, MD: Paul Brookes Pub. Co.

Teasdale, G. & Jennett, B. (1974). Assessment of coma and impaired consciousness: A practical scale. *Lancet, 2*, 81–84.

Theodoros, D.G. & Murdoch, B.E. (1994). Laryngeal dysfunction in dysarthric speakers following severe closed-head injury. *Brain Injury, 8*, 667–684.

Theodoros, D.G., Murdoch, B.E., & Chenery, H.J. (1994). Perceptual speech characteristics of dysarthric speakers following severe closed head injury. *Brain Injury, 8(2)*, 101–124.

Theodoros, D.G., Murdoch, B.E., & Stokes, P. (1995). Variability in the perceptual and physiological features of dysarthria following severe closed head injury: An examination of five cases. *Brain Injury, 9(7)*, 671–696.

Theodoros, D.G., Shrapnel, N., & Murdoch, B.E. (1998). Motor speech impairment following traumatic brain injury in childhood: A physiological and perceptual analysis of one case. *Pediatric Rehabilitation, 2(3)*, 107–122.

Thomsen, I.V. (1984). Late outcome of severe blunt head injury: A ten to fifteen year second follow-up. *Journal of Neurology, Neurosurgery and Psychiatry, 38*, 713–718.

Thompson-Ward, E.C. & Theodoros, D.G. (1998). Acoustic analysis of dysarthric speech. In B.E. Murdoch (Ed.), *Dysarthria: A Physiological Approach to Assessment and Treatment* (pp. 102–129). Cheltenham: Stanley Thornes.

Van Dongen, H.R., Catsman-Berrevoets, C.E., & van Mourik, M. (1994). The syndrome of cerebellar mutism and subsequent dysarthria. *Neurology, 44*, 2040–2046.

van Mourik, M., Catsman-Berrevoets, C.E., Paquier, P.F., Yosef-Bak, E., & van Dongen, H. R. (1997). Acquired childhood dysarthria: Review of its clinical presentation. *Pediatric Neurology, 17(4)*, 299–307.

Weismer, G. (1984). Acoustic descriptions of dysarthric speech: Perceptual correlates and physiological inferences. *Seminars in Speech and Language, 5*, 293–313.

Wit, J., Maassen, B., Gabreels, F.J.M. & Thoonen, G. (1993). Maximum performance tests in children with developmental spastic dysarthria. *Journal of Speech and Hearing Research, 36*, 452–459.

Wit, J., Maassen, B., Gabreels, F.J.M. & Thoonen, G., & de-Swart, B. (1994). Traumatic versus perinatally acquired dysarthria: Assessment by means of speech-like maximum performance tasks. *Developmental Medicine and Child Neurology, 36*, 221–229.

Ylvisaker, M. (1986). Language and communication disorders following pediatric head injury. *Journal of Head Trauma Rehabilitation, 1*, 48–56.

Ylvisaker, M. (1992). Communication outcome following traumatic brain injury. *Seminars in Speech and Language, 13(4)*, 239–251.

Yorkston, K.M. & Beukelman, D.R. (1981). *Assessment of Intelligibility of Dysarthric Speech*. Austin, Texas: Pro-Ed.

Ziegler, W. & von Cramon, D. (1986). Spastic dysarthria after acquired brain injury: An acoustic study. *British Journal of Disorders of Communication, 21*, 173–187.

Zimmerman, R.A., Bilaniuk, L.T., Bruce, D., Dolinskas, C., Obrist, W., & Kuhl, D. (1978). Computed tomography of pediatric head trauma: Acute general cerebral swelling. *Radiology, 126*, 403–408.

CHAPTER
Eight

Treatment of Dysarthria Following Traumatic Brain Injury

Deborah G. Theodoros and Bruce E. Murdoch

Introduction

The management of dysarthria in adults and children following traumatic brain injury (TBI) is a complex and extended process that should be considered within a broad perspective, encompassing an awareness of the individual's basic deficits, and the effects of these impairments on his/her quality of life. The rehabilitation of dysarthria following TBI involves an understanding of the physiological impairments that affect speech production, the impact of that impairment on speech intelligibility, and the degree of disability evident in the individual's attempts to communicate in a variety of social and physical settings. Furthermore, an awareness of the limitations imposed upon the TBI individual by society, with respect to access to services and opportunities, and to fulfilling personal and vocational roles is a necessary component of a comprehensive rehabilitative approach (Yorkston, 1996; Yorkston, Strand, & Kennedy, 1996). Treatment planning for the TBI dysarthric speaker should be considered on a long-term basis, with programs tailor-made to suit the needs of the individual.

Despite the complexity of the task of rehabilitating dysarthric speakers following TBI, there are numerous reports in the literature that have documented positive improvements in speech and overall communication in these individuals. The majority of these studies have involved the treatment of adult dysarthric speakers, with only a few reports of treatment of TBI children evident in the literature. Furthermore, most of the treatment strategies used for the TBI pediatric population with dysarthria have been adapted from those techniques developed for adults. As yet, insufficient research has been conducted to develop a range of treatment approaches specific to children with dysarthria following TBI.

The following sections of this chapter will outline the research findings in relation to the treatment of dysarthria following TBI, describe a framework for intervention in the TBI population, and detail an extensive range of treatment techniques and management strategies currently available to address the different components of the intervention model.

Treatment Efficacy in Dysarthria Following TBI

A number of studies detailing the treatment of dysarthric speakers following TBI have been documented in the literature. These studies have highlighted: the treatment of specific aspects of speech and/or communication; multicomponent physiological approaches to treatment; recovery of functional communication many years postinjury; the issue of timing and extent of intervention; complicating factors that impinge on rehabilitation; and the treatment of dysarthria post-TBI in the pediatric population. As noted by Yorkston (1996), group treatment studies of dysarthric speakers post TBI are low in number due to the diversity in the type and severity of dysarthria in this population, which precludes the use of one particular form of treatment for all TBI dysarthric speakers. Even less frequent are studies reporting on the effects of treatment on dysarthric speech disturbances following TBI in the pediatric population (Ylvisaker & Urbanczyk, 1990). The studies conducted to date, however, have demonstrated mostly positive outcomes for TBI dysarthric speakers in relation to speech production per se and general communicative effectiveness, with a strong trend indicating that impressive changes in speech can be achieved many years posttrauma (Yorkston, 1996). Such evidence suggests that long-term follow-up of persons with dysarthria following TBI is warranted and should be incorporated into treatment planning.

Most of the treatment-related investigations are single case studies that have targeted a particular aspect of speech production and/or communication, using a range of behavioral, physiological, acoustic, and prosthetic approaches (Bellaire, Yorkston, & Beukelman, 1986; Beukelman & Yorkston, 1977; Bougle, Ryalls, & Le Dorze, 1995; Brand, Matsko, & Avart, 1988; Draizar, 1984; Enderby & Crow, 1990; Goldstein, Ziegler, Vogel, & Hoole, 1994; Kuehn & Wachtel, 1994; Light, Beesley,

Table 8-1. Single case studies of treatment of dysarthria following TBI.

Reference	Subjects	Treatment Focus	Nature of Treatment	Outcome
Bellaire, Yorkston, & Beukelman, (1986)	1 case mild dysarthria	Breath patterning	↑ number of words per breath; ↑ frequency of pauses without inhalations	Improved speech naturalness
Beukelman & Yorkston, (1977)	1 case severe dysarthria	Rate & intelligibility	Alphabet supplementation	↓ rate & ↑ speech intelligibility
Bougle, Ryalls, & Le Dorze (1995)	2 cases mild-to-moderate ataxic dysarthria	Fundamental frequency modulation using two types of therapy	Behavioral (auditory feedback) & instrumental (visual feedback)	↑ frequency modulation; therapies equivalent
Brand, Matsko, & Avart (1988)	1 case moderate-to-severe dysarthria	Palatal lift retention	Topical anesthetic to reduce sensory feedback	Eliminated retention problem
Draizar (1984)	1 case severe dysarthria	Control of posterior tongue & velar function during swallowing & articulation	Electromyographic feedback	↑ coordination velar function & posterior tongue movement; ↓ dysphagia
Enderby & Crow (1990)	4 cases severe dysarthria	Oral/motor function	Oral motor exercises	Improvement began long-term (24–30 months) post-TBI
Goldstein, Ziegler, Vogel, & Hoole (1994)	1 case severe dysarthria	Velopharyngeal incompetence Lingual motor control	Palatal lift Electropalatography	↑ speech intelligibility
Kuehn & Wachtel (1994)	2 cases moderate dysarthria	Velopharyngeal function	Continuous positive airway pressure (CPAP) therapy	↓ hypernasality
Light, Beesley, & Collier (1988)	1 case severe dysarthria	Functional communication	Augmentative & alternative (AAC) systems	Development natural speech & ↑ communication abilities

(continues)

Table **8-1**. (*continued*)

Reference	Subjects	Treatment Focus	Nature of Treatment	Outcome
Murdoch, Pitt, Theodoros, & Ward (1999)	1 child severe dysarthria	Speech breathing	Visual biofeedback of chest wall movement	Improved speech breathing pattern
Murdoch, Sterling, & Theodoros (1995)	2 cases moderate dysarthria	Coordination of chest wall movement	Visual biofeedback of chest wall movement	↑ respiratory coordination
Nemec & Cohen (1984)	1 case severe dysarthria	Facial hypertonia & mandibular closure	Electromyographic biofeedback	Improved monitoring of muscular tension & ↑ mandibular closure
Stewart & Rieger (1994)	1 case severe dysarthria	Nasal emission	Use of nasal obturator	↓ nasal emission; Improved regulation of nasal airflow
Stringer (1996)	1 case dysarthria	Prosody	Visual biofeedback of pitch (VisiPitch)®	↑ pitch range

↑ = Increased/improved; ↓ = Decreased; TBI = traumatic brain injury.

& Collier, 1988; Murdoch, Pitt, Theodoros, & Ward, 1999; Murdoch, Sterling, Theodoros, & Stokes, 1995; Nemec and Cohen, 1984; Stewart & Rieger, 1994; Stringer, 1996). Table 8-1 outlines a number of single case treatment studies reported in the literature that have targeted mainly one aspect of speech production in a TBI dysarthric speaker, giving the type of treatment used in the study and the outcome of this intervention.

In other studies, a multicomponent physiological approach has been used to improve speech and communication, and swallowing, following TBI (Aten, 1988; Harris & Murry, 1984; McHenry, Wilson, & Minton, 1994; Netsell & Daniel, 1979; Workinger & Netsell, 1992). Netsell and Daniel (1979) reported marked improvements in the speech intelligibility of a 20-year-old TBI man with severe flaccid dysarthria following a treatment approach in which the velopharyngeal, respiratory, laryngeal, and articulatory subsystems of the speech mechanism were targeted consecutively for therapy. Since velopharyngeal function was severely impaired, the subject underwent trials of biofeedback therapy using visual feedback of velar position and degree of nasal airflow, in an attempt to gain control of velopharyngeal musculature. Since this form of treatment was found to be unsuccessful, the subject was fitted with a palatal lift prosthesis, which subsequently prevented excessive nasal air flow. Following the fitting of the palatal lift, the subject's respiratory function was treated using a U-tube manometer to increase subglottal pressure. The hypofunctioning laryngeal activity identified in this subject was targeted for treatment using visual biofeedback of glottal airflow. Following therapy, glottal airflow and perceived breathiness were reduced, while loudness was noted to increase by approximately 25%. An auditory feedback signal that was proportional to the voltage of surface electromyography (EMG) was used to increase lip strength in this subject. After only three treatment sessions, his force of lip closure increased from 10 to 30 grams. Tongue function was improved by exerting an opposing force upwards against a tongue depressor, repeatedly, three times per day. Following this form of therapy, the movement of the dorsum of the subject's tongue had improved to such an extent that he was able to produce velar sounds. At discharge, the subject's speech had improved from a 5%–10% to a 95% intelligibility level, his voice was breathy and hypernasal, and his loudness was only slightly reduced. At 3 years postdischarge, the subject had maintained his intelligibility level and was gainfully employed in a service industry.

In a similar case of a young 18-year-old female with severe flaccid dysarthria, McHenry et al. (1994) adopted a multisystem approach to treatment. This young woman demonstrated severely reduced speech intelligibility that was due to inefficient speech breathing strategies, weak vocal fold adduction, poor velopharyngeal function, and reduced posterior tongue strength. Therapy was conducted three times per week and targeted respiratory, laryngeal, velopharyngeal, and articulatory components of the speech mechanism within speech contexts. The subject was instructed and encouraged to increase physiological effort and exaggerate inspiration prior to speech to compensate for inadequate laryngeal and velopharyngeal valving. To overcome laryngeal hypofunction, the subject was instructed to increase the number of syllables per breath to reduce breathiness, and to substantially increase loudness to facilitate vocal fold adduction. Once optimal vocal quality was established, therapy focused on the development of vocal control and the maintenance of increased effort. Despite several attempts to modify and fit a palatal lift to reduce nasal airflow, this strategy was unsuccessful in this case. Therapy was refocused towards increasing vocal effort, which was noted to reduce nasal resonance and air emission. Articulation therapy was used to elicit the phonemes /k/ and /g/ in various contexts and improve posterior tongue elevation. Following 7 months of therapy, and at 3 months postdischarge, the subject had made improvements in all components of the speech production mechanism. Speech intelligibility was rated as being understood more than half the time 3 months postdischarge, compared to being rated as almost unintelligible pretreatment. Moderate improvements across all physiological systems were apparent, although no system returned to normal function. Inspiratory volumes had increased to twice pretherapy levels, while vocal intensity increased 14 dB. Laryngeal resistance was found to increase to near normal levels 3 months post-discharge, with optimal vocal quality close to normal and only minimally breathy. With the palatal lift in position, velopharyngeal resistance had increased to half that of normal values. Acoustically, nasalance values were within normal limits. Following therapy, objective measures of tongue strength revealed that the subject was able to approximate all target forces. The subject achieved the production of posterior tongue sounds and all blends with 80% accuracy in unstructured conversational speech by the end of therapy.

Improvements in speech and communication effectiveness have been demonstrated in TBI dysarthric speakers long after recovery had been expected to occur, indicating that the management of the dysarthric speech disturbance in individuals following TBI should remain long-term and proactive (Aten, 1988; Beukelman & Garrett, 1988; Enderby & Crow, 1990; Harris & Murry, 1984; Keatley & Wirz, 1994; Keenan & Barnhart, 1993; Light et al., 1988; Workinger & Netsell, 1992). These findings are exemplified in a study by Workinger and Netsell (1992), who reported the restoration of intelligible speech in a 28-year-old male head injured client, 13 years post-TBI. Assessment indicated the presence of a severe mixed dysarthria characterized by poor speech intelligibility during conversation, significantly reduced phonation time and respiratory support for speech, a strained-strangled vocal quality with limited voicing of sounds, and severe velopharyngeal incompetence and hypernasality. Lip and tongue movements during consonant and vowel productions were adequate. In this case, a multicomponent approach to intervention was adopted to address velopharyngeal incompetence, respiratory support, and poor vocal fold adduction. Following 9 months of therapy, the subject was able to communicate functionally without a communication board, and his conversational speech was considered to be 80% to 90% intelligible. Similarly, Harris and Murry (1984) reported the case of a 44-year-old man with severe flaccid dysarthria and aphagia, who, 7 years post-TBI, regained his ability to swallow and demonstrated improvements in speech intelligibility, following 9 weeks of intensive oromotor treatment.

The issues of timing and extent of intervention for dysarthric speakers following TBI have been further highlighted in severely injured individuals (Enderby & Crow, 1990; Keenan & Barnhart, 1993; Light et al., 1988). Enderby and Crow (1990), in their study of four severely dysarthric patients following TBI, raised the issue of the timing of intervention during the course of recovery. These investigators found that improvements in bulbar function in these patients were minimal in the first 18 months postinjury, despite regular therapy to address these impairments. After the cessation of treatment to improve bulbar function, two subjects were found to improve 24 months and 30 months post-TBI, respectively. All subjects demonstrated the most substantial changes in their bulbar function approximately 48 months postinjury. Enderby and Crow (1990) proposed that a better recovery may be facilitated if specific motor/articulation therapy was introduced at a more favorable time, when the speech systems were more physiologically responsive, and when this form of therapy was not competing for attention with other demands on the patient. In their study of the development of yes/no systems in 82 individuals with severe TBI, Keenan and Barnhart (1993) highlighted the importance of ongoing intervention or consultation with the TBI patient, because of the high variability in the rate of development of these communicative systems across their group of subjects, and the changing nature of recovery following TBI. Similarly, Light et al. (1988) highlighted the need for adopting an ongoing assessment-treatment model during the development of an appropriate communication system for a TBI child.

In many cases with dysarthria following TBI, the rehabilitation process is complicated by a range of nonspeech issues that may impede treatment progress. McHenry and Wilson (1994) reported on the case of a 34-year-old TBI male with a moderate-to-severe dysarthria, who also demonstrated reduced cognitive abilities, exacerbated negative premorbid personality characteristics, and psychosocial factors such as postinjury psychosis. Although this patient had achieved dramatic decreases in speech rate and an immediate improvement in intelligibility using a pacing board, he failed to continue with treatment due to his nonacceptance of the structure imposed on his lifestyle, and his drug abuse. The complicating factors associated with each dysarthric speaker must be considered, therefore, when planning intervention to ensure that the treatment provided is maximized within this context.

As previously mentioned, there is a paucity of studies in the literature that have investigated the effects of treatment on children with acquired dysarthria following TBI. An early study by Light et al. (1988) reported on a transition through the use of multiple alternative and augmentative (AAC) systems over a 3-year period, during the rehabilitation of a 13-year-old child with TBI who initially presented without oral communication. The case study illustrated an ongoing assessment-intervention model in which the child's needs were assessed, goals for intervention were determined, the nature and extent of facilitator support identified, and training for the child's facilitators initiated. Over a 3-year period, the child's communication systems were regularly adjusted in line with the child's requirements, and technical advances. More than 3 years after her head injury, the child recovered functional speech. This recovery seemed to have been facilitated by the AAC systems. During this rehabilitative period, it was recognized by the rehabilitation team that the child not only required an appropriate communication system, but also that she needed to develop the appropriate interaction strategies to ensure that she was an efficient and effective communicator in various social contexts (Light et al., 1988).

A recent study by Murdoch et al. (1999) reported on the effectiveness of real-time continuous visual biofeedback in the treatment of speech breathing disorders in a 12-year-old male child with persistent dysarthria following severe TBI. In this study, the efficacy of traditional and physiological biofeedback methods for modifying abnormal speech breathing patterns were compared through the use of an A-B-A-B single subject research design, which allowed for two exclusive periods (eight sessions) of each type of therapy. Visual biofeedback of rib cage excursion was provided to the child using the Respitrace® system. The results of this study indicated that real-time continuous visual biofeedback techniques were effective in modifying speech breathing patterns in this case, and were superior to traditional therapeutic techniques targeting the same deficits. In particular, the subject was able to use visual biofeedback of rib cage excursion to modify abnormal breathing patterns to achieve more natural speech breathing. The subject demonstrated an increase in phonation time, a decrease in voice onset latencies, and, to some extent, a decrease in rib cage paradoxing. Murdoch et al. (1999) concluded that physiological biofeedback techniques are potentially useful for the treatment of speech breathing disorders in the pediatric dysarthric population and may have application in the treatment of other aspects of abnormal speech production evident in these children.

A Framework for Intervention

Although dysarthria following TBI is the end result of neuropathophysiological deficits in the various components of the speech production mechanism, the management of this speech disorder must move beyond the treatment of the basic impairment alone, to address the communicative limitations of this disorder on the individual, in relation to the emotional, social, and vocational aspects of life. Indeed, Hartley (1992) stressed the importance of persons with TBI communicating not only adequately, but also appropriately in all life contexts. Worrall (2000) advocated the use of a model of disablement as a framework for the management of neurogenic communication and swallowing disorders, to describe the process of disablement or functioning and the effects of the individual's environment on communicative ability, and to provide some consistency in the terminology used across disciplines. To this end, a framework for intervention in dysarthria following TBI is required to encompass the functional limitations of this disorder and the impact of such a communication impairment on the individual's capacity to perform desirable roles in society.

A global conceptual framework for intervention in chronic disorders, which has application to dysarthria following TBI, is the *International Classification of Impairments, Activities, and Participation* (ICIDH-2) developed by the World Health Organization (WHO) (World Health Organization, 1997). This particular classification system has been derived from a revision of the original framework the *International Classification of Impairments, Disability, and Handicap* (World Health Organization, 1980), and reflects a more positive concept of disablement. The somewhat negative terms of *disability* and *handicap* have been replaced with *activity limitation* and *participation restriction*, respectively. The term *impairments* relates to either body functions or body structures. Dysarthria is coded as an impairment of function, while structures of the speech mechanism are identified as impaired structures, using this classification (Worrall, 2000). The *activity* aspect of the ICIDH-2 relates to the individual's everyday life activities and includes communication activities (understanding messages, communicating messages, and using communication devices) and interpersonal behaviors (initiating social contact, relating to a spouse or partner, and maintaining friend and peer relationships; Worrall, 2000). *Participation* refers to the individual's degree of participation in personal maintenance; mobility; exchange of information; social relationships; education; work; leisure; and spirituality; and economic, community, and civic life. This dimension also refers to society's role in facilitating or hindering the individual's participation (Worrall, 2000).

While the ICIDH-2 (World Health Organization, 1997) provides an appropriate and widely recognized framework on which to base intervention for dysarthria following TBI, Yorkston et al. (1996) proposed a conceptual framework for the assessment and treatment of dysarthria that provides a more detailed practical model for intervention. This framework is based on a revision of the original ICIDH (World Health Organization, 1980) by the Institute of Medicine (1991) and contains five parameters: pathophysiology, impairment, functional limitation, disability, and societal limitation. In this model, impairment and functional limitation are seen as separate entities rather than being placed within the same category, as in the ICIDH-2, and pathophysiology has been included as another dimension. This five-parameter model for dysarthria allows for a clearer delineation of the different aspects of intervention that are possible across a broad perspective of management. As applied to dysarthria, Yorkston (1996) and Yorkston et al. (1996) described these five parameters of the framework as follows:

- Pathophysiology: Pathophysiology is an interruption or interference of normal physiological processes and structures involving the central and peripheral nervous systems.

- *Impairment*: This refers to motor speech impairment in which there are slow, weak, imprecise, and uncoordinated movements of the speech musculature, resulting in deficits in respiration, phonation, resonance, and articulation.

- *Functional Limitation*: The functional limitation experienced by the individual due to motor speech impairment is a reduction in speech intelligibility and rate, and the presence of abnormal prosodic patterns.

- *Disability*: The disability associated with dysarthria involves the reduced ability to function in communicative situations that require natural, understandable, and efficient speech. As a result, the individual may be limited in the ability to perform activities and roles within a social and physical environment.

- *Societal Limitation*: This dimension involves the restrictions (social policy) or barriers (structures or attitudinal) placed on the dysarthric speaker that limit fulfillment of roles or deny access to opportunities and services.

This framework for intervention in dysarthria proposed by Yorkston (1996) and Yorkston et al. (1996) may be readily applied to dysarthric speakers following TBI and will be the model adopted in this chapter.

Having established an overall framework for intervention, the clinician must then determine a clinical management plan for each case that is specifically designed to target the communication needs of the individual. Such planning involves identifying the general goals or directions of treatment for the case, consideration of a variety of internal and external factors that are unique to that individual, and the identification of techniques or strategies to reduce impairment, functional limitation, disability, and societal limitations. A clinical management plan for a TBI person with dysarthric speech should be flexible and responsive to different stages of recovery and the changing communicative needs of the individual, and remain proactive in the long-term. Currently, the treatment of children with dysarthria following TBI involves adaptation of the techniques and strategies employed in the management of dysarthria in the adult population, to suit the developmental and cognitive function of this particular clinical group.

Determining Treatment Goals

Within a framework of intervention, the general goals of treatment/management need to be determined in relation to the severity of the dysarthric speech disturbance post-TBI. Yorkston, Beukelman, Strand, and Bell (1999) stressed that "'normal' speech is rarely a realistic goal for individuals with dysarthria" (p. 266). Indeed, realistic goal setting is crucial for a successful outcome from intervention.

In the case of a mildly impaired dysarthric speaker following TBI, in which speech is intelligible but not as natural and efficient as a normal speaker, the degree of disability that this speech disturbance causes for the individual needs to be determined. For example, in the case of an unskilled laborer who returns to employment following a head injury, a mild dysarthric speech disturbance is not likely to have a significant impact on that individual's work situation, while a teacher with a similar speech disorder will experience a considerable degree of disability in the classroom. A mild dysarthria in a child following TBI is not likely to result in a marked disability at an early age but may have a significant effect on the individual during adolescence and young adult life because of societal barriers and attitudes. Where necessary, the treatment of a mild dysarthric speech disturbance should focus on optimizing the naturalness of speech (Yorkston et al., 1999; See Chapter 8, "Reducing Functional Limitation").

For those head-injured persons who exhibit a moderate dysarthria, however, speech is not consistently intelligible, and therefore, a considerable functional limitation is imposed on these speakers. Treatment, therefore, should be focused on improving speech intelligibility through a variety of compensatory techniques (Yorkston et al., 1999; See Chapter 8, "Reducing Functional Limitation"). Some of these techniques, such as prosthetic devices, although effective in improving speech intelligibility, may not be acceptable to some individuals, particularly the adolescent and young adult head-injured population, and different treatment techniques or approaches may need to be selected. In some cases, treatment may also need to target underlying physiological impairments to improve motor speech control and reduce the impact of physiological impairment on speech intelligibility (See Chapter 8, "Reducing Impairment").

A number of adults and children with TBI will present with a severe degree of dysarthria resulting in an inability, or marked reduction in their capacity, to communicate verbally. For these individuals, the initial goal of treatment should be to establish a functional means of communication to reduce the level of disability. In many cases, AAC approaches may be required to achieve this (Yorkston et al., 1999). In this situation, the clinician will need to determine treatment methods for increasing communication efficiency (See Chapter 8, "Reducing Disability"), be immediately responsive to any changes in communicative function, and play a major role in educating family and other professionals in the communication approach being implemented and used by the individual. In the pediatric TBI population, a severe dysarthria may be apparent for only a short time in some children in the initial stages of recovery, and then improve rapidly. In these cases, the clinician needs to monitor communicative function closely and adjust approaches accordingly. It is often the case that individuals with severe dysarthria following TBI also demonstrate severe physical and cognitive disabilities due to the overall severity of the injury. These concomitant impairments must be considered when determining the most optimal functional communication systems. Although a TBI adult or child with severe dysarthria may require an alternate means of communication in the initial stage of recovery, reducing the physiological impairment should also be an important goal of treatment. By facilitating motor control for speech, the individual may make a transition to independent use of speech at a later stage of recovery (Yorkston et al., 1999).

Other Considerations in the Management of Dysarthria Post-TBI

Inherent within any broad concept of management of dysarthria post-TBI is the need to consider a range of developmental, psychosocial, educational, cognitive, vocational, economic, and social factors that are unique to the individual. In the case of an adult with dysarthria following TBI, premorbid characteristics relating to personality, lifestyle, level of education, and vocational history may have a significant impact on the rehabilitation process in either a positive or negative direction. For the adolescent individual with TBI, a number of social-emotional-behavioral and cognitive-academic-vocational issues need to be considered during the early, middle, and late stages of adolescence (Ylvisaker & Feeney, 1995). In the pediatric population, the effect of an acquired speech disorder on the developmental continuum of speech and language must be considered (Murdoch & Hudson-Tennent, 1994). The child's phonological development prior to the onset of the dysarthria and any developmental components in the speech disorder need to be identified if appropriate treatment goals are to be determined (Murdoch, Ozanne, & Cross, 1990).

For both adults and children, the level of cognitive function post-TBI may have a substantial impact on intervention, with attention, concentration, and memory deficits impeding the individual's ability to stay on task, to learn and maintain new compensatory strategies, and to self-monitor and adjust speech output. Other psychosocial factors, such as poor motivation for treatment, an inability to accept postinjury impairments, and a reluctance to utilize certain compensatory techniques because of their "less than normal connotation," will have an impact on the degree of disability or handicap experienced by the individual, and seriously impinge on treatment outcome (McHenry & Wilson, 1994). Economic and social factors may have a significant influence on the individual's commitment to a rehabilitation program.

Reducing Impairment

Because dysarthria is a speech disorder resulting from neurological impairment that affects the muscular control of the speech production mechanism, the aim of this level of intervention is to reduce the degree of neuromotor dysfunction in the subsystems of the speech mechanism (i.e., respiratory, laryngeal, velopharyngeal, and articulatory systems). Those working to reduce the motor dysfunction/impairment evident in dysarthric speakers should incorporate the principles of motor control and learning in the therapeutic process to ensure positive outcomes (McNeil, Robin, & Schmidt, 1997).

Schmidt (1988) has defined motor learning as a process in which an individual acquires the ability to produce skilled actions. Such motor learning is achieved through practice and experience. McNeil et al. (1997) highlighted the importance of distinguishing between performance during practice (acquisition) and learning (retention). The fact that an individual is performing well during a treatment session does not necessarily mean that this improved performance will result in learning in the long-term, and factors that facilitate performance may have little or no effect, or a negative effect, on retention. For motor learning to be effective and achievable, the cognitive functions of attention and memory are required. Poor attention will affect all aspects of information processing during learning, while impaired long-term memory will impede the storage of information. These factors need to be considered by the clinician in determining an individual's candidacy for motor learning tasks (McNeil et al., 1997). A motor learning program for a person with dysarthria following TBI should be designed with a number of prepractice and practice principles in mind (McNeil et al., 1997; Schmidt, 1988). In the prepractice phase of the program, the clinician needs to establish motivation for learning. This parameter of learning may require the clinician to outline the importance of the learning task (e.g., need to practice tongue movements to be able to produce speech sounds) and set goals to be achieved at the end of the task (e.g., 90% accuracy). During prepractice, it is necessary for the person to be fully informed as to the nature of the skill that is to be learned and the ways in which this learning will be achieved. McNeil et al. (1997) emphasized the importance of not overinstructing the person since this could overload the individual's attentional system. Modeling and demonstration of the task to be learned should occur during the prepractice phase, as well as verbal pretraining. During this process, all stimuli to be targeted in the treatment session are demonstrated to the individual. Prepractice sessions should also include information on how a movement is produced, preferably through visual representations rather than verbal instructions, and a prepractice reference of correctness (McNeil et al., 1997).

A number of basic principles pertaining to the actual practice component of motor learning need to be considered. These include the importance of the quality and amount of practice, and the type and structure of feedback (knowledge of results and knowledge of performance; Schmidt, 1988, 1991). During the practice session, it is essential that practice be variable so that generalization and carry-over to speech is facilitated. McNeil et al. (1997) recommended the use of random practice throughout a session, whereby block practices on a particular skill are interspersed randomly with each other to facilitate learning. The timing and manner of delivery of the knowledge of results (i.e., feedback on the outcome of movement) to the patients must also be determined by the clinician. Long delay intervals in providing this feedback may inhibit learning, while a summary feedback of results is considered to be preferable to immediate feedback of results on each performance, because the latter tends to provide too much information (Schmidt, 1991). Principles similar to those mentioned above for knowledge of results feedback apply to knowledge of performance feedback given to individuals during motor learning (McNeil et al., 1997).

When working to reduce impairment in motor speech function in TBI individuals with dysarthria, effective motor learning may be difficult or impossible to achieve in the early stages of recovery in some cases because of attentional and memory deficits and poor physical status in these patients. The timing of this form of intervention, therefore, is critical to success, and it may need to be delayed to a later period of recovery, when the individual is more cognitively and physically receptive, as indicated by Enderby and Crow (1990).

A large range of treatment techniques have been developed to address the physiological impairment underlying dysarthria (Theodoros & Thompson-Ward, 1998). These techniques include behavioral and instrumental methods that target dysfunction in the respiratory, laryngeal, velopharyngeal, and articulatory subsystems.

Treatment of Respiratory Dysfunction

Depending on the type of respiratory dysfunction exhibited by the TBI individual, treatment aims to establish and maintain: an appropriate posture for speech breathing; an adequate breath supply/capacity for speech; a regular inspiratory-expiratory pattern of breathing whereby inspiration is initiated rapidly, followed by a slow expiratory phase; consistent and adequate subglottal pressure for phonation; and adequate expiratory breath control during speech (Theodoros & Thompson-Ward, 1998). The range of behavioral and instrumental techniques designed to improve respiratory function are outlined in Table 8-2.

Treatment of Laryngeal Dysfunction

Laryngeal dysfunction following TBI may result in disorders of vocal fold adduction (hyperadduction and hypoadduction), phonatory instability, and phonatory incoordination (Theodoros & Thompson-Ward, 1998). When hyperadduction of the vocal folds occurs following TBI, as in the case of spastic dysarthria, treatment is aimed at reducing the degree of vocal fold adduction and laryngeal resistance to airflow through the glottis, to establish normal vocal fold vibratory patterns. In contrast, the treatment of hypoadduction of the vocal folds post-TBI involves enhancing the adduction of the vocal folds through physiologically effortful activities. Determining the presence of either hyperadduction or hypoadduction of the vocal folds in persons following TBI is critical to treatment planning, in that the treatment techniques used in the management of these laryngeal behaviors are diametrically opposed and, therefore, may be harmful if incorrectly applied. The treatment of phonatory instability, which manifests perceptually as glottal fry, diplophonia, vocal tremor, and ventricular phonation (Ramig & Scherer, 1989), aims to increase the steadiness and clarity of phonation by modifying patterns of vocal fold adduction, phonatory airflow, and breath control. Techniques for reducing laryngeal impairment are outlined in Table 8-2.

Table 8-2. Treatment techniques for reducing respiratory, laryngeal, velopharyngeal, and articulatory impairment in dysarthria following TBI.

Impairment & Technique	Description	References
Respiratory		
• Establish & maintain optimal posture	• Person supported in chair/wheelchair by pillows, etc.	• Netsell & Rosenbek (1985), Rosenbek & LaPointe (1991)
• Instruction re normal process of respiration	• Establish appropriate inspiratory/expiratory pattern (i.e., rapid inspiration followed by slow, controlled expiration) • Auditory, visual, & tactile cues of movement of rib cage & abdomen during inspiration & expiration	• Theodoros & Thompson-Ward (1998)
• Providing abdominal support during exhalation	• Push against abdomen during exhalation	• Rosenbek & La Pointe (1991)
• Inspiratory checking	• Requires deep inspiration followed by slow exhalation • Makes use of passive recoil of lungs	• Netsell & Hixon (1992)
• Breath control exercises	• Maximum phonation tasks involving vowel prolongation • Serial speech tasks of increasing length performed on one breath • Establishing optimal breath groups (number of syllables produced comfortably on one breath)	• Moncur & Brackett (1974)
• Accent Method	• Breathing exercises designed to assist voicing control • Emphasis on transferring respiratory effort to abdominal region during speech	• Kotby (1995)

(continues)

Table 8-2. (*continued*)

Impairment & Technique	Description	References
Respiratory		
• U-tube manometer	• U-shaped thin plastic tubing filled with colored water & marked with centimeter gradations to indicate movement of water • Individual blows into one end of tubing & displaces the level of water • Normal speech—need to maintain 5 to 10 cms water for 5 seconds (Netsell & Rosenbek, 1985)	• Rosenbek & La Pointe (1991)
• Glass and straw system	• Glass filled with water, with straw secured to side of glass to a depth of 5 cm • Individual required to blow a steady stream of bubbles • If able to do this, then person is generating sufficient respiratory pressure	• Hixon, Hawley, & Wilson (1982)
• Respiratory kinematic feedback	• Respitrace® used to display simultaneous but independent movements of rib cage & abdomen during speech • Useful for improving incoordination of respiratory muscles, respiratory-phonatory timing, & breath control; increasing lung volumes; & facilitating abdominal breathing	• Murdoch et al. (1999); Murdoch et al. (1995) • Thompson-Ward, Murdoch, & Stokes (1997)

(*continues*)

Table 8-2. (*continued*)

Impairment & Technique	Description	References
Laryngeal		
• Techniques to reduce vocal fold hyperadduction	• Chewing method • Yawn-Sigh technique • Gentle voice onsets • Oral resonance & voice projection therapy • Phonation at high lung volumes, which results in passive abduction of vocal folds due to downward pull of trachea by lowered diaphragm	• Boone & McFarlane (1988) • Smitheran & Hixon (1981)
• Techniques to increase vocal fold adduction	• Pushing, pulling, lifting exercises performed simultaneously with phonation • Hard glottal onset exercises • Postural adjustment of head (turn head to affected side to decrease distance between vocal folds) • Use higher pitch • Lee Silverman Voice Treatment (LSVT) Program. Designed to increase vocal fold adduction, using increased physiological effort and production of loud voice	• Aronson (1990); Boone & McFarlane (1988) • Ramig, Bonitati, Lemke, & Horii (1994)

(*continues*)

Table 8–2. (*continued*)

Impairment & Technique	Description	References
Laryngeal		
• Techniques to improve phonatory stability	• Exercises to increase respiratory-phonatory coordination (e.g., initiation of phonation at beginning of exhalation)	• Yorkston et al. (1988)
	• Maximum duration vowel phonation exercises	• Ramig, Mead, & DeSanto (1988)
	• Breath control exercises involving frequent inspirations & production of fewer syllables per expiration	• Linebaugh (1983)
	• Techniques to enhance phonatory effort & vocal fold adduction	• Ramig & Scherer (1989)
• Accent Method	• Aims to create optimal balance between expiration and vocal fold power, and coordination between phonation and resonating cavities	• Kotby (1995)
	• Abdominal-diaphragmatic breathing simultaneously with accentuated rhythmic phonation at different tempos	
	• Appropriate for each form of laryngeal dysfunction	
• Visual biofeedback of pitch, vocal intensity, & duration of phonation	• VisiPitch®, VisiSpeech®, Speech Viewer®	• Yorkston et al., (1988); Johnson & Pring (1990); Bougle et al. (1995)
• Visual biofeedback of respiratory-phonatory coordination	• Respitrace (provides feedback of breath control) & VisiPitch (feedback of phonation)	• Yorkston et al. (1988)
	• Strain-gauge respiratory kinematic system in conjunction with a throat accelerometer	• Thompson-Ward et al. (1997)

(*continues*)

Table 8-2. *(continued)*

Impairment & Technique	Description	References
Laryngeal		
• Visual biofeedback of vocal fold movement	• Videolaryngoscopy	• Bastian (1987)
• Visual biofeedback of subglottal pressure & airflow	• Air pressure and airflow transducers	• Netsell & Daniel (1979); Simpson, Till, & Goff (1988)
• Auditory feedback of degree of laryngeal tension	• Electromyography. Surface electrodes placed over cricothyroid region of larynx to record tension. Individual monitors tension through auditory feedback	• Prosek, Montgomery, Walden, & Schwartz (1978)
Velopharyngeal		
• Increase palatal awareness	• Palatal massage. Palate is massaged in anterior-posterior and medial-lateral directions & elevated during production of non-nasal sounds.	• Rosenbek & La Pointe (1991)
• Use of pressure, icing, brushing, or vibration on velum	• Prolonged icing • Pressure to muscle insertion points • Slow & irregular brushing & stroking	• Dworkin & Johns (1980)
• Increase vocal effort	• Increasing physiological effort results in a decrease in velopharyngeal orifice area	• McHenry (1997)
• Visual biofeedback of levels of nasalance (ratio of nasal to oral acoustic output)	• Nasometer® • Threshold levels of nasalance may be set during therapy.	• Theodoros & Thompson-Ward (1998)
• Visual biofeedback of velar muscle activity	• Electromyography • Surface electrodes placed under chin, in front of hyoid bone to record electrical activity of glossopalatine muscles during oral facilitation procedures & speech tasks	• Draizar (1984)

(continues)

Table 8-2. (*continued*)

Impairment & Technique	Description	References
Velopharyngeal		
• Visual biofeedback of nasal & throat vibrations	• Accelerometry • Miniature accelerometers attached to side of nose & throat to detect vibrations of acoustic energy • Visual feedback to observe nasal/non-nasal contrasts	• Stevens, Kalikow, & Willemain (1975)
• Continuous Positive Airway Pressure (CPAP) therapy	• An air pressure flow device delivers positive air pressure to nasal cavity via a mask. • Air pressure provides resistance for soft palate to work against during speech tasks • Increases palatal strength & decreases hypernasality	• Kuehn & Wachtel (1994)
Articulatory		
• Alter muscle tone	• Hypertonia—jaw shaking, chewing method & progressive relaxation • Hypotonia—increase physiological effort	• Boone & McFarlane (1988); Rosenbek & La Pointe (1991)
• Increase muscle strength	• Isotonic (repetitive movements without resistance) & isotonic (movements against resistance) exercises for lips, tongue, & jaw • 5–10 repetitions at a time	• Rosenbek & La Pointe (1991); Dworkin (1991)
• Improve control & direction of articulatory movement	• Specific speech & nonspeech exercises for lips, tongue, & jaw, designed to facilitate coordination & direction of movements. Movements performed to set rhythm	• Dworkin (1991)

(*continues*)

Table 8-2. (continued)

Impairment & Technique	Description	References
Articulatory		
• PROMPT (Prompts for Restructuring Oral Muscular Phonetic Targets) therapy	• Tactile technique in which a structured set of finger placements on face & neck provide feedback to the individual about the articulatory position to move toward during speech • Cues speaker about muscular tension, duration of production, & continuance	• Square-Storer & Hayden (1989)
• Visual biofeedback of articulatory muscle tension, strength, endurance, & fine motor control	• Electromyography—muscle tension & strength • Lip & tongue pressure transducers—strength, endurance, & fine motor control	• Draizar (1984); Nemec & Cohen (1984); Netsell & Daniel (1979); • Robin, Somodi, & Luschei (1991); Thompson, Murdoch, Theodoros, & Stokes (1996)
• Visual biofeedback of tongue placement	• Electropalatography—Artificial palate embedded with miniature electrodes • Provides visual representation of location & timing of tongue placement against palate during speech	• Hardcastle, Gibbon, & Jones (1991); Goozee, Murdoch, & Theodoros (1999)

A wide variety of techniques are used to target phonatory incoordination, which may affect voice onset-offset, voiced-voiceless contrasts, and prosodic aspects of speech (Kent, 1988; Kent & Rosenbek, 1982; Ramig & Scherer, 1989; Titze & Durham, 1987; Weismer, 1984; Yorkston, Beukelman, & Bell, 1988). The treatment goals for this aspect of laryngeal dysfunction include: facilitating synchronization of phonation and exhalation to reestablish voice onset-offset; improving the coordination between the laryngeal and articulatory subsystems of the speech mechanism to improve the production of voiced-voiceless contrasts; and improving the control of subglottal pressure, vocal fold tension, pitch and loudness variation, and pitch level and duration of phonation to improve the prosodic aspects of speech. Although the treatment of phonatory incoordination may be seen as addressing a specific disturbance in laryngeal function, within the framework of intervention proposed in this chapter, treatment of this aspect of laryngeal function is considered to enhance the speech signal itself, and therefore, speech intelligibility. As a result, the specific techniques and strategies to improve phonatory incoordination will be dealt with in the section on reducing functional limitation (See Chapter 8, "Reducing Functional Limitation").

Treatment of Velopharyngeal Dysfunction

Depending on the type of dysarthric speech disturbance evident following TBI, velopharyngeal dysfunction may be manifest as either a reduced ability to elevate the soft palate, or intermittent or inappropriate velar opening due to poor coordination. Individuals with spastic or flaccid dysarthria are more likely to present primarily with reduced velar elevation, while those persons with ataxic dysarthria are more likely to demonstrate impaired velar coordination. Techniques available to improve velar movement and coordination during speech are documented in Table 8-2.

Treatment of Articulatory Dysfunction

Following TBI, physiological impairment of the lips, tongue, and jaw may be evident to varying degrees. These impairments include reductions in the strength, rate, range, and control of articulatory movements during speech and abnormalities of muscle tone (e.g., spasticity or flaccidity). It should be noted that these deficits may occur differentially across the articulatory system, with some components of the articulatory system (e.g., the tongue) being more impaired than others (Theodoros, Murdoch, & Stokes, 1995). Detailed assessment of articulatory function, therefore, is important for determining treatment goals. Treatment of the articulatory dysfunction at the impairment level in persons following TBI is focused on normalizing muscle tone, increasing muscle strength, and improving the control and direction of movement of the articulators (Theodoros & Thompson-Ward, 1998), utilizing behavioral, and instrumental techniques (See Table 8-2).

Reducing Functional Limitation

Impairment in the motor subsystems of the speech mechanism results in the production of a degraded acoustic speech signal, which manifests as a reduction in speech intelligibility (i.e., the degree to which the acoustic signal is understood by the listener; Yorkston et al., 1996). According to the current model of intervention for dysarthric speakers following TBI, reduced speech intelligibility is the functional limitation resulting from physiological impairment of the speech mechanism, and from the compensatory strategies employed by the speaker in response to this impairment (Yorkston et al., 1996). The aim of this level of intervention is to reduce the functional limitation in dysarthric speakers with TBI by maximizing speech intelligibility through a variety of compensatory strategies. For those TBI individuals with dysarthria who are poor candidates for motor retraining of physiological impairment because they have cognitive deficits, the development of compensatory strategies to enhance intelligibility will be an important focus of intervention, together with strategies to reduce the degree of disability in different communicative environments.

Improving speech intelligibility for a dysarthric speaker post-TBI may involve the adoption of a number of compensatory strategies based on behavioral, instrumental, and prosthetic approaches to treatment, which are designed to enhance the speech signal per se, not the physiological impairment underlying the speech disturbance. These strategies may include altering stress patterns; improving intonation, rate control, and volume; and altering articulatory patterns to increase speech intelligibility. Examples of these techniques and strategies are detailed in Table 8-3.

Reducing Disability

At this level of intervention, the goal of treatment is to optimize communication in natural settings (Hustad, 1999). Disability resulting from dysarthria may be reduced by improving the individual's ability "to function in physical and social contexts that require understandable, efficient, and natural sounding speech" (p.18; Yorkston et al., 1999). Inherent within this level of intervention is the concept of "comprehensibility" of speech, which refers to the adequacy of speech, performance in a social context (Yorkston et al., 1996). Comprehensible speech is a consequence of information being adequately received through the speech signal (i.e., adequate speech intelligibility), together with signal-independent information such as semantic and syntactic context, situational and orthographic (alphabet supplementation) cues, and gestures or illustrators (Hustad, 1999; Yorkston et al., 1996). A relationship exists between these two sources of information in such a way that when the speech signal is rich in information (i.e., high intelligibility), the transmitted message is comprehensible even if there is only limited contextual information. However, if the speech signal is poor, as in the case of severe dysarthria, then the contextual information is crucial for comprehension of the message being transmitted between, or among, the communication partners (Hustad, 1999; Yorkston et al., 1996).

Reducing the disability of the speech impairment involves the participation of both the dysarthric speakers and their communication partners (Yorkston et al., 1999). The communication partner must play an active role in the communicative exchange by receiving and interpreting the speech signal, and by providing feedback and response to the message (Hustad, 1999).

Table 8-3. Treatment techniques for reducing functional limitation and enhancing speech intelligibility in dysarthria following TBI.

Technique	Description	References
• Improving stress patterning	• Contrastive stress drills. Core sentence of drill exercise consists of two or more components that are differentiated in meaning by varied stress patterns	• Rosenbek & La Pointe (1991); Yorkston et al. (1999); Robertson & Thomson (1984)
• Improving intonation	• Establishing and/or improving breath group capacity and pattern • Decrease uniformity of breath group to reduce monotony of pitch, pause without inhalation • Contrastive intonation drills	• Yorkston et al. (1988) • Bellaire et al. (1986) • Rosenbek & La Pointe (1991)
• Rate control	• Controlled reading tasks. Each word presented one at a time • Speech linked to hand tapping at a predetermined rate • Rhythmic cuing. Words to be read presented in a rhythmic manner by clinician • Computerized rhythmic cuing—PACER. Regulates speech rate during reading while allowing naturalness of speech to be maintained • Delayed auditory feedback (DAF). Results in reduction of speech rate & improvements in vocal intensity, fundamental frequency variability, pause time, & speech intelligibility Average delay 50 msecs. • Pacing board. Speaker required to place finger in separate slots on a board as words are spoken • Alphabet board. Speaker identifies first letter of each word, thus slowing rate of speech as each letter is located • Increasing vocal effort may indirectly reduce speech rate e.g., LSVT program • Establishing appropriate phrasing and breath patterning may decrease rate • Improving pitch & loudness variation & stress patterning may decrease rate	• Rosenbek & La Pointe (1991) • Yorkston et al. (1988) • Beukelman, Yorkston, & Tice (1988) • Hanson & Metter (1983) • Helm (1979) • Beukelman & Yorkston (1978); Crow & Enderby (1989) • Ramig, Pawlas, & Countryman (1995) • Yorkston et al. (1999) • Simmons (1983)

(continues)

Table 8-3. (*continued*)

Technique	Description	References
• Visual feedback of parameters of stress, intonation, & rate (duration, intensity, pitch)	• VisiPitch® • Speech Viewer®	• Bougle et al. (1995)
• Improving articulation (compensated speech intelligibility)	• Speaker required to make adjustments to speech movement patterns to produce an acceptable speech outcome. Specific speech movements not taught. • Contrastive production & intelligibility drills • Voiced-voiceless contrasts. Exaggerating aspiration of voiceless sounds, increasing vowel duration before voiced sounds, increasing duration of voiceless plosives as compared to voiced cognate • Establish or normalize articulatory targets	• Yorkston et al. (1988, 1999) • Rosenbek & La Pointe (1991); Yorkston et al. (1999) • Kearns & Simmons (1988)
• Prosthetic enhancement of speech intelligibility (vocal intensity, resonance, articulation)	• Increase intensity of speech signal using: (a) voice amplifier, (b) Edinburgh Masker—delivers white noise to speaker, resulting in increase in vocal intensity • Improve resonance of speech signal using palatal lift • Improve articulation using a bite block, which is positioned between the teeth to stabilize the jaw	• Allen (1970); Adams & Lang (1992) • Yorkston et al., (1988); Netsell & Rosenbek (1985) • Netsell (1985)

Treatment for TBI individuals with dysarthria at this level of intervention, therefore, involves enhancing the communicative effectiveness of these speakers by developing a range of speaker and partner communicative strategies, as well as strategies to facilitate communicative interaction (See Table 8-4). Speaker strategies may include: alerting the partner prior to transmission of the message, setting the topic, using grammar to enhance the message, using gestures, using turn maintenance signals, timing of important communication exchanges, and selecting a conducive environment for the communication exchange (Hustad, 1999). Partner strategies to enhance communication with a dysarthric speaker require the partner to alter behavior to compensate for the degraded speech signal. Strategies that may be useful for a communication partner to adopt include: maintaining topic identity, paying attention to the speaker, and identifying and consolidating clues (Hustad, 1999). To enhance the communication interaction per se, both the speaker and the partner should determine the methods by which they will manage communication breakdowns, and the rules by which interaction will proceed (Hustad, 1999).

At this level of intervention, augmentative and alternative communication (AAC) systems and strategies may play an important role in reducing the disability encountered by severely dysarthric children and adults following TBI, in performing social roles and activities. Light et al. (1988) stressed that the process of implementing and maintaining AAC systems in the head-injured population may differ from that used in other communicatively disordered clinical groups. In particular, Light and colleagues suggested that AAC systems should be implemented early in recovery to reduce the individual's frustration and to promote interaction and participation in a rehabilitation program. Light et al. (1988) also recommended that there is a need for ongoing reassessment to identify the changing communicative needs and skills of the individual so that AAC systems may be modified accordingly. Since it is possible for some individuals to recover natural speech many years post-TBI, Light et al. (1988) proposed that AAC programs should be integrated with other specific therapeutic techniques to facilitate the recovery of speech.

A large number of AAC systems have been developed that may have application to communicatively impaired individuals following TBI. The reader is referred to an extensive bibliography pertaining to AAC systems and strategies compiled by Silverman (1993). A relatively simple AAC device to enhance the comprehensibility of speech that may be useful for TBI dysarthric speakers is alphabet supplementation. With this system, the individual points to the first letter of each word while simultaneously speaking (i.e., the communication partner is provided with signal-independent information in the form of orthographic cues to aid comprehension; Hustad, 1999). This type of AAC device may be effectively used by the pediatric population since it involves minimal use of literacy skills, requiring only an awareness of the first letter of the word. Alphabet boards may be complemented by the addition of words referring to frequently used topics and situations that the individual may indicate to the communication partner prior to speaking. Communication boards may also include spoken word and phrase dictionary lists. The speaker points to the word or phrase prior to, or simultaneously with, speaking (Hustad, 1999).

Table 8-4. Treatment techniques to reduce disability and enhance comprehensibility of speech and communication in dysarthric speakers following TBI.

Strategies and Techniques	Description	References
Speaker Strategies		
• Prepare the partner	• Alert communication partner of intention to transmit message.	• Hustad (1999)
• Indicate how communication will occur	• Speaker points to first letter of word as spoken. • Communication partner asked to repeat each word or sentence after it is spoken • Communication partner to ask for clarification as soon as communication is not understood	• Duffy (1995)
• Identify context and topic of conversation	• Speaker identifies contextual cues (e.g., person's name, food items, activity etc.). • Speaker explicitly identifies topic of conversation, particularly when changing topics within an interaction.	• Dongilli (1994); Yorkston, Dowden, & Beukelman (1992); • Duffy (1995); Hustad (1999)
• Modify content and length of utterance	• Speaker either simplifies content of utterance or elaborates. • Speaker reduces the use of idiomatic expressions and uses more literal expressions. • Speaker reduces or increases length and grammatical complexity of utterance.	• Duffy (1995); Vogel & Miller (1991) • Duffy (1995) • Dongilli (1994); Hustad (1999)
• Use gestures	• Use gesture concurrently to supplement speech	• Garcia & Cannito (1996a, 1996b); Hustad (1999)
• Use turn maintenance signals	• Adopt a consistent signal to indicate initiation of a turn in conversation (e.g., leaning forward, raising hand etc.)	• Hustad (1999)
• Time important communication exchanges	• Communicate when energy levels are high.	• Hustad (1999)
• Select a conducive environment for communication	• Avoid distracting, noisy environments.	• Hustad (1999)

(continues)

Table 8-4. *(continued)*

Strategies and Techniques	Description	References
Communication Partner Strategies		
• Maintain topic identity	• Partner should be equally responsible for maintaining topic	• Hustad (1999)
• Pay attention to speaker	• Maintain visual and auditory attention while reducing distractions as much as possible. • Be positioned in front of speaker	• Hustad (1999)
• Piece clues together	• May need to piece together fragments of information comprehended during conversation	• Hustad (1999)
Enhancing Communication Interaction Strategies		
• Manage communication breakdowns	• Communication partner requests repetition. • Speaker offers occasional pauses to allow partner to ask for clarification, or asks partner if message has been understood. • Speaker rephrases the message. • Misunderstood words or phrases are repeated one at a time. • Shadowing—partner repeats each word or phrase after the speaker • Partner periodically summarizes his/her interpretation of what has been said. • Explicit cues to facilitate improved comprehension (e.g., slow down, speak louder, give the first letter etc.)	• Duffy (1995); Hustad (1999)
• Establish interaction rules	• Determine mutually agreeable rules or communication signals for use during interaction (e.g., when communication breakdown has occurred, turn-taking etc.).	• Hustad (1999)

(continues)

Table 8-4. (*continued*)

Strategies and Techniques	Description	References
Alternative and Augmentative Communication (AAC)		
• Residual speech & AAC	• Alphabet supplementation. Speaker points to first letter of a word as it is spoken. • Spoken word & phrase dictionaries. Lists of these words and phrases added to the communication board. Speaker points to word or phrase prior to, or simultaneously with, word being spoken.	• Hustad (1999)
• Other AAC systems	• Extensive range of AAC systems available	• Silverman (1993)

Where comprehensibility of speech is markedly reduced and a significant break-down in communication occurs, the mode of communication should be changed to another format (e.g., writing, gesture etc.). Traumatically brain injured persons with severe dysarthria may also improve their comprehensibility by providing some form of context for their communication such as photograph albums or collections of remnants associated with daily experiences (e.g., tickets, programs, menus etc.). This type of material greatly assists in the communication of complex and specific information (Beukelman & Mirenda, 1998; Hustad, 1999).

For the child with a severe dysarthria following TBI, improving communicative effectiveness in various social contexts requires modification of the strategies out-lined for adults. For example, for very young children whose literacy skills have not yet developed, the alphabet board may be modified so that the individual letters are represented pictorially, as well as orthographically. Dowden (1997) has outlined a number of modified strategies to enhance communication specifically for children. These strategies include: enhancing natural communication strategies, managing the dynamics of communication breakdowns, setting the context for common and unusual topics, alternative strategies for predictable vocabulary for ambulatory chil-dren, alternative strategies for unpredictable vocabulary, familiarizing new commu-nication partners (e.g., babysitters, teachers etc.), and various strategies to promote adequate communication in the future (e.g., regular opportunities for the child to communicate with unfamiliar partners and about new topics and events, and an emphasis on literacy development).

Reducing Societal Limitation

Reducing the limitations that society imposes on the TBI dysarthric speaker and increasing the individual's life participation, involves providing opportunities for communication and access to services and experiences. Social policies and barriers that limit fulfillment of social, educational, and vocational roles need to be altered and/or eliminated (Yorkston, 1996, Hustad, 1999). Societal limitations may be con-sidered under two broad categories: the effect of environment on opportunities for communication, and the perceived reaction of others (Hustad, 1999). Four types of social barriers that may affect children and adults with dysarthria following TBI include: *policy* barriers, which are the result of legislative decisions; *practice* barriers, which consist of inflexible procedural processes; *attitude* barriers, whereby an indi-vidual presents a barrier to participation; and a *knowledge* barrier, which occurs as a result of lack of information (Hustad, 1999). These types of societal barriers are illustrated in the following example of a severely dysarthric TBI child, Tim.

Tim, a 10-year old boy, acquired a severe dysarthria following a motor vehicle accident. Physically, he was confined to a wheelchair with spastic quadriplegia. The comprehensibil-ity of his speech was adequate for basic social communication with the aid of an alphabet board. Cognitively, Tim was functioning quite well despite some reduction in attention and memory. He lived down the road from a local school that he had attended prior to the acci-dent. Following a period of hospitalization and rehabilitation, Tim and his parents requested that he be allowed to return to school and a normal routine. On application to his school, however, Tim's parents were informed that their son would not be accepted because of his disabilities and that he would be required to attend a special school a considerable distance from home (policy barrier). *After considerable appeals to the authorities, Tim was eventually allowed to attend his local school with the assistance of a care-giver for a trial period of one term. At school, however, Tim was restricted in his opportunities to participate in everyday activities of his class because of structural limitations of the school, which prevented him from accessing the computer and library facilities. As a result, he was unable to participate in the class activities in these areas, and no alternate arrangements were organized to facilitate this process* (practice barrier). *Although Tim was assisted by a caregiver, his teacher was reluctant to allow him to be involved in a number of class activities due to his communication difficulty* (attitude barrier). *In particular, his teacher tended to assign activities to Tim that were well below his cognitive level, leading to frustration, boredom, and attention-seeking behavior* (knowledge barrier). *Social interactions with his peers were also limited due to the children's perception that he was "scary" and "stupid"* (knowledge barrier). *No attempts were made by the school to assist Tim in integrating into the school community* (practice barrier).

To reduce the limitations placed on Tim, allowing him to participate in a regular educational routine, intervention would be required to address each barrier confronting him. With respect to the policy barrier, the speech pathologist, other health professionals, and family support groups might need to advocate on behalf of the family for Tim to remain in a mainstream school in the long term. With respect to the limited opportunities provided to Tim for interaction and communication with his peers, practical solutions would need to be introduced to overcome these barriers (e.g., provision of a wheelchair ramp, moving class activities to a more accessible venue, etc.). The inappropriate attitude of the teacher and students could be addressed by providing appropriate information to both the teacher and students as to the nature of Tim's disability. In particular, the teacher needs to be more fully informed as to Tim's level of cognitive functioning. A proactive program aimed at the social integration of Tim into the classroom, and the school in general, would also need to be initiated.

Determining the type and degree of societal limitation imposed on a person with dysarthria following TBI requires consideration of a range of factors specific to that individual (e.g., emotional, psychosocial, academic, developmental, vocational, etc.). The framework of intervention proposed for the management of individuals with dysarthria following TBI does not imply that there is a linear relationship among the different levels of the model such that the degree of severity at one level predicts a corresponding degree of severity at another level (Hustad, 1999). Indeed, two young head-injured individuals with similar levels of impairment in the speech mechanism, and comparable levels of speech intelligibility and communicative disability, may experience very different limitations in attaining and performing their desired roles in society. For example, one young man, who had just completed his second year of a law degree at the time of his accident experienced major difficulties in fulfilling his ambitions, due to a number of barriers and societal attitudes experienced throughout the remainder of his university life and during the early stages of his career. His slowed cognitive processes and impaired speech made it difficult for him to meet the required criteria for oral performance in this field of study. Following graduation, he was confronted by attitudinal barriers that precluded him from obtaining his desired employment. In contrast, a young man with a similar degree of dysarthric speech disturbance was able to return to his previous employment on a farm, where his communication skills and level of cognitive functioning did not affect his day-to-day activities, which were very routine in nature.

To date, the role of the speech pathologist in affecting the societal limitations imposed on TBI individuals with a dysarthric speech disturbance has been minimal. The intervention framework proposed in this chapter, and others such as the ICIDH -2 (WHO, 1997) herald a new phase in the management of communication disorders of this nature for the speech pathologist, other health professionals, and government agencies.

Case Report

The following case report provides a clinical example of the application of the framework for intervention for dysarthric speakers following TBI proposed in this chapter.

Jacob is a 26-year-old accountant who suffered a TBI following a motor vehicle accident, 9 months prior to assessment. On admission to the hospital, Jacob recorded a Glasgow Coma Score of 5, indicating the presence of a severe head injury. He remained in a coma for 4 months. Radiological investigation involving magnetic resonance imaging (MRI) revealed bilateral subcortical hemorrhages and multiple contusions.

Assessment of motor speech function revealed the presence of a moderate spastic-ataxic dysarthria. Perceptually, Jacob's speech was characterized by a reduction in speech intelligibility, impairments in consonant precision and breath support for speech, hypernasality and strained-strangled vocal quality, reduced pitch and loudness variation and rate of speech, and impaired stress patterning. Physiological evaluation of the speech mechanism revealed dysfunction in all subsystems of the speech mechanism. Kinematic assessment of respiratory function revealed the presence of impaired coordination of chest wall movements during speech breathing and a reduction in the number of syllables produced per breath. Assessment of laryngeal aerodynamics indicated a hyperfunctional pattern of laryngeal activity, involving high laryngeal airway resistance and reduced phonatory airflow. Accelerometric evaluation of velopharyngeal function revealed the presence of increased nasality during the production of non-nasal utterances. Reductions in tongue strength and rate of repetitive tongue movements during nonspeech tasks were identified, while lip function was found to be mildly impaired in relation to strength and rapid movement.

Prior to his accident, Jacob had completed a university degree and was employed in a large firm of accountants. His employers remained supportive of him throughout his rehabilitation and were keen to assist him in returning to his previous position within the firm. Jacob was married, and his wife and family were also very supportive of him. Physically, Jacob was making good progress and was likely to achieve independent mobility with the aid of a cane.

Table 8-5 outlines a management plan for Jacob, based on the framework for intervention previously detailed in this chapter. Goals for reducing impairment, functional limitation, disability, and societal limitations are identified, and examples of strategies to achieve these goals are provided.

Table 8-5. Management plan for Jacob, who has a moderate spastic-ataxic dysarthria following TBI.

Goals	Suggested Strategies
REDUCING IMPAIRMENT	
• *Reduce physiological dysfunction in the respiratory, laryngeal, velopharyngeal, and articulatory subsystems of speech mechanism*	
Respiratory function	
• Improve coordination of chest wall movements • Improve breath control for speech	• Visual biofeedback of chest wall movements • Maximum vowel phonation tasks • Serial speech tasks of increasing length on one breath • Establish optimal breath groups • Accent method
Laryngeal function	
• Reduce vocal fold hyperadduction	• Visual biofeedback of air pressure and airflow • Phonation at high lung volumes to achieve passive abduction of vocal folds • Chewing method, yawn-sigh, gentle voice onset techniques • Accent method • Visual/auditory biofeedback of laryngeal tension (electromyography)
Velopharyngeal function	
• Increase strength & movement of soft palate in speech & nonspeech activities	• Continuous Positive Airway Pressure (CPAP) therapy • Visual biofeedback of nasalance during speech (e.g., Nasometer)
Articulatory function	
• Increase tongue strength and rate of movement	• Isotonic & isometric tongue exercises • Speech & nonspeech exercises to facilitate an increase in rate of tongue movement • Visual biofeedback of tongue pressures and rate of movement (e.g., pressure transducers)

(continues)

Table 8-5. (*continued*)

Goals	Suggested Strategies
REDUCING FUNCTIONAL LIMITATION	
• *Enhance acoustic speech signal and increase speech intelligibility*	
• Improve stress & intonation patterns	• Visual feedback of stress & intonation parameters (intensity & pitch) using the VisiPitch®
	• Contrastive stress & intonation drills
	• Increase flexibility of breath grouping to reduce monotony of pitch
• Increase rate of speech	• Speech rate regulated through hand tapping, rhythmic cuing, & PACER
• Improve articulation	• Compensated speech intelligibility tasks (e.g., contrastive production & intelligibility drills to normalize articulatory targets).
REDUCING DISABILITY	
• *Enhance comprehensibility of speech and communication*	
• Increase communication partner's awareness of context & topic of conversation	• Jacob to practice the method of identifying contextual cues & explicitly identifying topic of conversation
• Manage communication breakdowns	• Jacob to practice altering content & length of utterances appropriately during conversation
	• Learn the use of specific cues to enhance comprehension (e.g., slow down, speak louder, use written communication)
	• Adopt a strategy of asking communication partner if message has been understood and a strategy of providing opportunities for the communication partner to request clarification
• Be aware of importance of maximizing communication at certain times and in certain environments	• Communicate when energy levels are high
	• Avoid noisy, distracting environments

(continues)

Table 8-5. *(continued)*

Goals	Suggested Strategies
REDUCING SOCIETAL LIMITATIONS	
• ***Increase opportunities for participation in social and vocational contexts by reducing barriers (policy, practice, attitudinal, knowledge)***	
• Improve family members, friends, and workplace colleagues awareness & understanding of Jacob's communication abilities & disabilities	• Provide information re: the nature of Jacob's communication status
• Increase communication partners' knowledge of techniques to assist in effective communication with Jacob in the workplace & in social situations to prevent isolation	Provide advice re: • Maintaining topic identity • Paying attention to Jacob when he is speaking • Being positioned in front of Jacob during conversation • Being prepared to piece parts of a conversation together • Requesting clarification if message not understood • Need to communicate in nondistracting environments • Strategies adopted by Jacob to communicate effectively & manage communication breakdowns
• Identifying appropriate client caseload in conjunction with employer	• Jacob may be assigned clients with whom he may communicate mainly through electronic communications (e.g., e-mail, etc.).
• Increase employer's awareness of need for additional support in some situations	• Impress upon employer the need to provide an assistant to Jacob in situations in which he is involved in complicated face-to-face interviews with clients

Evaluating Intervention

The framework for intervention in the management of individuals with dysarthria following TBI proposed in this chapter provides a model for evaluating treatment efficacy. Independent measurement of impairment, functional limitation, disability, and integration into society potentially provides opportunities to document the impact of treatment (Yorkston et al., 1999). For example, a decrease in functional limitation in the presence of a nonprogressive impairment, such as occurs in a head injury, suggests that treatment was effective. In contrast, measures of disability that remain unchanged following therapy indicate that improvements in functional communication have not been achieved, despite positive changes in speech intelligibility.

Treatment efficacy studies involving highly heterogeneous populations, such as TBI individuals, lend themselves to the adoption of single subject experimental designs, which can be used to identify which factors (e.g., treatment techniques) alter a target behavior (McNeil & Kennedy, 1984; McReynolds & Kearns, 1983). This type of research design has application to the clinical model of service delivery, allowing clinicians to evaluate the efficacy of therapeutic techniques with minimal disruption to the individual's treatment program (Kearns & Simmons, 1990; Theodoros & Thompson-Ward, 1998).

In evaluating the efficacy of treatment at the level of impairment, an extensive range of physiological assessment methods are now available to identify changes in the impairment of the subsystems of the speech mechanism following treatment. These forms of assessment of articulatory, velopharyngeal, laryngeal, and respiratory function have been described in Chapters 3, 4, 5, and 6. In addition, physical clinical assessments of speech subsystem function, such as the Frenchay Dysarthria Assessment (FDA; Enderby, 1983) and other nonstandardized clinical assessments may be used in conjunction with instrumental methods.

In determining the effectiveness of treatment to enhance speech intelligibility, perceptual ratings of speech production and intelligibility tests provide qualitative and quantitative assessment. Although a perceptual rating of overall speech intelligibility may be obtained from a speech sample, standardized measures of speech intelligibility, incorporating measures of speaking rate, provide a more meaningful index of the severity of the functional limitation (Yorkston et al., 1999). Clinical measurement of speech intelligibility and rate may be achieved through the use of any one of a number of intelligibility tests developed by Yorkston and Beukelman and colleagues (See Chapter 2). Phonetic contrast errors and single-word intelligibility may be identified using the phonetic intelligibility test designed by Kent, Weismer, Kent, & Rosenbek (1989).

Few assessments are currently available to determine the effectiveness of treatment to reduce the disability of the speech disturbance. Evaluation of treatment efficacy at this level of intervention involves determining the degree of comprehensibility of speech and functional communication that has been achieved following therapy. Enderby and John (1997) developed the Therapy Outcome Measure (TOM) to provide speech pathologists with a broader approach to monitoring communication disorders beyond impairment. The outcome measure consists of four dimensions: impairment, disability/activity, handicap/participation, and well-being. The core 11-point ordinal scale has descriptors developed for a specific communication disorder such as dysarthria. The five-point rating scale of the disability component of the TOM may be used to evaluate the treatment efficacy in relation to the TBI dysarthric speaker's functional communication skills. Briefly, the ratings for this dimension include: inability to communicate in any way; occasionally able to make basic needs known with familiar persons; limited functional communication, consistently able to make basic needs known but heavily dependent on cues and context; consistently able to make needs known, less dependent on cues and context; able to be understood most of the time by any listener although requiring some special consideration; able to communicate effectively in all situations (Enderby & John, 1997).

The ultimate aim of a management plan for a dysarthric speaker following TBI is for the individual to reintegrate into and participate in society with a level of communicative effectiveness that is sustainable. Achieving this endpoint of the management plan is the culmination of all other levels of intervention. Hustad, Beukelman, and Yorkston (1998) have suggested that societal limitation may be measured in relation to the level of perceived communicative effectiveness of a speaker in typical communication situations (i.e., the perceived success with which the speaker interacts and exchanges information). A method of evaluating communication effectiveness, using a questionnaire, has been developed by Sullivan, Beukelman, and Gaebler, cited in Hustad (1999). This questionnaire aims to determine how effectively the speaker communicates in various social situations and to identify the most frequently or important communication situations for the speaker. The speaker or a family member is required to rate these situations on a seven-point equal-appearing interval scale. Sample situations include: having a conversation with a few friends, being part of a conversation in a noisy environment, speaking in front of a small group without a microphone, and communicating at work.

The handicap component of the TOM for dysarthria (Enderby & John, 1997) may be used to evaluate a dysathric speaker's participation in society. Briefly, the ratings for this scale include: inability to fulfill any social, educational or family role and no social integration; limited social integration, socially isolated, contributes to some decisions; some social integration and self-confidence; self-confidence and autonomy emerging, makes decisions, some limited integration; mostly confident, difficulty achieving in some situations; achieving potential, autonomous and unrestricted, able to fulfill social, educational, and family roles. Broader scales available to measure the social participation of head-injured individuals include the Craig Handicap Assessment and Reporting Technique (CHART; Whiteneck, Charlifue, Gerhart, Overholser, & Richardson, 1992), the Community Integration Questionnaire (CIQ; (Willer, Rosenthal, Kreutzer, Gordon, & Rempel, 1993) and the Functional Life Scale (FLS; Sarno, Sarno, & Levita, 1973).

Summary

The management of an individual with a dysarthric speech disturbance following a TBI is an intrinsically complicated process that addresses not only the speech impairment per se, but also the complexities of communicative interaction within a social context. The practical framework for intervention presented in this chapter provided a model for treatment across a continuum from the physiological bases of the disorder to the broader application of communication skills in society.

Given the diversity of neurological impairment following TBI, treatment programs need to be specifically designed for each individual to meet his/her unique characteristics and needs, to be responsive to the changing communicative and physical status of the individual during recovery, and to remain proactive in the longterm. Although there is an extensive range of treatment techniques and strategies available for the treatment of adults with dysarthria following TBI, these methods will continue to require modification for use with the pediatric population until more specific techniques are developed for this younger clinical group. An essential dimension of any management plan, however, is the evaluation of all aspects of intervention. Such evaluation is achievable within the framework presented in this chapter.

The proposed intervention model provides a broad perspective of the treatment of dysarthria following TBI, and in doing so, also provides insight into an extension of the role of the speech pathologist in managing this speech disorder. It is commonly acknowledged that a dysarthric speech disturbance resulting from TBI has a significant impact on the quality of life of these individuals and their families, and on the resources of the community. Research into the development of more effective treatment techniques and management strategies is urgently required to address this debilitating communication disorder and produce more positive functional outcomes for individuals following traumatic brain injury.

References

Adams, S.G. & Lang, A.E. (1992). Can the Lombard effect be used to improve low voice intensity in Parkinson's disease? *European Journal of Disorders of Communication, 27*, 121–127.

Allen, C.M. (1970). Treatment of nonfluent speech resulting from neurological disease—treatment of dysarthria. *British Journal of Disorders of Communication, 5*, 3–5.

Aronson, A.E. (1990). *Clinical voice disorders: An interdisciplinary approach.* Third edition. New York: Thieme.

Aten, J.L. (1988). Spastic dysarthria: Revising understanding of the disorder and speech treatment procedures. *Journal of Head Trauma Rehabilitation, 3*, 63–73.

Bastian, R.W. (1987). Laryngeal image biofeedback for voice disorder patients. *Journal of Voice, 1*, 279–282.

Bellaire, K., Yorkston, K.M., & Beukelman, D.R. (1986). Modification of breath patterning to increase naturalness of a mildly dysarthric speaker. *Journal of Communication Disorders, 19*, 271–280.

Beukelman, D.R. & Garrett, K.L. (1988). Augmentative and alternative communication for adults with acquired severe communication disorders. *Augmentative and Alternative Communication, 4*, 104–121.

Beukelman, D.R. & Mirenda, P. (1998). *Augmentative and alternative communication: Management of severe communication disorders in children and adults.* Second edition. Baltimore: Brookes.

Beukelman, D.R. & Yorkston, K.M. (1977). A communication system for the severely dysarthric speaker with an intact language system. *Journal of Speech and Hearing Disorders, 42*, 265–270.

Beukelman, D.R. & Yorkston, K.M. (1978). Communication options for patients with brainstem lesions. *Archives of Physical Medicine and Rehabilitation, 59*, 337–340.

Beukelman, D.R., Yorkston, K.M., & Tice, B. (1988). *Pacer/Tally.* Tucson, AZ: Communication Skills Builders.

Boone, D.R. & McFarlane, S.C. (1988). *The Voice and Voice Therapy*. Fourth edition. Englewood Cliffs, NJ: Prentice Hall.

Bougle, F., Ryalls, J., & Le Dorze, G. (1995). Improving fundamental frequency modulation in head trauma patients: A preliminary comparison of speech-language therapy conducted with and without IBM's Speech Viewer. *Folia Phoniatrica Logopaedia, 47,* 24–32.

Brand, H.A., Matsko, T.A., & Avart, H.N. (1988). Speech prosthesis retention problems in dysarthria: Case report. *Archives of Physical Medicine and Rehabilitation, 69,* 213–214.

Crow, E. & Enderby, P. (1989). The effects of an alphabet chart on the speaking rate and intelligibility of speakers with dysarthria. In K.M. Yorkston & D.R. Beukelman (Eds.), *Recent Advances in Clinical Dysarthria* (pp. 99–107). Boston: College-Hill Press.

Dongilli, P. (1994). Semantic context and speech intelligibility. In J. Till, K. Yorkston, & D. Beukleman (Eds.), *Motor Speech Disorders: Advances in Assessment and Treatment* (pp. 175–192). Baltimore: Brookes.

Dowden, P.A. (1997). Augmentative and alternative communication decision making for children with severely unintelligible speech. *Augmentative and Alternative Communication, 13,* 48–58.

Draizar, D. (1984). Clinical EMG feedback in motor speech disorders. *Archives of Physical Medicine and Rehabilitation, 65,* 481–484.

Duffy, J.R. (1995). Managing the dysarthrias. In J.R. Duffy, *Motor Speech Disorders: Substrates, Differential Diagnosis, and Management* (pp. 389–416). St. Louis, MO: Mosby.

Dworkin, J.P. (1991). *Motor Speech Disorders: A Treatment Guide.* St. Louis, MO: Mosby-Yearbook, Inc.

Dworkin, J.P. & Johns, D.F. (1980). Management of velopharyngeal incompetence in dysarthria: A historical review. *Clinical Otolaryngology, 5,* 61–74.

Enderby, P. (1983). *Frenchay Dysarthria Assessment.* San Diego: College-Hill Press.

Enderby, P. & Crow, E. (1990). Long-term recovery patterns of severe dysarthria following head injury. *British Journal of Disorders of Communication, 25,* 341–354.

Enderby, P. & John, A. (1997). *Therapy Outcome Measures (Speech and Language Therapy).* London: Singular Publications.

Garcia, J.M. & Cannito, M.P. (1996a). Influence of verbal and nonverbal context on sentence intelligibility of a speaker with dysarthria. *Journal of Speech and Hearing Research, 39,* 750–760.

Garcia, J.M. & Cannito, M.P. (1996b). Top down influences on the intelligibility of a dysarthric speaker: Addition of natural gestures and situational context. In D. Robin, K. Yorkston, & D. Beukelman (Eds.), *Disorders of Motor Speech* (pp. 89–104). Baltimore: Brookes.

Goldstein, P., Ziegler, W., Vogel, M., & Hoole, P. (1994). Combined palatal-lift and EPG-feedback therapy in dysarthria: A case study. *Clinical Linguistics and Phonetics, 8,* 210–218.

Goozee, J.V., Murdoch, B.E., & Theodoros, D.G. (1999). Electropalatographic assessment of articulatory timing characteristics in dysarthria following traumatic brain injury. *Journal of Medical Speech-Language Pathology, 7,* 209–222.

Hanson, W.R. & Metter, E.J. (1980). DAF as instrumental treatment for dysarthria in progressive supranuclear palsy: A case report. *Journal of Speech and Hearing Disorders, 45,* 268–275.

Hardcastle, W.J., Gibbon, F.E., & Jones, W. (1991). Visual display of tongue-palate contact: Electropalatography in the assessment and remediation of speech disorders. *British Journal of Disorders of Communication, 26,* 41–74.

Harris, B. & Murry, T. (1984). Dysarthria and aphagia: A case study of neuromuscular treatment. *Archives of Physical Medicine and Rehabilitation, 65,* 408–412.

Hartley, L.L. (1992). Assessment of functional communication. *Seminars in Speech and Language, 13,* 264–279.

Helm, N.A. (1979). Management of palilalia with a pacing board. *Journal of Speech and Hearing Disorders, 44,* 350–353.

Hixon, T., Hawley, J., & Wilson, J. (1982). An around the house device for the clinical determination of respiratory driving pressure: A note on making simple even simpler. *Journal of Speech and Hearing Disorders, 47,* 413.

Hustad, K.C. (1999). Optimizing communicative effectiveness: Bringing it together. In K.M. Yorkston, D.R. Beukelman, E.A. Strand, & K.R. Bell, *Management of Motor Speech Disorders in Children and Adults* (pp. 483–541). Austin, TX: Pro-Ed.

Hustad, K.C., Beukleman, D.R., & Yorkston, K.M. (1998). Functional outcome assessment in dysarthria. *Seminars in Speech and Language, 19,* 291–302.

Institute of Medicine (1991). *Disability in America: Toward a National Agenda for Prevention.* Washington: National Academy Press.

Johnson, J.A. & Pring, T.R. (1990). Speech therapy and Parkinson's disease: A review and further data. *British Journal of Disorders of Communication, 25,* 183–194.

Kearns, K.P. & Simmons, N.N. (1988). Motor speech disorders: The dysarthrias and apraxia of speech. In N.J. Lass, I.V. McReynolds, J.L. Northern, & D.E. Yoder (Eds.), *Handbook of Speech-Language Pathology and Audiology* (pp. 592–621). Toronto: B.C. Decker.

Kearns, K.P. & Simmons, N.N. (1990). The efficacy of speech-language pathology intervention: Motor speech disorders. *Seminars in Speech and Language, 11,* 273–295.

Keatley, A. & Wirz, S. (1994). Is 20 years too long? Improving intelligibility in long standing dysarthria: A single case treatment study. *European Journal of Disorders of Communication, 29,* 183–202.

Keenan, J.E. & Barnhart, K.S. (1993). Development of yes/no systems in individuals with severe traumatic brain injuries. *Augmentative and Alternative Communication, 9,* 184–190.

Kent, R.D. (1988). The dysarthric or apraxic client. In D.E. Yoder & R.D. Kent (Eds.), *Decision Making in Speech-Language Pathology* (pp. 156–157). Philadelphia: B.C. Decker.

Kent, R.D. & Rosenbek, J.C. (1982). Prosodic disturbance and neurologic lesion. *Brain and Language, 15,* 259–291.

Kent, R.D., Weismer, G., Kent, J.F., & Rosenbek, J.C. (1989). Toward phonetic intelligibility testing in dysarthria. *Journal of Speech and Hearing Disorders, 54,* 482–499.

Kotby, M.N. (1995). *The Accent Method of Voice Therapy.* San Diego: Singular Publishing.

Kuehn, D.P. & Wachtel, J.M. (1994). CPAP therapy for treating hypernasality following closed head injury. In J.A. Till, K.M. Yorkston, & D.R. Beukelman (Eds.), *Motor Speech Disorders: Advances in Assessment and Treatment* (pp. 207–212). Baltimore: Paul H. Brookes.

Light, J., Beesley, M., & Collier, B. (1988). Transition through multiple augmentative and alternative communication systems: A three-year case study of a head injured adolescent. *Augmentative and Alternative Communication, 4,* 2–14.

Linebaugh, C.W. (1983). Treatment of flaccid dysarthria. In W. H. Perkins (Ed.), *Current Therapy of Communication Disorders: Dysarthria and Apraxia* (pp. 59–67). New York: Thieme.

McHenry, M.A. (1997). The effect of increased vocal effort on estimated velopharyngeal orifice area. *American Journal of Speech-Language Pathology, 6,* 55–61.

McHenry, M. & Wilson, R. (1994). The challenge of unintelligible speech following traumatic brain injury. *Brain Injury, 8,* 363–375.

McHenry, M.A., Wilson, R.L., & Minton, J.T. (1994). Management of multiple physiological deficits following traumatic brain injury. *Journal of Medical Speech-Language Pathology, 2,* 58–74.

McNeil, M.R. & Kennedy, J.G. (1984). Measuring the effects of treatment for dysarthria: Knowing when to change or terminate. *Seminars in Speech and Language, 5,* 337–357.

McNeil, M.R., Robin, D.A., & Schmidt, R.A. (1997). Apraxia of speech: Definition, differentiation, and treatment. In M.R. McNeil (Ed.), *Clinical Management of Sensorimotor Speech Disorders* (pp. 311–344). New York: Thieme.

McReynolds, L.V. & Kearns, K.P. (1983). *Single Subject Experimental Design in Communicative Disorders.* Baltimore: University Park Press.

Moncur, J.P. & Brackett, I.P. (1974). *Modifying Vocal Behavior.* New York: Harper & Row.

Murdoch, B.E. & Hudson-Tennent, L.J. (1994). Speech disorders in children treated for posterior fossa tumors: Ataxic and developmental features. *European Journal of Disorders of Communication, 29,* 379–397.

Murdoch, B.E., Ozanne, A.E., & Cross, J.A. (1990). Acquired childhood speech disorders: Dysarthria and dyspraxia. In B.E. Murdoch (Ed.), *Acquired Neurological Speech/Language Disorders in childhood* (pp. 398–341). London: Taylor & Francis.

Murdoch, B.E., Pitt, G., Theodoros, D.G., & Ward, E.C. (1999). Real-time continuous visual biofeedback in the treatment of speech breathing disorders following childhood traumatic brain injury: Report of one case. *Pediatric Rehabilitation, 3,* 5–20.

Murdoch, B.E., Sterling, D., Theodoros, D.G., & Stokes, P.D. (1995). Physiological rehabilitation of disordered speech breathing in dysarthric speakers following severe closed head injury. In J. Fourez and N. Page (Eds.), *Treatment Issues and Long-Term Outcomes,* pp. 137–145. Brisbane: Australian Academic Press.

Nemec, R.E. & Cohen, K. (1984). EMG biofeedback in the modification of hypertonia in spastic dysarthria: Case report. *Archives of Physical Medicine and Rehabilitation, 65,* 103–104.

Netsell. R. (1985). Construction and use of a bite block for use in evaluation and treatment of speech disorders. *Journal of Speech and Hearing Disorders, 50,* 103–106.

Netsell, R. & Daniel, B. (1979). Dysarthria in adults: Physiologic approach to rehabilitation. *Archives of Physical Medicine and Rehabilitation, 60,* 502–508.

Netsell, R. & Hixon, T.J. (1992). Inspiratory checking in therapy for individuals with speech breathing dysfunction. *Journal of the American Speech and Hearing Association, 34,* 152.

Netsell, R. & Rosenbek, J.C. (1985). Treating the dysarthrias. In J. Darby (Ed.), *Speech and Language Evaluation in Neurology: Adult Disorders* (pp. 363–392). Orlando, FL: Grune & Stratton.

Prosek, R.A., Montgomery, A.A., Walden, B.E., & Schwartz, D.M. (1978). EMG biofeedback in the treatment of hyperfunctional voice disorders. *Journal of Speech and Hearing Disorders, 43,* 282–294.

Ramig, L.O., Bonitati, C.M., Lemke, J.H., & Horii, Y. (1994). Voice treatment for patients with Parkinson's disease: Development of an approach and preliminary efficacy data. *Journal of Medical Speech-Language Pathology, 2,* 191–209.

Ramig, L.O., Mead, C.L., & DeSanto, L. (1988). Voice therapy and Parkinson's disease. *Journal of the American Speech and Hearing Association, 30,* 128.

Ramig, L.O., Pawlas, A.A., & Countryman, S. (1995). *The Lee Silverman Voice Treatment.* Iowa City: National Center for Voice and Speech.

Ramig, L.O. & Scherer, R.C. (1989). Speech therapy for neurologic disorders of the larynx. In A. Blitzer, M.F. Brin, C.T. Sasaki, S. Fahn, K.S. Harris (Eds.), *Neurologic Disorders of the Larynx* (pp. 163–181). New York: Thieme.

Robertson, S.J. & Thomson, F. (1984). Speech therapy in Parkinson's disease: A study of the efficacy and long term effects of intensive treatment. *British Journal of Disorders of Communication, 19,* 213–224.

Robin, D.A., Somodi, L.B., & Luschei, E.S. (1991). Measurement of strength and endurance in normal and articulation disordered subjects. In C.A. Moore, K.M. Yorkston, & D.R. Beukelman (Eds.), *Dysarthria and Apraxia of Speech: Perspectives on Management* (pp. 173–184). Baltimore: Paul H. Brookes.

Rosenbek, J.C. & La Pointe, L.L. (1991). The dysarthrias: Description, diagnosis, and treatment In D. Johns (Ed.), *Clinical Management of Neurogenic Communication Disorders* (pp. 97–152). Boston: Little, Brown & Co.

Sarno, J.E., Sarno, M.T., & Levita, E. (1973). The functional life scale. *Archives of Physical Medicine and Rehabilitation, 54,* 214–220.

Schmidt, R.A. (1988). *Motor Control and Learning: A Behavioral Emphasis.* Second edition. Champaign: Human Kinetics.

Schmidt, R.A. (1991). *Motor Learning and Performance: From Principles to Practice.* Champaign: Human Kinetics.

Silverman,F.H. (1993). *Comprehensive Bibliography on Augmentative and Alternative Communication: A Key to the AAC Literature for Clinicians and Researchers.* Greendale: CODI Publications.

Simmons, N.N. (1983). Acoustic analysis of ataxic dysarthria: An approach to monitoring treatment. In W.R. Berry (Ed.), *Clinical Dysarthria* (pp. 283–294). San Diego: College-Hill Press.

Simpson, M.B., Till, J.A., & Goff, A.M. (1988). Long-term treatment of severe dysarthria: A case study. *Journal of Speech and Hearing Disorders, 53,* 433–440.

Smitheran, J.R. & Hixon, T.J. (1981). A clinical method for estimating laryngeal airway resistance during vowel production. *Journal of Speech and Hearing Disorders, 46,* 138–146.

Square-Storer, P.A. & Hayden, D.C. (1989). PROMPT treatment. In P. Square-Storer (Ed.), *Acquired Apraxia of Speech in Adults* (pp. 190–219). London: Taylor & Francis.

Stevens, K.N., Kalikow, D.N., & Willemain, T.R. (1975). A miniature accelerometer for detecting glottal waveforms and nasalization. *Journal of Speech and Hearing Research, 18,* 594–599.

Stewart, D.S. & Rieger, W.J. (1994). A device for the management of velopharyngeal incompetence. *Journal of Medical Speech-Language Pathology, 2,* 149–155.

Stringer, A.Y. (1996). Treatment of motor aprosodia with pitch biofeedback and expression modelling. *Brain Injury, 10,* 583–590.

Theodoros, D.G., Murdoch, B.E., & Stokes, P.D. (1995). A physiological analysis of articulatory dysfunction in dysarthric speakers following severe closed head injury. *Brain Injury, 9,* 237–254.

Theodoros, D.G. & Thompson-Ward, E.C. (1998). Treatment of dysarthria. In B.E. Murdoch (Ed.), *Dysarthria: A Physiological Approach to Assessment and Treatment* (pp. 130–175). Cheltenham: Stanley Thornes (Publishers) Ltd.

Thompson, E.C., Murdoch, B.E., Theodoros, D.G., & Stokes, P.D. (1996). Physiological assessment of interlabial contact pressures in normal and neurologically impaired adults. In J. Ponsford, P. Snow, & V. Anderson (Eds.), *Proceedings of the 5th Conference of the International Association for the Study of Traumatic Brain Injury and the 20th Conference of the Australian Society for the Study of Brain Impairment* (pp. 259–266). Brisbane: Academic Press.

Thompson-Ward, E.C., Murdoch, B.E., & Stokes, P.D. (1997). Biofeedback rehabilitation of speech breathing for an individual with dysarthria. *Journal of Medical Speech-Language Pathology, 5,* 277–288.

Titze, I.R. & Durham, P.L. (1987). Passive mechanisms influencing fundamental frequency control. In T. Baer, C. Saski, & K. Harris (Eds.), *Laryngeal Function in Phonation and Respiration* (pp. 34–319). Boston: College-Hill Press.

Vogel, D. & Miller, L. (1991). A top-down approach to treatment of dysarthric speech. In D. Vogel & M. Cannito (Eds.), *Treating Disordered Speech Motor Control* (pp. 87–109). Austin, TX: Pro-Ed.

Weismer, G. (1984). Articulatory characteristics of Parkinsonian dysarthria: Segmental and phrase-level timing, spirantization, and glottal-supraglottal coordination. In M.R. McNeil, J.C. Rosenbek, & A.E. Aronson (Eds.), *The Dysarthrias: Physiology, Acoustics, Perception, Management* (pp. 101–130). San Diego: College-Hill Press.

Whiteneck, G.G., Charlifue, S.W., Gerhart, K.A., Overholser, J.D., & Richardson, G.N. (1992). Quantifying handicap: A new measure of long-term rehabilitation outcomes. *Archives of Physical Medicine and Rehabilitation, 73,* 519–526.

Willer, B., Rosenthal, M., Kreutzer, J.S., Gordon, W.A., & Rempel, R. (1993). Assessment of community integration following rehabilitation for traumatic brain injury. *Journal of Head Trauma Rehabilitation, 8,* 75–87.

Workinger, M.S. & Netsell, R. (1992). Restoration of intelligible speech 13 years post-head injury. *Brain Injury, 6,* 183–187.

World Health Organization (WHO) (1980). *International Classification of Impairments, Disabilities, and Handicaps.* Geneva: World Health Organization.

World Health Organization (WHO) (1997). *ICIDH-2 International Classification of Impairments, Activities, and Participation* [http://www.who.ch/programmes/mnh/mnh/ems/icidh/icidh.html].

Worrall, L.E. (2000). A conceptual framework for a functional approach to acquired neurogenic disorders of communication and swallowing. In L.E. Worrall & C.M. Frattali (Eds.), *Neurogenic Communication Disorders: A Functional Approach* (pp. 3–18). New York: Thieme.

Ylvisaker, M. & Feeney, T.J. (1995). Traumatic brain injury in adolescence: Assessment and reintegration. *Seminars in Speech and Language, 16*, 32–44.

Ylvisaker, M. & Urbanczyk, B. (1990). The efficacy of speech-language pathology intervention: Traumatic brain injury. *Seminars in Speech and Language, 11*, 215–226.

Yorkston, K.M. (1996). Treatment efficacy: Dysarthria. *Journal of Speech and Hearing Research, 39.* S46–S57.

Yorkston, K.M., Beukelman, D.R., and Bell, K.R. (1988). *Clinical Management of Dysarthric Speakers.* Boston: Little, Brown & Co.

Yorkston, K.M., Beukelman, D.R., Strand, E.A., & Bell, K.R. (1999). *Management of Motor Speech Disorders in Children and Adults.* Austin, TX: Pro-Ed.

Yorkston, K.M., Dowden, P.A., & Beukelman, D.R. (1992). Intelligibility as a tool in the clinical management of dysarthric speakers. In R.D. Kent (Ed.), *Intelligibility in Speech Disorders: Theory, Measurement, and Management* (pp. 265–286). Amsterdam: John Benjamins.

Yorkston, K.M., Strand, E.A., & Kennedy, M.R.T. (1996). Comprehensibility of dysarthric speech: Implications for assessment and treatment planning. *American Journal of Speech-Language Pathology, 5*, 55–66.

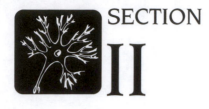

SECTION

II

Language Disorders Following Traumatic Brain Injury

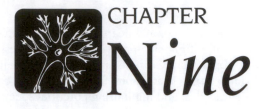

CHAPTER
Nine

Linguistic Deficits in Adults Subsequent to Traumatic Brain Injury

Fiona J. Hinchliffe, Bruce E. Murdoch, and Deborah G. Theodoros

Introduction

In recent times little attention has been paid to the linguistic impairments that occur following traumatic brain injury (TBI). This is because it is apparent that individuals with TBI often display minimal deficits on standardized tests of primary language function, in the presence of debilitating difficulties in the communicative activities of daily life. Rather than experiencing specific language problems, TBI individuals frequently encounter cognitive-communication disorders, which are considered to arise from impairments in linguistic and metalinguistic skills as well as from impairments in nonlinguistic cognitive functions such as attention, memory, reasoning, and perception discrimination (American Speech-Language-Hearing Association, 1991). To what extent the underlying language and cognitive impairments influence the endpoint communicative skill is not fully understood. Also unclear is the interaction between cognitive and linguistic impairment following TBI.

The goal of any investigations into communication disorders following TBI is to contribute information that will ultimately improve the effectiveness of the therapeutic management of this population. Current assessment and treatment of individuals with TBI is rightfully targeted at improving the level of communicative activity that the person is engaged in and minimizing potential social isolation (see Chapter 12). At the same time, an understanding of the component processes that underpin communicative activity is necessary for well-informed therapy planning.

This chapter endeavors to present detailed recent information concerning nature of the linguistic and cognitive processes that are thought to underpin communication skill. It is complemented by the next chapter, which presents recent investigations into noninteractive and interactive discourse production following TBI.

Language Disorders Reported in Adults Following TBI: A Historical Review

Disorders of language are a frequent legacy of TBI. Proficiency in language processing and production is fundamental to successful communication, which, in turn, is essential for psychosocial well- being. Loss or impairment of the ability to communicate may be a crucial factor in determining the quality of survival of individuals who have suffered TBI (Najenson, Sazbon, Fiselzon, Becker, & Schechter, 1978).

In the last 25 years there have been significant attempts to elucidate the nature of the communication disorders that are frequently a devastating consequence of TBI. During this time the characterization of the linguistic sequelae of TBI has constituted an area of controversy. This controversy has, in part, been due to the inherent variability of the TBI population, the inconsistencies in methodological parameters used in investigations, and the differences in the theoretical perspectives or the nomenclature adopted by the researchers.

In the 1970s many researchers used nomenclature associated with aphasia to classify the observed linguistic deficits in individuals with TBI (Groher, 1977; Heilman, Safran, & Geschwind 1971; Levin, Grossman, & Kelly, 1976; Luria, 1970; Thompsen, 1975). In doing so, the incidence of aphasia was found to be relatively rare when large series of consecutive cases were studied. In one of the most widely noted studies in the literature, Heilman et al. (1971) examined 750 consecutive acute admissions and diagnosed only 2% (13 cases) as having aphasia. Of these, nine cases were classified as having anomic aphasia, which was defined as fluent speech with relatively intact comprehension and repetition in the presence of verbal paraphasia and impaired object naming. The remaining four cases were found to exhibit fluent paraphasic speech, poor comprehension, and impaired repetition, characteristic of Wernicke's aphasia.

The definition of anomic aphasia used by Heilman et al. (1971) corresponded to the amnestic aphasia described by Thompsen (1975), who also found verbal paraphasia and anomia to be the most common symptoms of language impairment in 12 out of 26 TBI patients without mass lesions. Thompsen, however, concluded that the "aphasia" described in her subjects was not an isolated disorder but part of a neuropsychological syndrome dominated by deficits of memory. Thompsen also alluded to the fact that, while aphasia was not constantly present, no patient in the group had normal language function and all displayed aphasic traits. This observation may have been possible because of the higher-level, nonstandardized tests Thompsen included in her assessment battery, namely, describing a series of thematic pictures, providing synonyms and antonyms, and explaining metaphors.

Levin et al. (1976) found aphasia to occur in 14% of 50 cases of mild-to-severe closed head injuries, with naming ability and verbal associative fluency proving to be the most prominent sequelae of TBI in terms of language impairment. These investigators could not explain the observed linguistic deficits by the presence of demonstrated left hemisphere lesions. Since it appeared that the diffuse effects of TBI were present in most subjects, the authors suggested that the linguistic defects may be considered as instances of general mental impairment.

Groher (1977) investigated the memory and language performance of 14 male TBI subjects as soon as they regained consciousness and then each month for 4 consecutive months. There was an initial reduction in gestural, verbal, and graphic skills, as measured by the Porch Index of Communicative Ability (Porch, 1967) and the Weschler Memory Scale Form I (Weschler, 1945). At this time, gestural language skills were the poorest, while verbal skills were superior, and all subjects were described as having marked anomia, displaying both literal and nominal paraphasic errors. After 4 months, graphic skills had become superior to verbal and gestural abilities, and all subjects had essentially functional communicative skills. Most improvement in language and memory function occurred during the first month after regaining consciousness, with continued gradual improvement noted throughout the subsequent 4 months. Groher believed that all the patients in his experimental group initially displayed confused language as described by Halpern, Darley and Brown (1973), as well as aphasia. Many of the inappropriate behaviors improved during the first month, and it is therefore likely that Groher was, in effect, assessing and describing the language and behavioral manifestations of what is now considered posttraumatic amnesia (PTA).

While these studies show some consistency in the description of linguistic features found to occur after TBI, it is difficult to directly compare them because of methodologic variables. The populations differed with respect to subject selection criteria, time postinjury of assessment, and consideration of posttraumatic amnesia, aetiology, pathology, and severity of injury. The inconsistent use of repeatable or standardized testing procedures, and differences in the definition of aphasia, add further limitations when comparing results. It is noteworthy, however, that most of these authors alluded to the interplay between general intellectual skills and language functioning in the TBI population.

In the 1980s the debate over how best to conceptualize and describe the language behavior following TBI intensified with the publication of a series of studies by Sarno (Sarno, 1980, 1984; Sarno, Buonaguro, & Levita, 1986). In her first paper, Sarno reported on the performance of 56 TBI patients on 4 subtests of the Neurosensory Centre Comprehensive Examination for Aphasia (NCCEA) (Spreen & Benton, 1969). Before testing, the patients had been divided into three groups on the basis of clinical observation: aphasia only (32%), dysarthria with subclinical aphasic disorder (38%), and subclinical aphasic disorder only (30%). The diagnosis of aphasia was limited to patients who "manifested specific deficits in the processing of information via the speech code" (p. 686), and the type of aphasia was classified according to Geschwind (1971) and Benson (1967). "Subclinical aphasia disorder" was defined as "evidence of linguistic processing deficits on testing in the absence of clinical manifestation of linguistic impairments" (p. 687). The results indicated that all TBI patients suffered some degree of linguistic impairment. In contrast to the earlier studies, a larger proportion of patients evidenced classical aphasic syndromes (32%). Of these, the most frequent syndrome was fluent aphasia (39%). Anomia, which was the predominant linguistic disorder found in earlier studies (Groher, 1977; Heilman et al., 1971; Levin et al., 1976; Thompsen, 1975), occurred in only two (11%) patients in Sarno's group. The subclinical aphasic group was the least impaired and evidenced deficits in the subtests of Visual Naming, Word Fluency and the Token Test.

In 1984, Sarno repeated her original study, assessing 69 TBI patients admitted to a rehabilitation center. In this series, no patient who was assigned to the aphasia group was considered anomic. In the subclinical group, there were deficits in specific linguistic processing tasks (Sentence Repetition, Word Fluency, Token Test) as well as a "general decrease in richness and complexity" of verbal processing (p. 478). The author concluded that diffuse brain damage, severe enough to cause coma, will result in some form of verbal impairment.

In a later study, Sarno et al. (1986) applied a similar but more extensive methodology to a group of 125 TBI patients. Once again, all subject groups displayed compromised verbal functions in the form of aphasia (29.6%), dysarthria (34.4%), and subclinical aphasia (36%). The authors concluded that a severity continuum of verbal impairment was present in TBI, with the subclinical group being the least impaired.

Sarno's (1980, 1984) perspective on linguistic impairment following TBI evoked some criticism by those concerned with the limitations of using the conceptual framework established by classic aphasia theory to explain the verbal deficits in the TBI population. Holland (1982) contested the appropriateness of applying aphasia-related principles and nomenclature to describing individuals who did not demonstrate the focal lesions that underpin the traditional aphasic syndromes. While Holland agreed that aphasia can and does exist following TBI, she argued that most often the language was not disturbed in a typically aphasic way. Rather, she asserted that the language problems in TBI occurred as a manifestation of more general memory and cognitive deficits. Holland considered that the language deficits observed following TBI could be best described as disorders of language use, rather than as disorders of language form typical of true aphasic language.

Braun and Baribeau (1987) further criticized the work by Sarno et al. (1986) and attempted to refute their findings of a relatively high incidence of aphasia within the TBI population. They administered a battery of neuropsychological tests to 41 patients who had suffered a severe TBI and found that tests of verbal functions were generally less affected by TBI than tests of attention and memory. These authors judged the presence or absence of aphasia by the subjects' performances on the Token Test (Short form) (Spellacy & Spreen, 1969) and concluded that the incidence of aphasia evidenced in their study (2%) contrasted with the findings of Sarno (1980, 1984) and Sarno et al. (1986). Braun and Baribeau (1987) argued that their findings did not support the existence of "subclinical aphasia" in TBI, but suggested that the verbal deficits were most likely a "reflection of underlying cognitive dysfunction" (p. 330).

As with Holland (1982), consideration of the pathophysiology underlying the neurobehavioral symptoms of TBI led Hagen (1984) to oppose the use of a traditional, aphasia-related conceptual framework when evaluating and diagnosing the verbal impairments in this population. In his benchmark deliberation on the topic, Hagen argued that an approach to diagnosing and treating language disorders that had been developed from knowledge and experience with other types of neurological impairments could not be successfully applied to TBI. He considered that the observed language disorder in TBI is "a secondary consequence of an underlying impairment, suppression, and/or disorganization of the nonlinguistic cognitive processes that support language processes" (p. 252). Hagen argued that the neuropathology of TBI disrupts cognitive processes such as attention, sequencing, memory, categorization, and associative abilities, and as a result the individual with a TBI has difficulty in organizing and integrating incoming information and is impaired in his/her capacity to interact efficiently and appropriately with the environment. This cognitive disorganization can be reflected in the person's language, which may be disorientated, disorganized, confused, stimulus bound, disinhibited, or reduced in initiation.

Thus, by the mid-to-late 1980s, it had become widely accepted that language problems following TBI occurred against a backdrop of cognitive deficits. Indeed, this conceptualization is central to the current thinking that the language deficits that emerge following TBI are either secondary to the cognitive disruptions that are common following TBI, or interdependent on disrupted cognitive processes (Chapman, Levin, & Culhane, 1995).

The Nature of Language Disturbances in People with TBI: A Contemporary Understanding

Performance on Standardized Language Assessments

The current conviction that cognitive impairment is the foundation of the communication deficits found after TBI has evolved through the realization that most TBI individuals display overall normal performance on conventional aphasia tests in the presence of aberrant functional communicative ability (Hagen, 1984; Holland, 1982; Levin, Grossman, & Rose, 1979; Milton, Prutting, & Binder, 1984; Prigatano, Roueche, & Fordyce, 1986; Thompsen, 1975). While their abilities on specific subtests, namely word finding, verbal fluency, and comprehension of complex commands, have consistently been found to be below normal, the overall performances are not usually impaired enough to meet the criteria of aphasia as specified by the tests used (Levin et al., 1976, 1979; Sarno et al., 1986). In addition, it has been observed that TBI subjects display qualitative differences in performance as compared to aphasics on standardized test batteries (Holland, 1982; Levin et al., 1979; Prigatano et al., 1986).

Consistent with the observation that communication problems exist after TBI in the presence of proficiency in tests of primary language function, it has been argued that the communication problems following TBI cannot be adequately measured using traditional clinical test batteries designed to measure comprehension and production of language in aphasics. Such tests focus on specific linguistic processes and are seen as insensitive to the broader communication deficits in TBI. Most standardized tasks fail to test language skill beyond the level of the sentence, and the use of highly structured tasks may disguise the functional difficulties observed in more natural communicative situations (Benjamin et al., 1989; Coelho et al., 1991a, 1991b; Ehrlich & Barry, 1989; Hagen, 1984; Milton et al., 1984; Parsons et al., 1989).

While standardized measures of language have been denounced as insensitive to deficits experienced by TBI patients, it is likely that the selected assessments have been insufficient and incomplete. Even in the more recent research, language measures used to determine the presence and severity of linguistic disorders in the TBI populations have often been limited to basic tests for aphasia (Coelho et al., 1991a; Ehrlich & Barry, 1989; Irvine & Behrmann, 1986; McDonald, 1992; McDonald & Pearce, 1995; McDonald & van Sommers, 1993; Payne-Johnson, 1986) or subtests from neuropsychological assessment batteries (Chapman et al., 1992; Hartley & Jensen, 1991). These types of tests are designed to assess primary language skill but fail to examine language comprehensively on more complex tasks. It is not surprising, therefore, that individuals with TBI have frequently been found to display facile performances on assessments of primary language function in the presence of poor communicative performances in social contexts.

Communicative competence requires operational language beyond the primary language process or symbolic level (Bloom & Lahey, 1978), and involves proficiency with metacognitive and metalinguistic operations (Baker, 1982; Wiig, 1984; Wiig & Becker-Caplan, 1984). Metalinguistic skill and the ability to consciously and efficiently access and manipulate the semantic system are linguistically-based operations requiring an intricate interplay of primary language processes, cognitive processes, and executive processes such as self-monitoring and social judgement. The contribution of linguistic proficiency, where linguistic proficiency includes facility with primary language and higher-level cognitive-linguistic operations, must receive greater emphasis in the systematic and holistic evaluation of communication competence in TBI.

The tendency to limit the assessment of language in subjects with TBI to aphasia batteries results in failure to systematically investigate the mature and functional linguistic system. As a result, several researchers have concluded, on the basis of performance on aphasia batteries or subtests of neuropsychological batteries, that language function after TBI is largely intact (Coelho et al., 1991a, 1991b,; Ehrlich & Barry, 1989; Hartley & Jensen, 1991,; Irvine & Berhmann, 1986; McDonald & Pearce, 1995; McDonald & van Sommers, 1993; Mentis & Prutting, 1987; Milton et al., 1984; Payne-Johnson, 1986).

In an effort to redress the inadequacy of the standardized language assessments often used in investigating TBI subjects, Hinchliffe, Murdoch, and Chenery (1998) examined 25 people who had suffered a severe TBI, using a test battery that allowed assessment of language function across different modalities and along a heirachy of complexity, structure, and predictability. The primary focus of the test battery, which is displayed in Table 9-1, was on oral language and it was based on the Hinchliffe, Murdoch, and Chenery (1998) conceptual model of verbal communicative competence, which is reproduced here in Figure 9-1. This model represents schematically the interplay between linguistic and other cognitive processes and emphasizes the contribution of a proficient language system to the achievement of communicative competence. In this model, a proficient language system embraces primary and higher-order linguistic functions. The test battery used by Hinchliffe, Murdoch, and Chenery (1998) therefore included tests that evaluate primary language processes, as well as tests designed to examine the integrity of linguistic skill on complex and linguistically demanding tasks.

***Table* 9-1.** Comprehensive language test battery for TBI subjects (Hinchliffe, Murdoch, & Chenery, 1998).

	Abbreviation
PRIMARY LANGUAGE TESTS	
Western Aphasia Battery	WAB
Spontaneous Speech	SS
Auditory Comprehension	AC
Repetition	WR
Naming	NAM
Reading Comprehension	RE
Boston Diagnostic Test of Aphasia	BDAE
Complex Ideational Material	IM
Reading Comprehension	RC
Boston Naming Test	BNT
Neurosensory Center Comprehensive Examination of Aphasia	NCCEA
Sentence Repetition	SR
Sentence Construction	SC
The Revised Token Test	TT
HIGHER ORDER LANGUAGE TESTS	
Test of Language Competence - Expanded	TLC-E
Ambiguous Sentences	AM
Listening Comprehension	LC
Oral Expression	OE
Figurative Language	FL
Remembering Word Pairs	RW
The Word Test - Revised	TWT
Associations	AS
Synonyms	SY
Semantic Absurdities	SA
Antonyms	AN
Definitions	DEF
Multiple Definitions	MD
The Test of Word Knowledge	TOWK
Conjunctions and Transitions	CAT
Wiig-Semel Test of Linguistic Concepts	WS
The Right Hemisphere Language Battery	RHLB
Metaphor Picture Test	MP
Metaphor Written Test	MW
Comprehension of Inferred Meaning	IN
Appreciation of Humor	HU
Lexical-Semantics	LS
Emphatic Stress	ES

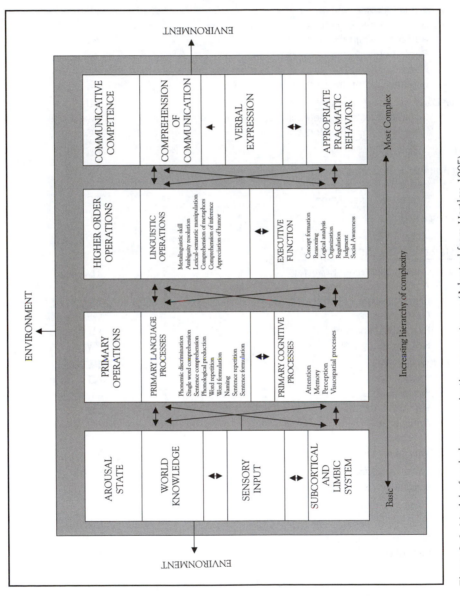

Figure 9-1. Model of verbal communicative competence (Adapted from Hartley, 1995)

The results indicated that, when compared with matched controls, individuals recovering from TBI had minor deficits in primary language function as measured by traditional tests of aphasia, but the differences in performance between the TBI subjects and their matched controls were further pronounced on language tasks, which are more demanding on metalinguistics and the lexical-semantic system.

Performance by TBI Subjects on Standardized Tests of Primary Language Function

The findings of Hinchliffe, Murdoch, and Chenery (1998) supported those of previous investigations that have identified, in groups of TBI subjects, deficiencies in confrontation naming, verbal associative tasks, auditory comprehension (Levin et al., 1976; Sarno, 1980, 1984; Sarno et al., 1986), and reading comprehension (Sarno, 1984). While their results revealed such deficits on rudimentary linguistic tasks, the subjects in the Hinchliffe, Murdoch, and Chenery sample did not display symptoms typical of the aphasic syndromes demonstrated by head-injured persons described in earlier research reports (Groher, 1977; Heilman et al., 1971; Levin et al., 1976; Sarno et al., 1986). Indeed, in describing the performance by the subject group on tests of naming (the Object Naming subtest of the WAB and the Boston Naming Test), Hinchliffe, Murdoch, and Chenery (1998) concluded that the TBI subjects had linguistic impairments that were qualitatively and quantitatively different from the impairments encountered by sufferers of focal cerebral lesions, but they were nonetheless deficient on these tasks when compared to non-brain-damaged controls. In particular, the error behavior on tests of naming did not reflect symptoms observed in the classic description of anomic aphasia (Geschwind, 1971). Instead, the error behavior of the TBI subjects resembled that of the normal control subjects, with delayed word retrieval and self-cueing of correct responses through semantic association and circumlocution.

Performance by TBI Subjects on Tests of Higher-Order Language Function

Standardized assessments of linguistic proficiency that test metalinguistic competence, integrative language skills, and the ability to manipulate the lexical-semantic system have been shown to discriminate consistently between TBI subjects and their matched controls (Hinchliffe, Chenery, & Murdoch, 1998). Error analysis of the performance by the subjects with TBI on subtests of the Test of Language Competence-Expanded edition, Level 2 (TLC-E) (Wiig & Secord, 1989) by Hinchliffe, Chenery, and Murdoch (1998) revealed key features of the higher-order language abilities after TBI.

The TBI subjects had difficulty recognizing and expressing alternate interpretations of ambiguities in sentences, reflecting inefficiency in achieving lexical access and shifting cognitive-linguistic set (Wiig, Alexander, & Secord, 1988). Difficulty on the TLC-E listening comprehension tasks revealed reduced ability to attend to salient information and integrate information in order to recognize plausible inferences or draw logical conclusions. The TLC-E was also shown to be a sensitive measure of the verbal planning and monitoring ability of individuals with TBI. The Oral Expression subtest of the TLC-E requires cognitive flexibility, conceptual integration, and lexical access and choice, as well as synthesis and monitoring of semantic, syntactic, and pragmatic variables (Bock, 1982; Wiig et al., 1988). Performance by the TBI subjects on this subtest was marked by response behavior suggestive of impulsivity and lack of reflection, evaluation, and planning. Because of such task behavior, the TBI subjects had difficulty in monitoring the linguistic integrity and relevance of the sentence and often produced sentences that were semantically, pragmatically, and/or syntactically deviant.

Hinchliffe, Murdoch, and Chenery (1998) also found the subjects with TBI in their study to be significantly less competent than matched control subjects in explaining the meaning of the metaphorical expressions included in the Figurative Language (FL) subtest of the TLC-E. This task requires the subjects to verbally interpret a metaphoric statement and then to match this statement to another expression denoting the same meaning. Previous investigators (Towne & Entwistle, 1993; Wiig & Secord, 1985) had found that TBI subjects who had attained relatively high levels of cognitive functioning, as measured by the Rancho Los Amigos Level of Cognitive Functioning Scale (LOCF; Hagen, 1984), were able to perform similarly to normal control subjects on this task. In contrast, Hinchliffe, Murdoch and Chenery (1998) found that despite relatively high LOCF scores, their subjects with TBI had difficulty transcending literal meanings in order to interpret the figurative expressions. Difficulty with interpreting figurative language may reflect reduced appreciation of the denotation of words (Zurif, Caramazza, Myerson, & Galvin, 1974) and diminished acceptance of connotative language (Gardner & Denes, 1973). The poor performance by the TBI group on this task could also be attributed to poor formulation of verbal explanation as well as failure to utilize contextual cues to determine the nonliteral meaning of the sentence.

The Word Test - Revised (Huisingh, Barrett, Bachman, Blagcen, & Orman,1990) was found to be sensitive to disorders of expressive vocabulary and semantic ability following TBI (Hinchliffe, Murdoch, & Chenery, 1998). The TBI group attained significantly lower scores than their matched controls on all the tasks that required them to make semantic associations, recognize and explain semantic incongruity, retrieve semantically similar or opposite words, recognize alternate meanings of words, and formulate explanations containing critical semantic elements in order to define nouns and verbs. Poor performances on these tasks reflect impaired verbal planning and reasoning; difficulty recognizing and expressing critical semantic attributes of words; poor organization, categorization, and recall of lexical items; and depressed mental flexibility.

Although little attention has been given to the impact of right hemisphere brain damage on the language function of people with TBI, it has been suggested that communicative behaviors seen in TBI patients resemble language disorders associated with right hemisphere damage (McDonald, 1993a). In TBI, the right and left cerebral hemispheres are equally vulnerable to damage, and it is well recognized that the right cerebral hemisphere has a significant role in normal language processing (Bryan, 1988, 1989; Code, 1987). Hinchliffe, Murdoch, and Chenery (1998) found that four of the six subtests of the Right Hemisphere Language Battery (RHLB; Bryan, 1989) proved to be difficult for the TBI subjects with TBI in their study. Performances on the Metaphor Picture Test (MP) revealed that the subjects with TBI were significantly less adept at comprehending figurative speech than the normal controls, even when supportive contextual cues were available. The subjects with TBI demonstrated a disruption in the comprehension of implicature and appreciation of connotative meaning (Winner & Gardner, 1977). This difficulty is consistent with the performance of the TBI group on the Figurative Language subtest of the TLC-E. The subjects with

TBI made significantly more errors on the Inferential Meaning test (IN) of the RHLB than their matched controls. This finding further attests to the apparent difficulty that TBI subjects encounter in appreciating the implicature in messages. It seems that the TBI subjects fail to utilize the information provided in order to draw a conclusion. It is uncertain as to whether the deficit lies in the failure to correctly perceive and attend to salient detail or in the failure to make use of the contextual information in order to make an inference.

The subjects with TBI attained a significantly poorer score than the control group on the Humor (HU) subtest of the RHLB. In this task the subjects heard an unfinished joke and were instructed to select an appropriate punch line to complete the joke. Right-hemisphere-damaged (RHD) patients have been found to perform poorly on this task and display a tendency to select irrelevant endings. This behavior is said to indicate that the RHD subjects appreciate that the joke must end in surprise, but they cannot determine the ending that is tied coherently with the body of the joke (Brownell, Michel, Powelson, & Gardner, 1983). The TBI subjects in the Hinchliffe, Murdoch, and Chenery (1998) study did not favor one type of ending in their erroneous selections. Poor performance on this task provides further evidence of failure by the TBI subjects to integrate across a narrative unit, attend to salient semantic information, and appreciate implied meaning.

There is evidence, therefore, that impairments in the language system following TBI can be delineated using standardized and sensitive measures of linguistic function. It is important, however, to use a test battery that appropriately reflects the complexity of the mature language system in order to delineate the nature of the language behavior of subjects with TBI. The use of a single language measure, such as naming, or measures of primary language function only, gives limited information as to the nature and extent of the language profile of the person with TBI and may lead to inappropriate generalizations regarding the entire language system following TBI (Chapman et al., 1995).

The use of a comprehensive battery of language measures provides a means to reliably assess improvements in language performance over time and a foundation on which to base understanding of the deficits realized in discourse behavior. Tests that tax the ability to integrate linguistic and nonlinguistic components of communication and metalinguistic ability have been shown to consistently discriminate between the present sample of TBI subjects and normal control subjects. These tests have the advantage of isolating linguistic and cognitive-linguistic tasks and assessing the ability of people with TBI to manipulate the semantic system under varying contextual constraints. Therefore, they provide the examiner with snapshots of an individual's ability to successfully use the fundamental components of language: language content, form, and use.

The Relationship Between Linguistic and Cognitive Functioning Following TBI

The management of individuals with TBI in a clinical setting involves a team of rehabilitation specialists. Clinicians strive to provide a comprehensive and integrated rehabilitation program based on the collective results of their specialist examinations and clinical observations. A frequent clinical challenge is to understand the interrelationship between the TBI person's performance in various specialist tests and the extent to which the performance in standardized tests reflects functional ability. There is, however, little available literature that guides clinical judgement or supports clinical observations regarding the interrelationship of clinical language and cognitive impairments following TBI.

It is well established philosophically that developmental language and cognition are entwined (Bloom & Lahey, 1978; Piaget & Inhelder, 1969; Vygotsky, 1962) and several aspects of cognition that may affect language have been identified (American Speech-Language-Hearing Association [ASHA], 1987). Characteristics of language behavior have also been described in relation to the stages of cognitive recovery following TBI by Malkmus (as cited in Kennedy & DeRuyter, 1991). While these well-grounded descriptions are based on extensive clinical observation, there is little empirical evidence resulting from attempts to delineate how deficits in language and cognitive processes coexist after TBI and subsequently affect communicative competence.

There have been some attempts to examine the relationship between scores on cognitive tests and discourse performances in the TBI population (Chapman, et al., 1992; Dennis & Barnes, 1990; Hartley & Jensen, 1991). Few, however, have examined the relationship between nondiscourse clinical measures of language and cognition. In an attempt to understand the impact of language and cognitive functioning on discourse behavior, Hartley and Jensen (1991) examined the association between the performance of 11 TBI subjects on the oral language subtests of the WAB, the Logical Memory and Digit Span subtests of the Weschler Memory Scale, Form I (Weschler, 1945), and measures of discourse function across three discourse tasks. The results showed the patterns of significant correlations between measures of discourse and the language and memory scores differed according to the discourse task. Significant correlations between the language and memory scores, however, occurred on only three occasions. These occurred between the Logical Memory score and the Spontaneous Speech Content, Speech Fluency, and Naming scores of the WAB.

Coppens (1995) found that the performance by TBI subjects on basic measures of language function could be dissociated from their performance on clinical measures of cognitive functioning. This conclusion was based on the results from a principal component analysis that yielded a two-factor model. One factor was considered representative of cognitive and visuospatial measures, whereas the other factor contained the language variables. It should be noted, however, that in some instances the differences in factor loadings was minimal and the resultant factor allocation debatable. The extent to which cognition and language can be dissociated from one another in such instances is, therefore, debatable.

In the effort to define the nature of the language and communicative impairments following TBI, there has been an abundance of investigations into the discourse behavior of TBI subjects. Recent reviews of this literature pertaining to functional discourse skills of TBI subjects have, however, identified the need for increased understanding of the underlying bases of discourse deficits (Chapman et al., 1995; Coelho, 1995). To achieve this, a comprehensive, conceptual approach that examines the complex interrelationships across cognitive and language functions at multiple levels is required.

The conceptual model of verbal communicative competence presented in Figure 9.1 represents schematically the interplay between linguistic and other cognitive processes and emphasizes the contribution of a proficient language system to the achievement of oral communicative competence. In this model, a proficient language system embraces primary and higher-order linguistic functions, which together with input from primary and higher-order cognitive processes, form the substratum of discourse ability and communicative competence. The model does not isolate language from cognition, but identifies the functions, at all levels, that are considered to be language operations.

Hinchliffe, Murdoch, and Chenery (1998) examined the interrelationships between performances on clinical measures of language and cognition following TBI. Comprehensive batteries of language and neuropsychological function that examine skills at multiple levels of function were administered to 23 subjects with severe TBI. The subtests were grouped according to the aspects of language or cognition they assessed, and correlational analyses were conducted to affirm these groupings. This resulted in the formation of a total of five language factors and four neuropyschological factors. The five language factors were considered to measure basic auditory comprehension, naming, lexical-semantic skill, sentential-semantic skill, and complex/integrative auditory comprehension. The four neuropsychology factors measured attention, memory and learning, visuospatial and visual memory, and oral fluency.

In order to detail the nature of the relationship between the language and neuropsychological factors, Pearson product-moment correlations for pairs of variables were performed on the five language and four neuropsychology factors (See Table 9-2). The correlations between language and neuropsychological factors illuminated to some extent the nature of the relationship between aspects of language and cognition.

The performance by the TBI subject group on tests of memory was found to correlate highly with the language factors representing auditory comprehension, lexical semantics, and sentential-semantics. Interestingly the memory factor was more strongly associated with the language factor representing basic auditory comprehension than with the factor representing higher-level comprehension of inferred information, abstract concepts, and metaphorical expressions. On consideration, this is not surprising, given that the basic auditory comprehension factor, although simpler conceptually, placed greater demand on immediate verbal memory and working memory than did the complex/integrative comprehension factor.

The basic auditory comprehension factor contained the Revised Token Test (McNeil & Prescott, 1978), which requires subjects to process auditory commands of increasing length and syntactic complexity. The scoring system for this test allows the measurement of the accuracy and efficiency of response behavior. A review of the error behavior apparent in the present TBI group revealed that more errors occurred on the longer commands, which contained a higher number of critical semantic elements. Often test scores were reduced by delayed response behavior, including self-correction, self-repetition of the command, and requests for repetition of the command.

These findings support earlier research (Coppens, 1995; Irvine & Behrmann, 1986), which found subjects with TBI to be deficient on the Token Test commands that were greater in length. While sentence comprehension requires both lexical and semantic competence (Butler-Hinze et al., 1990), one can accept that impaired auditory-verbal memory would contribute to inefficiency and inaccuracy on this task (Reitan & Wolfson, 1987).

Table 9-2. Correlations between performances by CHI subjects on language and neuropsychological factors.

	FAC	FNAM	FLSEM	FSENT	FCOMP	FATT	FMEM	FVIS	FOF
FAC	1.000								
FNAM	0.456	1.000							
FLSEM	0.745**	0.497*	1.000						
FSENT	0.676**	0.723**	0.737**	1.000					
FCOMP	0.487*	0.801**	0.608**	0.785**	1.000				
FATT	0.585*	0.132	0.688**	0.489*	0.351	1.000			
FMEM	0.622**	0.547*	0.622**	0.688**	0.537*	0.597*	1.000		
FVIS	0.253	0.011	0.424	0.559*	0.529*	0.396	0.328	1.000	
FOF	0.416	0.311	0.464	0.559*	0.529*	0.396	0.458	0.118	1.000

Note: * = Significant $p < 0.01$; ** = Significant $p < 0.001$; FAC = Basic auditory comprehension factor; FNAM = Naming factor; FLSEM = Lexical-semantic factor; FSENT = Sentential-semantic factor; FCOMP = Complex/integrative language factor; FATT = Attention factor; FMEM = Verbal memory and learning factor; FVIS = Visual memory and visuospatial factor; FOF = Oral fluency factor.

The factor representing attention correlated strongly with the language factor representing lexical-semantic manipulation, and to a lesser extent with the factors representing sentential-semantics and basic auditory comprehension (see Table 9-2). The tasks in the lexical-semantic factor were four subtests from TWT-R, including Synonyms, Antonyms, Associations, and Definitions. These tasks were designed to yield information about the subject's ability to recognize and express the critical semantic attributes of their lexicon (Huisingh et al., 1990). Poor performances on these tasks may therefore reflect difficulty recognizing and expressing critical semantic attributes of words, poor semantic memory, poor semantic organization, and/or reduced efficiency of access to semantic memory.

Several researchers (Goldstein, Levin, Boake, & Lohrey, 1990, Haut & Shutty, 1992; Levin & Goldstein, 1986) have examined semantic processing in TBI groups. These investigations have consistently found less-efficient semantic processing but the absence of a specific deficit in the accessing and recognition of semantic relations by TBI subjects. They speculated that, while TBI subjects retain the capacity to engage semantic processes, they require greater cognitive effort and additional attentional resources to do so. Reduced attentional mechanisms may therefore underlie the reduced efficiency with which semantic analysis can occur (Goldstein et al., 1990). In the present study, the high correlation between the neuropsychological factor representing complex attentional processing on offline tasks and the lexical-semantic factor, supports the notion of an association between attentional skills and semantic processing. Schmitter-Edgecombe, Marks, and Fahy (1993), on the other hand, found that increasing attentional processing demands on a semantic priming task did not affect the ability of the TBI group to process semantic information and access the semantic network. It may be, however, that the attentional demands applied to the task designed by Schmitter-Edgecombe et al. (1993) did not sufficiently tax the attentional resources of the TBI subjects in order to display their deficits in attention-driven processes.

It is interesting to note that the oral fluency factor, which consisted of the COWAT, did not correlate highly with the language factors, and was not even weakly associated with the performance on the other neuropsychological factors. This finding has interesting clinical implications, considering that the COWAT is often used to represent testing for language function in research and clinical environments. Clinically, this further emphasizes the need to examine language beyond lexical retrieval and highlights the inadequacy of making assumptions about the integrity of the language system based on contextual lexical retrieval skills.

There is, therefore, evidence to suggest an influential association between the cognitive processes of memory and attention, and ability with linguistic manipulations following TBI. The data available to date is, however, insufficient to determine whether the relationship between cognitive deficits and language impairment is linear or causative. Recent evidence suggests that a clearer understanding of the relationship between language and cognitive disturbances in TBI may be best achieved through the establishment of homogeneous groups within the TBI population (Chapman, et al.,1995; Coppens, 1995; Peach, 1992). The identification of subgroups of TBI subjects with common profiles of language and cognitive deficits may assist in the defining of cognitive and language associations following TBI.

While impairment in cognitive functioning following TBI is unquestionable and pervasive, it can be argued that the impairments in the linguistic system are real, clinically identifiable, and should be considered fundamental to breakdown in communicative competence.

Variability in Language Outcomes Following TBI: A Case for Subgroups

A major difficulty faced by investigators of TBI is the hallmark heterogeneity of its neurobehavioral sequelae. High degrees of individual variability have been frequently described by investigators of language and discourse abilities in TBI subjects (Groher, 1977; Hartley & Levin, 1990; Levin et al., 1976; Sarno et al., 1986). Peach (1992) has highlighted the fact that many conclusions regarding the integrity of the language system following TBI have been based on the collective performance of heterogeneous groups of TBI subjects. His study controlled for neurological heterogeneity in an attempt to isolate the effects of predominantly diffuse neurological damage on language function following TBI. Peach found that some subjects in his sample displayed definite language impairment on language subtests in the absence of focal lesions as identified by computed tomograpy (CT) scan.

Several investigators have suggested that the discourse profiles of TBI subjects can be distinguished according to pathophysiological features. Hartley and Jensen (1992) described three distinct patterns of discourse behaviors, which they proposed reflected different patterns of neuropathological damage after TBI. Chapman et al. (1992) also identified discourse profiles in children with TBI, which resembled the discourse behaviors of people with circumscribed frontal lesions. McDonald (1993b) proposed that the discourse behaviors observed in TBI groups are attributable to the deficits in frontal lobe functioning, as indicated by performances on neuropsychological tests. Elsewhere, McDonald and Pearce (1995) acknowledge that consideration of the group performance of a TBI sample on a discourse task may dilute distinct performance patterns within the group. Collectively, these findings highlight the need to establish homogeneous subgroups with respect to language function within the TBI population.

Reliable grouping of TBI subjects on the basis of neuropathological features for the purposes of examining their communication profiles is problematic. Subgrouping based on lesion focus may be limited by the availability of sensitive neuroradiological techniques. Studies have shown that CT scanning and, to a lesser extent, magnetic resonance imaging (MRI), fail to detect many focal lesions following TBI (Goldenberg, Oder, Spatt, & Podreka, 1992; Wilson & Wyper, 1992). In addition, the findings of these neuroimaging techniques have not always been found to correlate with clinical signs (Goldenberg et al., 1992; Levin, Williams, Eisenberg, High, & Guinto, 1992; Vilkki, Holst, Ohman, Servo, & Heiskanen, 1992).

Through the study of focal brain function, the existence of certain brain-behavior relationships have been well described and understood. The same research however, warns that even for the most highly circumscribed functions such as language, anatomoclinical correlations are not absolute, and a focal lesion can manifest itself very differently in distinct individuals (Basso, Lecours, Moraschini, & Vanier, 1985). It appears that there may exist interindividual differences in brain organization for cognition. Such differences are further influenced by a unique set of intrinsic and extrinsic factors and result in diverse patterns of language skill and communicative style (Joanette, Ska, Poissant, & Beland, 1992). Intrinsic factors, such as sex and handedness, along with extrinsic factors, including premorbid language ability, personality, speaking style, and demographic features affecting sociolinguistic characteristics, are all influential components in achieving communicative competence following TBI.

A priori subgrouping of TBI samples based on severity indicators would also be problematic since severity scales, such as the Glasgow Coma Scale (GCS), have been demonstrated to be unreliable predictors of language function (Groher, 1977; Levin et al., 1976; Sarno et al., 1986). Recently, Coppens (1995) proposed that a more relevant approach to examining subgroups within a TBI sample would be to classify the TBI subjects in a similar way to aphasics, that is, according to their pattern of linguistic and cognitive symptomatology, independent of severity levels. Coppens' study identified four distinct groups with differing patterns of cognitive-linguistic performance. He distinguished memory from other cognitive functioning and found one group to demonstrate largely visuospatial-cognitive impairment, another to have language-memory impairments, a third group to demonstrate globally depressed skills, and a fourth group to display poor language performance in the presence of relatively good cognitive, visuospatial, and discourse skills. Coppens' findings indicated that while interactions between cognition and language skills existed in some cases, low cognitive scores were not necessarily indicative of low language scores. Coppens argued that the performance of one group, with high overall language scores in the presence of poor scores on general cognition and visuospatial tasks, indicated that language skill and cognition can be dissociated in TBI. The presence of another group in Coppens' study, however, which demonstrated globally depressed scores, supported the notion of global disorganization of language and cognition following TBI (Hagen, 1984; Wiig et al., 1988).

Hinchliffe, Murdoch, Chenery, Baglioni, and Harding-Clark (1998) used hierarchical cluster analysis in order to determine whether their sample of 23 subjects with severe TBI were universally impaired on cognitive-linguistic tasks or consisted of individuals who possessed pockets of preserved ability. In addition, they conducted a Q-type factor analysis (McKeown & Thomas, 1988) in order to determine whether there existed subgroups of TBI subjects who possessed similar cognitive-linguistic profiles independent of the severity of dysfunction. The cluster analysis revealed that the TBI subjects in this sample were not universally impaired on language and neuropsychological factors. Four subgroups emerged from the analysis, which varied in their patterns of impairment across the language and neuropsychological factors. The groups were described as "close to normal language", "attention and visual impairment", "global impairment with spared visual skills" and "global impairment with spared memory." All four subgroups differed significantly from the control subjects on the lexical-semantic, sentential-semantic, complex comprehension, oral fluency, and attention factors. These factors were therefore found to be consistently impaired and could be said to represent the cardinal cognitive-linguistic impairments following TBI.

The first subgroup derived from the analysis represented the group of TBI subjects who were generally operating at levels close to the normal controls. When impairment was present, it was mild in comparison with the other TBI subgroups and was confined to the cardinal impairments. This illustrates that the functional areas that appear most vulnerable to disruption in this sample of subjects with severe TBI are tasks that involve lexical-semantic access and manipulation, complex auditory comprehension, and attentional processes.

Deficits in sentential-semantics as well as lexical-semantics were further apparent in comparison to the normal naming and mild auditory comprehension problems of the "attention and visual impairment" subgroup members. These subgroup members had marked deficits in tasks requiring attentional processing. Deficits in memory were also present, but not as remarkable as the attentional impairment.

The two "global impairment" subgroups saw a general decline in language function. In one subgroup, however, this was accompanied by comparatively superior visuospatial abilities. While members of this subgroup displayed problems across the language system, their performances on the factors pertaining to auditory comprehension were noticeably worse than the other three subgroups. The decline in performance by these group members on the comprehension factor was accompanied by a marked decrease in performance on the memory factor and attentional factor tasks.

In general, subjects in the "global impairment with spared memory" subgroup displayed poor performances on the language factors when compared with the other subgroups. In contrast to the other two impaired subgroups, however, this subgroup was not as impaired on the neuropsychological factors of attention and memory. This result substantiates the suggested relationships between memory and auditory comprehension skills, and between attentional and lexical-semantics skills.

These results contrast with earlier studies (Heilman et al., 1971; Levin et al., 1976; Thompsen, 1975) in that a naming disorder, as measured mainly by confrontation naming tests, was neither a constant nor prominent feature of the impairment patterns in the present TBI group. While the TBI sample as a whole displayed impaired performance on naming when compared to controls, this difference was in fact accounted for by a portion of the TBI sample only. Similarly, performances on tasks relating to visuospatial facility, visual memory, short-term verbal recall, verbal learning, and auditory processing of simple information were not uniformly deficient. The subgroups that did show deficits in these areas were generally more severely impaired on all aspects of language and neuropsychological function. It may be considered, therefore, that tests of naming, basic auditory comprehension, and memory may be useful in alerting the clinician to the global nature and severity of impairment experienced by the individual with TBI. In the same light, restricting assessment to these primary tests of language could, however, fail to delineate the deficiencies in higher-order linguistic operations in some individuals.

The language and neuropsychological factors that were consistently impaired in this sample of TBI subjects included tasks that measured (a) the application of metalinguistic competence, (b) integrative language and reasoning skills, (c) divergent production and mental flexibility, and (d) semantic judgement, organization and retrieval (Huisingh et al., 1990; Wiig & Secord 1989, 1992). Along with impairments in these areas, each subgroup in this sample experienced deficits in tests requiring sustained and controlled attention and concentration. Together, these deficits represent the cardinal cognitive-linguistic impairments following TBI in this sample. The cooccurrence of higher-order attentional deficits and impairments in higher-order linguistic operations supports suggestions that maximum sustained attention and concentration is required to participate in verbal logical reasoning and interactive verbal behavior (Adamovich, 1990).

Given that the cluster analysis revealed that the subjects with TBI were not universally impaired in language and neuropsychological functions, the Q-type factor analysis was applied to investigate the presence of patterns or profiles of impairment. This technique has been used elsewhere in the examination of subgroups of TBI subjects (Coppens, 1995). Hinchliffe, Murdoch, Chenery, Baglioni, and Harding-Clark (1998) reported that the results of the Q-type factor analysis confirmed the major outcome of the cluster analysis: that is, that performances on the higher-order linguistic operations, namely those that involve lexical-semantics, sentential-semantics, complex comprehension, and oral fluency, along with performances on the neuropsychological attentional factor tasks are constantly impaired. The profiles of the Q-sorted groups reveal that the relative relationships between these factors change across the groups but do not tend to contribute to the distinction between groups. As with the cluster analysis, it is the performance on naming, memory, and visually related tasks that best highlight the differences between the groups.

The Q-sorted grouping conducted by Hinchliffe, Murdoch, Chenery, Baglioni and Harding-Clark (1998) revealed five contrasting patterns of linguistic and neuropsychological impairment in their sample of TBI subjects. Q-subgroup 1 displayed relatively preserved naming and verbal memory scores in the presence of relatively impaired visuospatial and visual memory skills. The reverse pattern occurred for subjects in Q-subgroup 2. This finding suggests a dissociation between performance on visually-related cognitive tasks and verbal memory and naming ability. The performance profiles in these groups suggest a possible dependency of naming skill on verbal memory skill.

The presence of Q-subgroup 5, however, contradicts this relationship and adds a further contrasting performance to Q-subgroups 1 and 2. Like Q-subgroup 1, Q-subgroup 5 members had relatively spared verbal memory skills but this was not accompanied by a relative sparing of naming ability. The memory tasks in the verbal memory factor involve the use of short-term storage of information and working memory (Lezak, 1995). These tasks, along with the tasks included in the naming and oral fluency factors, also involve the activation of semantic memory. Speed of access to semantic memory has been found to be impaired in TBI subjects (Baddely, Harris, Sunderland, Watts, & Wilson, 1987). It may be that a deficit in semantic memory is underpinning the apparent disorders on the naming, oral fluency, and verbal memory factors.

Q-subgroups 3 and 4 collectively could correspond to Coppens' (1995) "global" group in that there did not appear to be any particular area of preserved skill. Q-subgroup 3 subjects can be considered to be globally impaired with dominant neuropsychological deficits. In contrast, subjects within Q-subgroup 4 may be best described as being globally impaired with dominant linguistic deficits.

The existence of a double dissociation between verbal memory and naming skills, strongly suggests the presence of distinct subgroups in the sample of TBI subjects used by Hinchliffe, Murdoch, Chenery, Baglioni, and Harding-Clark (1998). It does not appear possible to conceptualize these subgroups as simply having cognitive disorders with or without subsequent language disorders (Hagen, 1984). Rather, it is the nature of the relationship between the various subsystems of cognition and language that effectively separated the groups. The results of the study by Hinchliffe, Murdoch, Chenery, Baglioni, and Harding-Clark (1998) confirm Coppens' conclusion that impairment in cognitive skills does not necessarily predict an equivalent degree of impairment in language skills. This assertion does not support the notion of global disorganization (Hagen, 1984; Wiig et al., 1988), which holds that language and communicative impairment will present as a manifestation of impaired cognitive abilities.

No subject in the Hinchliffe, Murdoch, Chenery, Baglioni, and Harding-Clark (1998) sample of subjects with severe TBI was spared verbal impairment, although the verbal impairment was not consistently evidenced in all tasks. This finding highlights the need to comprehensively examine the linguistic system so that the higher-order language operations are investigated. These linguistic functions, which subsume facility with pragmatic communication and discourse (Dennis & Barnes, 1990; Wiig & Secord, 1989) were found to be constantly impaired.

Summary

Investigations of the language function of people recovering from TBI have consistently shown that subjects with TBI perform relatively well, and in a manner different from that of individuals with focal neurological lesions, on aphasia test batteries. TBI subjects tend to display minor deficits on tasks involving naming, verbal associative skills, and basic auditory and reading comprehension. While TBI subjects have been found to be deficient in these areas when compared to non-brain-damaged control subjects, examination of the TBI subjects' response behavior and error patterns support the notion that TBI subjects have linguistic impairments that are qualitatively and quantitatively different from those encountered by sufferers of focal cerebral lesions.

Standardized tests that assess metalinguistic competence, integrative language skills, and the ability to manipulate the semantic system under varying contextual constraints have been found to consistently discriminate between TBI and control subject groups. In addition, subjects with TBI have been found to be impaired on tasks requiring complex attention, verbal memory and learning, executive function, and visual memory and visuospatial skills.

It appears that there are be some aspects of linguistic and cognitive function that may be constant across samples of people with severe TBI. These cardinal impairments include deficits in lexical-semantic and sentential-semantic skills, complex auditory comprehension, oral fluency, and attentional processes. Deficits in the primary language processes of basic auditory comprehension and naming, and in the cognitive tasks involving verbal memory, visual memory and visuospatial skills are neither constant nor prominent features of impairment in TBI. It is possible that these areas may be generally less vulnerable to impairment following TBI, and the presence of such deficits may well serve to distinguish TBI subjects in terms of severity and profile type. Indeed, the presence of these deficits in the cognitive-linguistic profile of TBI subjects may indicate generalized impairment and increased severity of dysfunction.

It is unlikely that the ability to perform cognitive and language tasks following TBI is dissociable. Neither does it appear that there is necessarily global disorganization of language and cognitive skills following TBI. Instead, it seems likely that there exist strong and consistent influential associations between aspects of linguistic proficiency and cognitive function. Performance by TBI subjects on tests of verbal memory and learning have been found to correlate highly with performances on tests involving auditory comprehension, lexical-semantics, and sentential-semantics. Additionally, performances on tests involving attentional processes have been found to correlate strongly with the ability to perform language tasks involving lexical-semantic manipulation, and to a lesser extent with tasks requiring sentential-semantic and basic auditory comprehension skills. The pattern of involvement of certain cognitive and language subsystems found to occur after TBI serves to distinguish TBI subjects and elucidates the existence of discrete subgroups within the heterogenous TBI population. While further research using larger samples of TBI subjects is required, there is enough evidence to suggest that future investigations should consider TBI as more than a unitary entity.

References

Adamovich, B. (1990). Information processing, cognition, attention and communication following closed-head injury. *Folia Phoniatre, 42*, 11–23.

American Speech-Language- Hearing Association (ASHA). (1987, June). Report of the subcommittee on language and cognition: The role of the speech-language pathologist in the habilitation and rehabilitation of cognitively impaired individuals. *American Speech and Hearing Association Journal*, 53–55.

American Speech-Language-Hearing Association. (1991). Guidelines for speech-language pathologists serving persons with language, socio-communicative and/or cognitive-communication impairments. *ASHA, 33*(Suppl. 5), 21–28.

Baddeley, A., Harris, J., Sunderland, A., Watts, K., &Wilson, B. (1987). Closed head injury and memory. In H. Levin, J. Grafman, H. Eisenberg (Eds.), *Neurobehavioral Recovery from Head Injury* (pp. 295–317). New York: Oxford University Press.

Baker, L. (1982). An evaluation of the role of metacognitive deficits in learning disabilities. *Topics in Learning and Learning Disabilities, 2,* 26–36.

Basso, A., Lecours, A.R., Moraschini, S., & Vanier, M. (1985). Anatomical correlations of the aphasias as defined through computerized tomography: Exceptions. *Brain and Language, 26,* 201–229.

Benjamin, L., Debinski, A., Fletcher, D., Hedger, C., Mealings, M., & Stewart-Scott, A. (1989). The use of the Bethesda Conversational Skills Profile in closed head injury. In V. Anderson & M. *Theory and Function: Bridging the Gap* (pp. 57–64). Melbourne: Australian Society for the Study of Brain Impairment.

Benson, D.F. (1967). Fluency in aphasia: Correlation with radioactive scan localization. *Cortex, 3,* 373–394.

Bloom, L. & Lahey, M. (1978). *Language Development and Language Disorders.* New York: Wiley.

Bock, J.K. (1982). Toward a cognitive psychology of syntax: Information processing contributions to sentence formulation. *Psychological Review, 89,* 1–47.

Braun, C.M. & Baribeau, J.M. (1987). Subclinical aphasia following closed head injury: A response to Sarno, Buonaguro and Levita. In R. Brookshire (Ed.), *Clinical Aphasiology, 17,* (pp.326–333). Minneapolis: BRK Publishers.

Brownell, H.H., Michel, D., Powelson, J., & Gardner, E. (1983). Surprise but not sensitivity to verbal humor in right hemisphere patients. *Brain and Language, 27,* 20–27.

Bryan, K. (1988). Assessment of language disorders after right hemisphere damage. *British Journal of Disorders of Communication, 23,* 111–125.

Bryan, K. (1989). *The Right Hemisphere Language Battery.* Southhampton: Far Communications.

Butler-Hinze, S., Caplan, D., & Waters, G. (1990). Characteristics of syntactic comprehension deficits following closed head injury versus cerebrovascular accident. *Journal of Speech and Hearing Research, 33,* 269–280.

Chapman, S., Culhane, K., Levin, H., Harward, H., Mendelson, D., Ewing-Cobbs, L., Fletcher, J., & Bruee, D. (1992). Narrative discourse after closed head injury in children and adolescents. *Brain and Language, 43,* 2–62.

Chapman, S., Levin, S., & Culhane, K. (1995). Language impairment in closed head injury. In S. Kirschner (Ed.), *Handbook of Neurological Speech and Language Disorders* (pp. 387–429). New York: Marcel Decker.

Code, C. (1987). *Language, Aphasia and the Right Hemisphere.* Chichester: John Wiley.

Coelho, C.A. (1995). Discourse production deficits following traumatic brain injury: A critical review of the recent literature. *Aphasiology, 9,* 409–429.

Coelho, C.A., Liles, B.Z., & Duffy, R.J. (1991a). Discourse analysis with closed head injured adults: Evidence for differing patterns of deficits. *Archives of Physical Medicine and Rehabilitation, 72,* 465–468.

Coelho, C.A., Liles, B.Z., & Duffy, R.J. (1991b). The use of discourse analyses for the evaluation of higher level traumatically brain-injured adults. *Brain Injury, 5,* 381–392.

Coppens, P. (1995). Subpopulations in closed head injury: Preliminary results. *Brain Injury, 9,* 195–208.

Dennis, M. & Barnes, M. (1990). Knowing the meaning, getting the point, bridging the gap and carrying the message: Aspects of discourse following closed head injury in childhood and adolescence. *Brain and Language, 39,* 428–446.

Ehrlich, J. & Barry, P. (1989). Rating communication behaviors in head-injured adults. *Brain Injury, 3,* 193–198.

Gardner, K. & Denes, G. (1973). Connotative judgements by aphasic patients on a pictorial adaption of the semantic differential. *Cortex, 9,* 183–412.

Geschwind, N. (1971). Current concepts: Aphasia. *North England Journal of Medicine, 284,* 645–656.

Goldenberg, G., Oder, W., Spatt, J., & Podreka, I. (1992). Cerebral correlates of disturbed executive function and memory in survivors of severe closed head injury: A SPECT study. *Journal of Neurology, Neurosurgery and Psychiatry, 55,* 362–368.

Goldstein, F., Levin, H., Boake, C., & Lohrey, J. (1990). Facilitation of memory performance through induced semantic processing in survivors of severe closed head injury. *Journal of Clinical and Experimental Neuropsychology, 12,* 286–300.

Groher, M. (1977). Language and memory disorders following closed head trauma. *Journal of Speech and Hearing Research, 20,* 212–223.

Hagen, C. (1984). Language disorders in head trauma. In A. Holland (Ed.), *Language Disorders in Adults: Recent Advances* (pp. 245–281). San Diego: College-Hill Press.

Halpern, H., Darley, F. L., & Brown, J. R. (1973). Differential language and neurologic characteristics in cerebral involvement. *Journal of Speech and Hearing Disorders, 38,* 162–173.

Hartley, L. (1995). *Cognitive-Communicative Abilities Following Brain Injury: A Functional Approach.* San Diego: Singular Publishing Group Inc.

Hartley, L. & Jensen, P.J. (1991). Narrative and procedural discourse after closed head injury. *Brain Injury, 6,* 271–281.

Hartley, L. & Jensen, P.J. (1992). Three discourse profiles of closed head injured speakers: Theoretical and clinical implications. *Brain Injury, 5,* 267–285.

Hartley, L., & Levin, H.S. (1990). Linguistic deficits after closed head injury: A current appraisal. *Aphasiology, 4,* 353–370.

Haut, M. & Shutty, M. (1992). Patterns of verbal learning after closed head injury. *Neuropsychology, 6,* 51–58.

Heilman, K.M., Safran, A., & Geschwind, N. (1971). Closed head trauma and aphasia. *Journal of Neurology, Neurosurgery and Psychiatry, 34,* 265–269.

Hinchliffe, F.J., Murdoch, B.E., & Chenery, H.J. (1998). Towards a conceptualization of language and cognitive impairment in closed head injury: use of clinical measures. *Brain Injury, 12,* 109–132.

Hinchliffe, F.J., Murdoch, B.E., Chenery, H.J., Baglioni, A.J., & Harding-Clark, J. (1998). Cognitive-linguistic subgroups in closed head injury. *Brain Injury, 12,* 369–398.

Holland, A.L. (1982). When is aphasia aphasia? The problem of closed head injury. In R. Brookshire (Ed.), *Clinical Aphasiology, Vol. 12* (pp. 345–349). Minneapolis: BRK Publishers.

Huisingh, R., Barrett, M., Bachman, L., Bagcen, C., & Orman, O. (1990). *The Word Test - Revised.* Illinois: Lingui Systems.

Irvine, L. & Behrmann, M. (1986). The communicative and cognitive deficits following closed head injury. *The South African Journal of Communication Disorders, 33,* 49–54.

Joanette, Y., Ska, B., Poissant, A., & Beland, R. (1992). Neuropsychological aspects of Alzheimer's disease: Evidence for inter- and intra- function heterogeneity. In F. Boller, Z. Khachaturain, M. Poncet, & Y. Christen (Eds.), *Heterogeneity of Alzheimer's Disease* (pp. 33–42). Berlin: Springer-Verlag.

Kennedy, M. & DeRuyter, F. (1991). Cognitive and language bases for communication disorders. In D. Beukelman & K. Yorkston (Eds.), *Communication Disorders Following Traumatic Brain Injury: Management of Cognitive, Language, and Motor Impairments* (pp. 123–190). Austin,TX: Pro-Ed.

Levin, H.S. & Goldstein, F.C. (1986). Organization of verbal memory after severe closed head injury. *Journal of Clinical and Experimental Neuropsychology, 8,* 643–656.

Levin, H.S., Grossman, R.G., & Kelly, P.J. (1976). Aphasia disorder in patients with closed head injury. *Journal of Neurology, Neurosurgery, and Psychiatry, 39,* 1062–1070.

Levin, H.S., Grossman, R.G., & Rose, S.E. (1979). Long term neuropsychological outcome of closed head injury. *Journal of Neurosurgery, 50,* 412–422.

Levin, H.S., Williams, D., Eisenberg, H., High, W., & Guinto, F. (1992). Serial MRI and neurobehavioral findings after mild to moderate closed head injury. *Journal of Neurology, Neurosurgery and Psychiatry, 55,* 255–262.

Lezak, M. (1995). *Neuropsychological Assessment* (3rd Ed.). New York: Oxford University Press.

Luria, A. (1970). *Traumatic Aphasia: Its Syndrome, Psychology and Treatment*. Mouton: The Hague.

Martin, A. (1990). Neuropsychology of Alzheimer's Disease: The case for subgroups. In M.F. Schwartz (Ed.), *Modular Deficits in Alzheimer-Type Dementia* (pp. 143–175). Cambridge, MA: MIT Press.

McDonald, S. (1992). Communication disorders following closed head injury: New approaches to assessment and rehabilitation. *Brain Injury, 6,* 283–292.

McDonald, S. (1993a). Viewing the brain sideways: Frontal versus right hemisphere explanations of non-aphasic language disorders. *Aphasiology, 7,* 535–549.

McDonald, S. (1993b). Pragmatic language skills after closed head injury: Ability to meet the information needs of the listener. *Brain and Language, 44,* 28–46.

McDonald, S. & Pearce, S. (1995). "The Dice Game" a new test of pragmatic language skills after closed head injury. *Brain Injury, 9,* 255–276.

McDonald, S. & van Sommers, P. (1993). Pragmatic language skills after closed head injury: Ability to negotiate requests. *Cognitive Neuropsychology, 10,* 297–315.

McKeown, B. & Thomas, D. (1988). *Q-Methodology.* Sage University paper series on quantitative applications in the social sciences, 07–066. Beverly Hills: Sage.

McNeil, M.R. & Prescott, T.E. (1978). *Revised Token Test.* Baltimore: University Park Press.

Mentis, M. & Prutting, C. (1987). Cohesion in the discourse of normal and head injured adults. *Journal of Speech and Hearing Research, 30,* 88–89.

Milton, S., Prutting, C., & Binder, G. (1984). Appraisal of communication competence in head injured adults. In R. Brookshire (Ed.), *Clinical Aphasiology, Vol. 14* (pp. 114–123). Minneapolis: BRK Publishers.

Najenson, T., Sazbon, L., Fiselzon, J., Becker, E., & Schechter, I. (1978). Recovery of communication functions after prolonged traumatic coma. *Scandinavian Journal of Rehabilitation Medicine, 10,* 15–21.

Parsons, C.L., Lambier, J., Snow, P., Couch, D., & Mooney, L. (1989). Conversational skills in closed head injury: Part 1. *Australian Journal of Human Communication Disorders, 17,* 37–46.

Payne-Johnson, J. (1986). Evaluation of communication competence in patients with closed head injury. *Journal of Communication Disorders, 19,* 237–249.

Peach, R.K. (1992). Factors underlying neuropsychological test performance in chronic severe traumatic brain injury. *Journal of Speech and Hearing Research, 35,* 810–818.

Piaget, J. & Inhelder, B (1969). *The Psychology of the Child.* New York: Basic Books.

Porch, B.E. (1967). *Porch Index of Communicative Ability.* Palo Alto, CA: Consulting Psychologists Press.

Prigatano, G., Roueche, J., & Fordyce, D. (1986). Nonaphasic language disturbances after brain injury. In G.P. Prigatano (Ed.), *Neuropsychological Rehabilitation After Brain Injury* (pp. 18–28). Baltimore: John Hopkins University Press.

Reitan, R.M. & Wolfson, D. (1987). Development, scoring and validation of the Neuropsychological Deficit Scale. In R.M. Reitan & D. Wolfson (Eds.),*Traumatic Brain Injury II: Recovery and Rehabilitation.* Tuscon, AZ: Neuropsychology Press.

Sarno, M. (1980). The nature of verbal impairment after closed head injury. *The Journal of Nervous and Mental Disease, 168 (11),* 685–692.

Sarno, M. (1984). Verbal impairment after closed head injury: Report of a replication study. *The Journal of Nervous and Mental Disease, 172 (8),* 475–479.

Sarno, M., Buonaguro, A., & Levita, E. (1986). Characteristics of verbal impairment in closed head injured patients. *Archives of Physical Medicine and Rehabilitation, 67,* 400–405.

Schmitter-Edgecombe, M., Marks, M., & Fahy, J. (1993). Semantic priming after severe closed head trauma: Automatic and attentional processing. *Neuropsychology, 7,* 136–148.

Spellacy, J.F. & Spreen, O. (1969). A short form of the Token Test. *Cortex, 5,* 390–397.

Spreen, O. & Benton, A. L. (1969). *Neurosensory Centre Comprehensive Examination for Aphasia: Manual for Directions.* Victoria, BC: University of Victoria.

Thompsen, I.V. (1975). Evaluation and outcome of aphasia in patients with severe closed head trauma. *Journal of Neurology, Neurosurgery and Psychiatry, 38,* 713–718.

Towne, R. & Entwistle, L. (1993). Metaphoric comprehension in adolescents with traumatic brain injury and adolescents with language learning disability. *Language, Speech and Hearing Sciences in Schools, 24,* 100–107.

Vilkki, J., Holst, P., Ohman, J., Servo, A., & Heiskanen, O. (1992). Cognitive test performances related to early and late computed tomography findings after closed-head injury. *Journal of Clinical and Experimental Neuropsychology, 14,* 518–532.

Vygotsky, L.S. (1962). *Thought and Language.* Cambridge, MA: The MIT Press.

Weschler, D. (1945). *Weschler Memory Scale Form 1.* New York: Psychological Corporation.

Wiig, E. (1984). Language disabilities in adolescents: A question of cognitive strategies. *Topics in Language Disorders, 4,* 41–58.

Wiig, E., Alexander, E., & Secord, W. (1988). Linguistic competence and level of cognitive functioning in adults with traumatic closed head injury. In H. Whitaker (Ed.), *Neuropsychological Studies of Nonfocal Brain Injury: Trauma and Dementia* (pp. 186-199). New York: Springer-Verlag.

Wiig, E. & Becker-Caplan, L. (1984). Linguistic retrieval strategies and word-finding difficulties among children with language disabilities. *Topics in Language Disorders, 4,* 1–18.

Wiig, E. & Secord, E. (1985). *Test of Language Competence.* Columbus, Ohio: Charles E. Merrill.

Wiig, E. & Secord, E. (1989). *Test of Language Competence-Expanded.* Columbus, Ohio: Charles E. Merrill.

Wiig, E. & Secord, E. (1992). *Test of Word Knowledge.* Columbus, Ohio: Charles E. Merrill.

Wilson, J. & Wyper, D. (1992). Neuroimaging and neuropsychological functioning following closed head injury: CT, MRI and SPECT. *Journal of Head Trauma Rehabilitation, 7,* 29–30.

Winner, E. & Gardner, H. (1977). The comprehension of metaphor in brain damaged patients. *Brain, 100,* 717–729.

Zurif, E.B., Caramazza, A., Myerson, R., & Galvin, J. (1974). Semantic feature representation for normal and aphasic language. *Brain and Language, 1,* 167–187.

CHAPTER

Ten

Discourse Production in Traumatic Brain Injury

Fiona J. Hinchliffe, Bruce E. Murdoch, and Deborah G. Theodoros

Introduction

Over the past decade the examination of communication deficits following traumatic brain injury (TBI) has been enhanced by the addition of discourse investigations. The impetus for looking beyond the status of the lexicon to discourse has arisen from the widely recounted failure of standardized language batteries to detect the subtle language deficits in individuals with TBI (Coelho, 1995; Snow, Douglas, & Ponsford, 1995). The fundamental criticism of such batteries is that they do not assess language function beyond the level of the sentence. As a result, TBI patients often display minimal problems on the most complex test tasks, giving the impression that their communication skills are functionally intact. The clinical presentation of the patient with TBI, however, is often contrary to the expected high level of competence delineated by the aphasia battery. In effect, it appears that the overestimated communicative performance of the TBI patient reflects the ceiling effect of aphasia batteries, which were designed to elucidate the disorders in elementary linguistic function experienced by sufferers of focal brain damage.

The observation that performances of TBI patients on standardized tests do not adequately explain the nature of their clinically observed communication problems was recognized by earlier researchers, who made an incidental comment on the notable impairments in conversation experienced by subjects with TBI (Levin, Grossman, & Kelly, 1976; Thompsen, 1975). Later, Prigatano, Rouche, & Fordyce (1986) described the characteristic phenomena of talkativeness, tangentiality, and peculiar phraseology observed in the conversational speech of TBI victims. This apparent impairment of communicative competence in nontest situations was aptly summarized by Milton, Prutting, & Binder (1984), who stated that, in contrast to aphasics, who are said to communicate better than they talk, TBI patients appear to talk better than they communicate. Developing from this perspective has been the recognition that the language assessment of TBI patients needs to be extended from static, process-specific measures to incorporate the use of language in its naturally occurring form.

There are generally four forms of discourse studied in the adult neurological population: narrative, procedural, and expository discourse, which are types of noninteractive discourse, and conversational discourse, which is interactive. Each discourse type is characterized by its own primary function and internal structure and organization (Clark & Clark, 1977) and each confronts the communicator with different cognitive and linguistic demands (Ulatowska & Chapman, 1989). The sections that follow summarize the literature relating to discourse ability in the TBI population. The discussion is presented in two parts: investigations of noninteractive discourse and investigations of interactive discourse. The interactive and noninteractive discourse genres present the speaker with different linguistic, cognitive, and communicative demands. As a result, the performance by TBI subjects on different discourse tasks needs to be considered with this in mind.

Noninteractive Discourse Ability in TBI

Noninteractive, or monologic, discourse includes narrative, procedural, and expository discourse tasks.

Narrative Discourse

A Framework for Narrative Discourse Analysis

Narration refers to storytelling, the retelling of story sequences, and the relating of personal experiences, and is a pervasive element of daily life. Through narrative thought, humans are able to represent and logically organize life events and internalize and comprehend life experiences (Westby, Van Dongen, & Maggart, 1989).

Although similar in many ways to conversational discourse, narratives have unique requirements and are expected to conform to a distinct structural organization. Narratives are assumed to include an orderly and logical presentation of information that adheres to the superstructure components of setting, complicating action, and resolution, and usually include introductory and closing statements (Roth & Spekman, 1986; Ulatowska & Chapman, 1989). A further distinction is the expectation that the speaker of a narrative maintains an oral monologue and the listener assumes a relatively passive role (Roth & Spekman, 1986).

Narrative discourse is a communicative function involving a complex interaction between cognitive and linguistic abilities, which may break down at a variety of levels (Patry & Nespoulous, 1990). The analysis of narrative discourse therefore needs to be conducted at multiple levels of performance (Coelho, 1995). Figure 10-1 represents a multilevel framework from which narrative discourse production can be represented and examined. It is based on Kintsch and van Dijk's propositional representation model (Kintsch & van Dijk, 1978; van Dijk & Kintsch, 1983) and Halliday and Hasan's (1976) model of text production.

Within this framework, narrative discourse production may be investigated from the two perspectives of surface structure and base structure. The surface structure of discourse production represents the output of words, which are organized into sentences. Analyses at this level focus on the quantity, syntactic complexity, and accuracy of verbal output.

The second level of representation is the base structure, or text base. The base structure is where the meaning of the text is represented, and it is said to be composed of a number of dissociable components that are hierarchically organized (Kintsch, 1974). The first component is the microstructure, which consists of a hierarchically organized list of micropropositions. Micropropositions are the smallest units of information and represent the individual ideas or the local information of the text (Fayol & Lemaire, 1993; Mross, 1990). Analysis at this level evaluates the quantity, type, and accuracy of the micropropositions.

Well-formed, cohesive discourse consists of micropropositions that share common arguments and therefore relate to each other in terms of meaning. Halliday and Hasan (1976) proposed that speakers ensure the continuity of meaning within a text by using certain types of linguistic devices—cohesive ties—which operate to conjoin meaning across sentences. This enables the interpretation of one linguistic element, such as a pronoun, which depends on another linguistic element in a preceding sentence, such as a noun. Thus cohesive ties provide the linguistic linkage necessary to achieve a unified, semantically coherent text, rather than a string of unrelated sentences. Halliday and Hasan (1976) identified five categories of cohesive techniques, including reference, substitution, ellipsis, conjunction, and lexical. The amount and pattern of use of each cohesive tie affects the cohesive quality of the discourse. Narratives that are deficient in the appropriate use of cohesive devices appear fragmented and difficult to follow. Analysis of cohesion involves the examination of the relative frequency with which a speaker chooses to use certain categories of linguistic markers to conjoin meanings in the text.

Macrostructure refers to the global semantic content of the discourse and is the part of the text base that represents the most important ideas in the text (Fayol & Lemaire, 1993; Mross, 1990). The macrostructure consists of a hierarchically ordered list of propositions (macropropositions), which are derived from micropropositions and yield the global meaning, theme, or gist of the text (van Dijk & Kintsch, 1983). The integrity of the macrostructure of the discourse can be assessed in terms of the presence or absence of propositions containing gist information or the ability to provide a title, summary, or moral of a story (Ulatowska & Chapman, 1989).

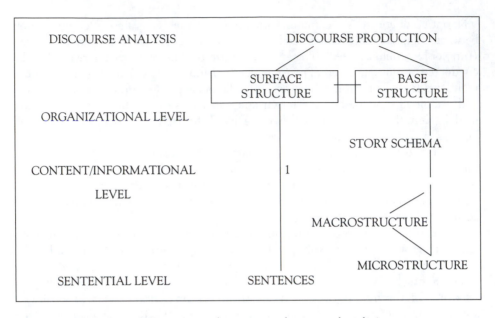

Figure 10-1. A framework for narrative discourse production and analysis

The third component of the base structure is the superstructure that corresponds to the way in which the text is organized. The superstructure is a form of abstract knowledge that specifies the elements of a particular discourse type but does not reflect its semantic content (Ulatowska & Chapman, 1989). Certain types of texts, such as reports or narratives, conform to a conventional superstructure, which operates as a framework for the macrostructure of the discourse (Mross, 1990). Story narratives conform to a regular internal structure that corresponds to the sequential arrangement of events in the story. This semantic structure, or story grammar, guides the comprehension and production of the logical relationships between people and events.

Researchers have identified critical or essential elements of the story grammar that must be present if the narrative is to be considered a story. These include a setting, a beginning or initiating event, a development, complicating action or attempt, and an ending or direct consequence (Labov, 1972; Mandler & Johnson, 1977; Stein & Glenn, 1979). Analysis of the story grammar may involve assigning the information units contained in the narrative to the superstructure component to which it belongs and examining the presence and absence of complete episodes within the narrative (Cannito, Hayashi, & Ulatowska, 1988; Stein & Glenn, 1979).

Elicitation of narrative discourse has been found to differentiate TBI subjects from control subjects (Biddle, McCabe, & Bliss, 1996; Coelho, 1995; Snow et al., 1995). Following is a summary of the recent studies on narrative discourse production deficits following TBI in adults. The summary addresses the findings and interpretations of reviewed investigations within the framework of the discourse analysis shown in Figure 10-1. It should be noted that most of the studies have been completed on relatively small subject samples, and in some cases control subjects have not been included.

Narrative Discourse in TBI

Surface Structure—Sentential Level Analysis

Productivity. The amount of language produced by subjects with TBI on narrative tasks has been measured by the number of words (Chapman et al., 1992; Glosser & Deser, 1990; Hartley & Jensen, 1991), number of syllables (Ehrlich, 1988), number of T-units—defined as an independent clause and all dependent clauses that modify it (Chapman et al., 1992; Liles, Coelho, Duffy, Zalagens, 1989; Snow et al., 1995; Wolfolk, Fucci, Dutka, Herberholz, & Latorre, 1992), and number of communication units (C-units)—defined as an independent clause with all its modifiers, and words per C-unit (Hartley & Jensen, 1991). Generally, investigations have not detected differences between TBI subjects and controls in the amount of verbal output elicited by narrative tasks (Ehrlich, 1988; Glosser & Deser, 1990; Liles et al., 1989; Snow et al., 1995). An exception has been the findings by Hartley and Jensen (1991), who found the subjects with TBI produced fewer words and shorter C-units on story retelling and story generation tasks.

Accuracy and efficiency. Accuracy of verbal output can be measured at the surface level by examining the number of *mazes* (Hartley & Jensen, 1991; Snow et al., 1995), *dysfluencies* (Biddle et al., 1996), *syntactic* and *lexical errors* (Glosser & Deser, 1990), or *hesitational phenomena* (Chapman et al., 1992). All these terms offer different labels for what are essentially episodes of erroneous verbal output, such as false starts, revisions, hesitations, filled pauses, paraphasias, and sound, syllable, or word repetitions. This output does not contribute to the communication of information.

Investigators who examined this parameter on narrative tasks found increased evidence of verbal disruption in the output of the subjects with TBI, compared with normal controls (Biddle et al., 1996; Glosser & Deser, 1990; Hartley & Jensen, 1991; Snow et al., 1995). Collectively these studies suggest that the inefficiencies observed in the output of subjects with TBI are measurable in terms of verbal disruptions.

Quality. The quality of verbal output at the surface level has been examined by investigating the complexity of the syntactic structures used in narrative expression. Several studies have used a ratio of subordination as an indicator of surface structure complexity. Generally, no detectable differences have been found in the syntactic structures used by the TBI subjects when compared to normal controls on narrative tasks (Chapman et al., 1992; Glosser & Deser, 1990; Liles et al., 1989). It appears, therefore, that knowledge and use of syntax is preserved following TBI.

Base Structure: Information/Content Level Analysis—Microstructure

Productivity. A small number of studies of TBI discourse have looked beyond the amount of verbal output to the amount of meaning conveyed or the propositional content of the output. Chapman et al. (1992) found that their group of subjects with severe TBI produced fewer propositions than the control group on a story retelling task. Similarly, Hartley and Jensen (1991) reported that their TBI group produced fewer target content units than controls on both story generation and story retelling tasks.

Contrasting findings were reported by Biddle et al. (1996), who found no difference in the total number of propositions generated by a group of 20 adult TBI subjects and their age-matched controls on a story generation task. Likewise, in terms of productivity, Ehrlich (1988) found no difference in the number of content units produced by 10 TBI subjects and matched controls on a picture description task.

It is difficult to conclude from these results whether subjects with TBI are proficient or have difficulty in representing the meaning of the discourse. Different methods of analyzing information content have been applied to an assortment of narrative tasks, which have been elicited within differing contexts.

Quality. The quality or nature of the propositional content in TBI narrative discourse has not been extensively examined. In one investigation, Biddle et al. (1996) considered whether the meaning of the narrative was represented by explicit and/or implicit propositions. Explicit propositions were defined as all propositions provided by the speaker. Implicit propositions represented information that had to be inferred by the listener. They found that while the TBI group produced nearly the same amount of explicit information as their matched controls, they also tended to leave more information implicit in their narratives. This contributed to more effort being required on behalf of the listener to make sense of the narrative.

Accuracy. The accuracy of information produced in a narrative was examined by Hartley and Jensen (1991), who found that on story retelling and generation tasks the TBI group produced more false or inaccurate information and had more problems with referential clarity than the control group. Further investigation (Hartley & Jensen, 1992) revealed that two subjects from the original group of 11 accounted for a large proportion of the TBI group's inaccuracy score. These two TBI subjects presented with a profile of confused discourse, in which a high amount of inaccurate content was a distinguishing feature. For the other subgroups of TBI subjects information was generally accurate.

Efficiency. The efficiency with which TBI subjects can impart informational content in narrative discourse has been infrequently examined. In their study involving children and adolescents, Chapman et al. (1992) examined the efficiency of information flow by evaluating the ratio of the amount of language (as measured by the total number of words) to the amount of information (as measured by the total number of propositions produced). Their findings revealed no significant difference between the subjects with TBI and their matched controls on this measure. In contrast, Ehrlich (1988) assessed efficiency by measuring the number of content units conveyed per minute and found his group of 10 TBI subjects were less efficient in conveying information than age-matched controls. Without using a specific measure of efficiency, other investigators have concluded that TBI discourse is characterized by inefficient expression, evidenced in reduced verbal output, inaccurate and diminished content, and increased difficulties with referential clarity (Hartley & Jensen, 1991, 1992). Again, it is difficult to draw conclusions from studies that are inconsistent in the techniques applied for narrative elicitation and quantification of informational efficiency.

Continuity of information—cohesion

Continuity of meaning in narrative discourse, as achieved through the use of cohesive devices, has frequently been examined in TBI. Mentis and Prutting (1987) were the first to examine amount and pattern of use of cohesive ties in the narrative discourse following TBI. They noted that their group of three adults with TBI produced fewer cohesive ties per sentence than the matched control subjects. Similarly,

Hartley and Jensen (1991) also noted that the narratives of 11 subjects with TBI contained significantly fewer cohesive ties per C-unit than those of the normal controls. These findings, however, are not supported by other studies, which found the number of cohesive ties produced by subjects with TBI to be the same as that of normal controls (Glosser & Deser, 1990; Liles et al., 1989; Wolfolk et al., 1992).

Differences in the pattern of use of cohesive ties by speakers with TBI have been reported. Mentis and Prutting (1987) examined collective data from narrative and procedural discourse and noted that the three TBI subjects used fewer lexical ties and a higher percentage of ellipsis and incomplete ties than the normal subjects. Liles et al. (1989) found the pattern of tie usage by four TBI subjects to be similar to that of normal subjects on a story retelling task but markedly different on a story generation task. In story generation, all of the subjects with TBI had a lower proportion of reference ties and a higher proportion of lexical ties. This cohesive style was thought to reflect the TBI subjects' tendency to refer directly to the stimulus picture and describe its features while failing to integrate and organize the information to form a continuous text.

Again, it must be stated that evidence of impairment in the capacity of TBI subjects to produce a cohesive narrative is inconclusive. The descriptive information available is based on narrative samples elicited under differing conditions and produced by a small number of subjects.

Base Structure: Information/Content Level Analysis—Macrostructure

There has only been one study (Chapman et al., 1992) that has examined the integrity of narrative macrostructure following TBI. These investigators established a set of 10 propositions based on the major setting, complicating event, and resolution information of the text. These core propositions were considered to represent the gist of the narrative. Results showed that the group of child and adolescent subjects with severe TBI ($n = 9$) were impaired in their ability to preserve the macrostructure when retelling the story. The group of mild/moderately injured TBI subjects ($n = 11$), however, were not deficient in this regard.

Base Structure: Organizational Level—Superstructure (Story Schema)

Organizational level analyses are concerned with the structural elements of a discourse without measuring any of the semantic content (Ulatowska & Chapman, 1989). Superstructure has been examined in three studies of TBI narrative discourse (Chapman et al., 1992; Coelho, Liles, & Duffy, 1991a; Liles et al., 1989). Chapman et al. (1992) used the story grammar analysis as described by Labov (1972) and found a group of subjects with severe TBI to be deficient in information organization because of failure to signal a new episode with setting information and omission of essential action information. Liles et al. (1989) and Coelho et al. (1991a) utilized the story grammar model proposed by Stein and Glenn (1979). Liles et al. (1989) found that on the retelling task, the subjects with TBI did not differ from the normal subjects in terms of production of complete episodes. On the generation task, however, three of the four TBI subjects were unable to produce a complete episode. Similarly, difficulty in episode production for generation tasks was reflected by one of the two TBI subjects studied by Coelho et al. (1991a). This subject produced a cohesive narrative but could not produce a complete episode when describing a picture. In contrast, the other subject was able to produce more complete episodes than those produced by the normal controls.

Summary of Findings from the Literature Investigating Narrative Discourse in Closed Head Injury

The investigations of narrative discourse skills following TBI have varied in choice of stimuli, type of analyses applied, and results achieved. In reviewing these studies, it is clear that definitive conclusions in relation to TBI discourse skills cannot be derived because of these inconsistencies. With most analyses being completed on small numbers of subjects it must be considered that the variations and vagaries of the discourse behaviors described, may simply be the result of individual variations in discourse skill and style, without necessarily representing a pathological state. While some investigations have identified apparently distinct patterns of discourse deficits in TBI (Coelho et al., 1991a; Hartley & Jensen, 1992), the existence of such patterns requires verification on larger subject groups. In larger group studies, however, it is essential to include systematic controls for markers of heterogeneity, including etiology, severity, time postonset of injury, coexisting deficits, and demographic features (Coelho, 1995).

Collectively, however, the results of these studies are testimony to what has long been anecdotally described. Subjects with TBI do appear to experience deficiencies of discourse production, but these deficiencies are diverse, difficult to define, and inconsistent. Multilevel analyses go some way to delineating the parameters of the discourse deficits experienced by this group. The Case File examples that follow illustrate the production of narrative discourse by two individuals with TBI. The discourse was elicited by a story retelling task, "The Businessman and the Tramp," which is reproduced in Appendix A. A multilevel analysis of discourse has been applied to the discourse samples and serves to delineate the features that underpin the overall effectiveness of the discourse.

The inconsistencies in results across studies may, in part, be related to the differences across tasks and the sensitivity of the tasks used. Some of the studies contrasted story retelling and story generation (Hartley & Jensen, 1991; Liles et al., 1989) and have concluded that story generation is a more challenging task. This finding is consistent with the effect of task elicitation in other brain-damaged populations (Ulatowska & Chapman, 1989) and normals (Shadden, Burnette, Eikenberry, & DiBrezzo, 1991). These studies, however, provide no evidence of any attempt to control for task complexity and sensitivity. It is difficult to conclude that one task is more difficult than another without consideration of the inherent syntactic, thematic, and information complexity of each task.

Case File Notes

Mark

Mark was a 22-year-old male who sustained a severe closed head injury in a motorcycle accident. He had completed 10 years of schooling with average grades in all subjects and superior grades in shop work. Mark had also completed 8 months of technical training in Marine and Motor Mechanics.

On formal language testing, Mark displayed spared basic auditory comprehension skills in the presence of impairments in naming, lexical-semantic manipulation, sentential-semantic processes, and complex auditory comprehension. On neuropsychological testing Mark displayed average to low-average performances on tasks of working memory and immediate auditory attention span. He was severely impaired in speed on tasks of selective attention.

Mark's narrative discourse was analyzed on multiple levels. At the level of surface structure, Mark's narrative was short, but contained sentences of adequate syntactic complexity, and was relatively free of verbal disruptions. Measures of information content revealed that Mark produced a narrative that was limited in the amount of propositional information it contained, and in the efficiency with which the information was conveyed. There were also a number of erroneous propositions. Also noted in Mark's narrative was the limited proportion of information relating to complication activity and an increased proportion of content relating to the resolution of the story. Mark's narrative contained a reduced number of cohesive ties per T-unit and a number of cohesive errors. The features of discourse identified by analysis are observable when reading the narrative, which is notably brief and devoid of detail, especially with regard to the main body of the story.

The Businessman and the Tramp

It's about a businessman who went to catch a train/ (um) The train wasn't there/ And he had his briefcase stolen by (ah) a tramp/ (um) He realized (it was) his briefcase was gone, picked up a plastic bag that the tramp left there and said "Somebody's delivered my lunch."

Ursula

Ursula was a 26-year-old female who suffered a severe closed head injury from a motor vehicle accident. Ursula had completed a tertiary education and was working as a project officer in a government department. Premorbidly she was considered to have excellent verbal communication skills.

For the most part, Ursula had little difficulty completing standardized language and neuropsychological test batteries. Indeed her scores on many language tests were above average, with a mild difficulty displayed on some lexical-semantic, sentential-semantic, and word fluency tasks. Apart from some evidence of attentional difficulty on one task, Ursula displayed a normal performance on neuropsychological tests.

When Ursula retold the narrative "The Businessman and the Tramp," discourse measures revealed a high level of verbal disruption, high verbal output, decreased amount of propositions, and decreased propositional production in relation to the amount of input. The discourse is presented on the following page and illustrates that Ursula was capable of conveying information that was generally accurate. The discourse is marked by verbal disruptions, which are primarily mazes and filler disruptions. The decreased efficiency of information production is illustrated well in the sample, which is unnecessarily wordy. Also illustrated here is the tendency to use a higher number of conjunctive cohesive ties as characterized by "and" at the beginning of sentences.

The Businessman and the Tramp

There was a busy and hungry businessman who was (um) going to catch a train/ And he sat down on a bench/ and he had his briefcase with him/ He (um) drew some papers out of the briefcase and (um) put the briefcase very carefully down beside him (um) on the bench as well/ He took some papers out of the briefcase and started to read them/ Along came a tramp and the tramp had just a crumpled paper bag with him. (And the tramp thought that this was a beautiful)…(he was he was obvi…) the businessman was obviously distracted/ and he thought it was a beautiful briefcase/ So (he replaced) he put the crumpled paper bag down and slid off very carefully the briefcase/ And the tramp walked around the train station showing everyone his beautiful briefcase/ And then (um) the businessman looked up and realized that his briefcase was gone / And (um) he looked in the crumpled paper bag that the tramp had left/ and he said "Oh! Someone's given me my lunch."

Procedural Discourse

Procedural discourse is a form of noninteractive discourse that involves explaining the sequence of actions required to complete a certain task or activity. Thus, the main function of procedural discourse is to accurately inform or instruct a listener in a precise and explicit manner (Ulatowska, Allard, & Chapman, 1990). Like narrative discourse, procedural discourse consists of a number of information units that are hierarchically organized. These information units are known as "steps" and can be classified as essential, optional, or target steps (Cannito et al. 1988; Ulatowska, Weiss-Doyal, Freedman-Stern, Macaluso-Hayes, 1983). The essential steps in a procedural discourse contain the information that is critical to the successful completion of the procedure. The information contained in the optional steps provides additional detail or clarification of the essential information. The target step informs the listener that the procedure is complete.

Procedural Discourse in TBI

In comparison to the number of investigations completed on narrative discourse following TBI, there have been relatively few studies investigating procedural discourse in this population. The studies that have been completed differ in terms of the techniques used to elicit the discourse and the analyses used to determine its adequacy. Speakers with TBI have been requested to describe how to play a favorite sport (Mentis and Prutting, 1987), how to buy groceries in a supermarket (Hartley and Jensen, 1991), or how to complete a familiar, goal-orientated task such as changing a tire or baking a cake (Coppens, 1995; Mentis & Prutting, 1987), making a sandwich, mailing a letter (Coppens, 1995), or withdrawing money from a bank (Snow, Douglas, & Ponsford, 1997a; Snow et al., 1995). In contrast, McDonald (1993) devised a task whereby the speaker had to describe an unfamiliar procedure, a board game, to a blindfolded listener who was unfamiliar with the game or its rules. In this way, the listener was truly naïve about the information to be conveyed, and the speaker could not rely on an assumption of shared world knowledge when describing the procedure.

The measures used to examine the quality of procedural discourse produced by TBI speakers have varied across investigations. Some have measured productivity in terms of speaking time, number of communication units, number of words

(Hartley & Jensen, 1991), number of syllables (Snow et al., 1995, 1997a), and number of T-units (Snow et al., 1995). Efficiency of verbal production has been evaluated by calculations of the amount of maze production (Snow et al., 1995, 1997a). The amount and accuracy of the information content produced by TBI subjects on procedural discourse tasks has been examined by measuring the number of essential and optional steps (Snow et al., 1995,1997a), the amount of target information (Hartley & Jensen, 1991; Snow et al.,1995), low content information (Snow et al., 1997a), and the amount of inaccurate content units and problems of reference (Hartley & Jensen, 1991). The cohesiveness of procedural discourse by subjects with TBI has also been investigated (Hartley & Jensen, 1991; Mentis & Prutting, 1987). Measures of pragmatic abilities have also been applied to procedural discourse production by subjects with TBI (Snow et al., 1995; 1997a).

The results of these investigations have varied, and comparisons of results across studies must consider differences in the nature of the tasks, numbers of subjects involved, and demographic qualities of the control groups used. When compared with a demographically similar control group, subjects with TBI have been found to produce procedural discourse that was normal in terms of amount of verbal output, and essential and "on-target" information, but which reflected poor topic maintenance and difficulty with information transfer (Snow et al., 1997a). Elsewhere, however, a group of subjects with TBI produced procedural discourse that was reduced in terms of verbal output, verbal efficiency, target content, and lexical cohesion (Hartley & Jensen, 1991). A reduction in the lexical cohesion of procedural discourse in TBI was also observed by Mentis and Prutting (1987), who, in addition, found that the subjects with TBI used an increased number of elliptical and incomplete ties when compared with normal control subjects. McDonald and Pearce (1995) found the TBI subjects to produce the same amount of propositional information, but this information differed from the control group in its quality. The subjects with TBI in McDonald's study produced more irrelevant and fewer essential propositions than the control subjects, and this, in turn resulted in disrupted sequencing of information.

Case File Notes

Gary

Gary was a 30-year-old male who fell from a horse while working as a farm manager on a cattle property. He suffered a severe closed head injury. Gary had completed 10 years of schooling and was a low-average achiever. On tests of language and neuropsychological function Gary displayed global cognitive-linguistic impairment characterized by poor auditory comprehension of logico-grammatical and logico-semantic relationships; poor lexical retrieval and semantic organization; pronounced impairment on lexical-semantic and sentential-semantic tasks; and moderate-severe impairments on tests of attention, verbal memory, and visuospatial functioning.

Gary's procedural discourse is strikingly sparse in output and essential informational content. His discourse reflects an overreliance on assumed shared knowledge and lack of referential and lexical cohesion.

> **Changing a light bulb**
>
> Get up to it first/ And you press it in/ And you give it just a (kwi) bit of a twist and /ka/
> And there's two hooks in there/ They come out/ And (that the old) that's the buggered
> on out/That's it.

Ursula

Ursula's history and cognitive-linguistic profile was described earlier. Her procedural discourse is a stark contrast to Gary's. It is wordy, but inefficient, conveying a great deal of propositional information but lacking the essential step of taking out the used light bulb. The listener can get lost in the detail.

> **Changing a light bulb**
>
> Well first you get a new light bulb that's the right number of watts for what you want, the
> brightness that you want/ You (um) probably have to stand on a chair because you're
> probably not tall enough to reach the light bulb/ If its on the ceiling or if it's on the lamp
> it's okay/(um) Now there are two different types of light bulbs/ We'll do the twist and
> swivel kind of one/ The sockets got two little holes that two little (um) things sticking
> out of the base of the light bulb have (have) to fit into/ So you have to find this (this)
> slot that those (those) little shoulders I guess they are can fit into/ Then you push the
> light bulb into it so that those things go along that slot/ and then you have to swivel it so
> that the light bulb stays in that position/ You can feel it you just (sw) swivel it around a
> little bit when you push it into the socket/ and you find the place that the little shoulders
> fit into/ And you push the bulb up/ And turn it so that it stays in position/ Then test
> it/And turn it on/And see if it's a good bulb/ And you're there.

Interactive Discourse Ability in TBI

The monologue genres described above offer much potential in the examination of aspects of discourse production. Day-to-day interactions involve the ability to relate both narratives and procedures within varying contexts. The assessment of ability to produce narrative and procedural discourse is therefore useful in the determination of an individual's communication skills. While the analyses outlined above are able to delineate the quality of micro- and macrolinguistic aspects of language production in connected discourse, they do not allow for the assessment of an individual's capacity to use language in certain contexts and cope with the dynamic aspects of communication. That is they are unable to assess the pragmatic skill of the speaker.

Pragmatics, which can broadly be defined as the use of language for communication within specific contexts, requires the interplay of linguistic skills (syntax, phonology, and semantics), with cognitive skills such as attention, memory, and executive skills. In addition pragmatic skill involves an understanding of and the ability to apply the social rules of language (Marsh, 1999). Pragmatic skill therefore entails sensitivity to the dynamic nature of the interaction, such as an awareness of the need to take turns, sustain and extend a conversation, observe politeness markers, meet the needs of the listener, and accurately understand verbal and nonverbal cues (Brown & Levinson, 1987; Clark, 1979, Clark & Schunk, 1980; Grice, 1975). The study of pragmatic ability, therefore, primarily serves to analyze the way a person interacts with others within various contexts.

Psychosocial Well-Being and Communication Skill Following TBI

The establishment and maintenance of healthy social relationships requires skilled social behavior. The ability to communicate effectively with different people in different contexts is central to attainment of adequate social skills. Difficulty in establishing psychosocial well-being following TBI represents a pervasive impediment to the social reintegration of individuals with TBI and affects their quality of life (Bond, 1976; Brown & Vandergoot, 1998; Galski, Tompkins & Johnston, 1998; Levin, Grossman, Rose, & Teasdale, 1979; Tate, Lulham, Broe, Strettles, & Pfaff, 1989; Willer, Rosenthal, Kreutzer, Gordon, & Rempel, 1993). Compromised psychosocial function can result from reduced emotional control and social perceptiveness, decreased self-regulation, increased stimulus-orientated behavior, and an impaired capacity for social learning (Lezak, 1978). In addition, persisting poor interpersonal communication skills have been identified as major contributing factors to social isolation and the resultant poor psychosocial outcome in the TBI population (Brooks, McKinlay, Symington, Beattie, & Campsie, 1987; Hartley, 1995; Marsh, 1999; Marsh & Knight, 1991; Marsh, Knight, & Godfrey, 1990; Newton & Johnson, 1985; Spence, Godfrey, & Bishara, 1993).

Earlier researchers made incidental comment on the notable impairments in conversation experienced by subjects with TBI (Levin et al., 1979; Thompson, 1975). The 1980s saw the development of a strongly held tenet that the problems of communication experienced following TBI are the manifestation of impairments in the broad-ranging cognitive and executive functions that support language and govern interactional behavior (Adamovich, 1990; Braun & Baribeau, 1987; Hagen, 1984; Holland, 1982; Mentis & Prutting, 1987). This belief, while lacking empirical support, was developed from well-grounded descriptions that realized the functional consequences of impairments in the cognitive processes such as attention and memory and the executive abilities such as planning, monitoring, abstraction, and inhibition.

TBI typically results in diffuse axonal injury with a preponderance of multifocal lesions in the temporal and frontomedial lobes. The resultant neurobehavioral effects potentially implicate every aspect of human thinking and behavior (Pang, 1989). While temporal lobe pathology following TBI is associated with disorders of memory and new learning, frontal lobe damage and diffuse axonal injury have been associated with loss of regulatory control over cognitive processes and affective and social behavior (Auberach, 1986). With lack of inhibitory control, the individual with TBI may produce excessive, tangential and inappropriate discourse that displays a lack of social perception, poor self-image, impaired self-analysis, and reduced ability to follow social rules (McDonald, 1993).

Alternately other individuals with TBI may demonstrate impoverished communication because of their inability to formulate and initiate goal-directed behavior and their reduced desire to express emotion or engage in social interaction (Auberach, 1986).

Recognition of the effect of impaired communication competence on the psychosocial well-being of the individual coincided with the postpositivist paradigmatic shift away from the measurement of isolated linguistic or cognitive processes towards the assessment and treatment of behavioral functions, conducted in naturalistic settings (Garrison, 1986). Hence, discourse analysis, and in particular, analysis of conversational discourse, has become recognized as being more robust in terms of sociolinguistic validity. Such an analysis has become recognized as a means by which to adequately capture the situationally valid, real-life account of the communication disorders following TBI, and this has led to a recent increase in investigations into conversational discourse and pragmatic language behavior following TBI.

Analysis of Conversational Discourse and the Study of Pragmatic Language in TBI

Apart from one study (Mentis & Prutting, 1987), investigations of conversational discourse in TBI have not involved the micro- and macrolinguistic analyses applied to narrative and procedural discourse. Instead, three main approaches have been adopted. The first has been to use a pragmatic framework to examine the overall quality of the interpersonal exchange. These investigations have employed profile analysis or checklist assessments. The second approach has examined specific aspects of the interpersonal exchange from a pragmatic perspective, while the third has addressed aspects of the structure of conversational exchanges in varying contexts.

Profile Analysis of Conversation Following TBI

With some exceptions (Ehrlich, 1988; Ehrlich & Barry, 1989; Friedland & Miller, 1998), the profile approaches to conversational production in TBI have largely been based on Grice's "cooperative principle of conversation" (Grice, 1975). This principle maintains that to promote successful conversation, speakers need to adhere to four maxims:

1. *Quantity*—make your contribution as informative as is required.
2. *Quality*—do not say what you believe to be false. Do not say that for which you lack adequate evidence.
3. *Relation*—be relevant.
4. *Manner*—avoid obscurity of expression and ambiguity; be brief and orderly in expression.

Other conversational profile analyses have been grounded in speech act theory (Searle, 1969). In general, global conversational profiles have been found to be of limited use in identifying the discourse features that discriminate TBI conversational discourse from non-TBI discourse.

Several studies of TBI conversation have used or modified Damico's Clinical Discourse Analysis (CDA), which assesses behaviors said to violate Grice's conversational maxims (Benjamin, Debinski, Fletcher, Hedger, Mealings, & Stewart-Scott, 1989; Jordan & Murdoch, 1990; Snow, Lambier, Parsons, Mooney, Couch, & Russell, 1987; Snow et al., 1995; Snow, Douglas, & Ponsford, 1997b). This analysis is considered clinically useful in that it has the potential to identify clusters of discourse errors, which in turn assists in defining treatment goals. Snow et al. (1995) used the CDA to compare the conversational discourse produced by three TBI subjects with the discourse produced by matched controls. Their results showed that the errors in Quality and Manner accounted for the bulk of the discourse errors produced by both groups of subjects. In general, however, Snow et al. (1995) found that this analysis was not sufficiently sensitive to discriminate between the discourse produced by TBI and non-TBI subjects. These findings supported those of Jordan and Murdoch (1990) and were confirmed in a later study by Snow et al. (1997b), where the bulk of the discourse errors for subjects in the clinical group and in two control groups occurred in the parameters of *nonspecific vocabulary*, *linguistic nonfluency*, and *revision behavior*. Snow et al. (1997b) refined the CDA by removing these parameters, producing the *Modified Clinical Discourse Analysis* (CDA-M). Using this measure, they were able to distinguish the TBI discourse from that of a control group's discourse. The TBI subjects were found to make significantly more overall errors than control subjects, with the TBI subjects making most errors in the parameters of *insufficient information*, *information redundancy*, and *failure to structure discourse*.

Linscott, Knight, and Godfrey (1996) reported on the construction of the Profile of Functional Impairment in Communication (PFIC), which they claim is based on Grice's pragmatic model of conversation, although the influence of Grice's theories on the final instrument may be somewhat remote. The PFIC assesses the adherence to 10 communication rules encompassing the parameters of *logical content*, *general participation*, *quantity*, *quality*, *internal relation*, *external relation*, *clarity of expression*, *social style*, *subject matter*, and *aesthetics*. The test instrument comprises 10 feature summary scales assessing severity of impairment, and 84 specific behavior items, assessing the frequency of specific communication impairments. To assess the psychometric properties of the scale, Linscott et al. (1996) rated videos of 21 subjects with severe TBI, individually interacting in an unstructured dialogue with a female confederate. The feature summary scales were found to have high concurrent validity and internal consistency. While the authors concluded that the scale is a useful measure for identification of specific impairments in clinical practice, there is, as yet, no research that inspects its ability to discriminate TBI discourse from normal conversational discourse.

Speech Act Theory (Searle, 1969) has also provided some theoretical basis for the development of pragmatic profile assessments used in TBI. Milton et al. (1984) analyzed the conversational skills of subjects with TBI, using the Prutting and Kirchner (197) Pragmatic Protocol. This protocol examines speech acts identified by Searle (1969), including the utterance act, the propositional act, and the illocutionary/perlocutionary act. Milton et al. (1984) compared the spontaneous, unstructured conversational discourse of five TBI subjects with five matched controls. Using descriptive statistics, Milton et al. (1984) found the subjects with TBI to have conversational problems with topic selection, topic introduction, topic maintenance, lack of specificity, and lack of conciseness. Penn and Cleary (1988) also used the Pragmatic Protocol to study six TBI subjects. The conversational difficulties experienced by their TBI sample were similar to those found by Milton et al. (1984), but Penn and Cleary (1988) also noted problems with turn-taking, intelligibility, prosody, and fluency.

Other studies examining the conversational production of subjects with TBI have used rating scales that have not been based on any stated theoretical foundation. For example, Ehrlich and Barry (1989) devised a five-point rating scale in an effort to quantify certain complex communication behaviors in TBI. Their rating scale examined six behaviors, including *intelligibility*, *eye gaze*, *sentence formation*, *coherence of narrative*, *topic*, and *initiation of communication*.

More recently, Friedland and Miller (1998) described a single case study in which Conversational Analysis (CA) was used to determine whether it was sensitive to the types of communication breakdown resulting from TBI. Conversational analysis details how an interaction is constructed by observing each speaker's contribution. It examines the parameters of turn-taking, breakdown repair, silences, and topic maintenance. For the case described, conversational analysis proved a sensitive tool for identifying and investigating pragmatic deficits.

Rating scales and checklists have, therefore, been used in efforts to delineate particular pragmatic behaviors of individuals with TBI. While these scales provide some clinical utility, they have not been widely tested and are at best only loosely based on theoretical foundations. It has also been suggested that the scales lack specificity in terms of identifying the aspect of discourse being judged (Togher, Hand, & Code, 1999).

Aspects of Interpersonal Conversational Exchange Following TBI.

In contrast to assessing the overall quality of conversation, several recent studies, mainly reported by McDonald and colleagues, have been designed to assess one specific aspect of communicative exchange that would be vulnerable to compromised frontal lobe functioning. In order to assess comprehension of conversational implicature, McDonald (1992) examined the ability of two TBI subjects to understand conventional indirect speech acts, and indirect speech acts in the form of sarcasm. The results showed that one TBI subject failed to detect both indirect speech acts, while the other subject had no difficulty interpreting direct speech acts but failed to detect sarcasm.

In a later study, McDonald assessed the ability of the same two TBI subjects to meet the informational needs of the listener (McDonald, 1993). This methodology was later refined to produce the "Dice Game" (McDonald & Pearce, 1995) as a means by which to assess the ability to formulate and express essential information in a logical sequence.

Elsewhere, McDonald and van Sommers (1993) examined the ability of the two TBI subjects to generate language that was appropriate to the specific context and utilized appropriate politeness strategies. In addition, they examined the TBI subjects' ability to communicate a social request indirectly, that is, the ability to communicate hints. Results showed that the TBI subjects demonstrated sensitivity to social context and were able to generate requests using politeness mechanisms. The TBI subjects did, however, have difficulty delivering hints, suggesting impaired problem solving and disrupted social communication skills.

More recently, McDonald has studied the ability of 15 TBI subjects and their controls to formulate requests that overcome listener reluctance (McDonald & Pearce, 1998). Formulating a request that addresses obstacles to listener compliance is thought to be more demanding than producing an indirect request. The subjects were given eight scenarios involving obstacles to listener compliance and were required to formulate a request that employed a strategy to overcome the obstacle. The findings revealed the TBI group used a lesser variety of strategies, and less frequently addressed the obstacles than the control subjects did. The TBI subjects were also found to make comments that were counterproductive to the attainment of the request. The authors suggested that this behavioral pattern reflects impairment in the executive capacity needed to produce adaptive and novel requests.

Analysis of the Structure of Conversational Exchanges in TBI.

Recent research, exemplified by the work of Togher and colleagues (Togher & Hand, 1998; Togher, Hand, & Code, 1996, 1997a, 1997b) has promoted the theory of Systemic Functional Linguistics (SFL) (Halliday, 1985; 1994) as a coherent model of language function in TBI. SFL examines the manner in which context influences language, and all language characteristics are described in terms of the functions they perform. This theory holds that each time a person speaks he/she makes a choice as to the content and manner of speech, and that the choice is influenced by the situational context and the power relationship with the communicative partner. SFL describes context as a combination of three dimensions: field, mode, and tenor. "Field" refers to the nature of the social interaction—e.g., a service encounter, a talk with a friend. "Tenor" refers to the participants in the interaction and the power relationship between them. "Mode" refers to the channel through which the information is being exchanged—e.g., oral or written.

Togher and colleagues have used SFL to examine the ability of people with TBI to complete common daily information exchanges with varying communicative partners. In one study (Togher, Hand, & Code, 1997a) five TBI adults, with identified inappropriate pragmatic behaviors and five matched controls were required to request information over the telephone from four different communicative partners—a familiar therapist, an information service, the police, and their mothers. The recorded exchanges were analyzed using exchange structure analysis, which examines the interaction between speaker and listener, which is said to be made up of "synoptic" and "dynamic" moves.

The results of the analysis revealed that communication partners interacted differently with TBI subjects as compared with controls. Differences were noted in the amount of information given and requested. Therapists gave more information to control subjects, just as mothers gave more information to their normal sons as compared with their head-injured sons. The information service and police, however, gave TBI and control subjects the same amount of information. In addition, therapists were more likely to ask questions of the control subjects than of the TBI subjects, and produced more dynamic moves with the TBI subjects than with the controls.

In a later study, Togher & Hand (1999) used a different type of exchange structure analysis—generic structure potential—to examine the structure of communicative interchanges with TBI subjects. Generic structure potential (GSP) analysis (Ventola, 1979) examines oral texts as genre, the structure of which is determined by the field and tenor of the interactions. GSP involves identifying "moves," which are semantic units of negotiable information presented by one speaker within an interactive turn. The analysis involves coding the moves according to the type of generic element being expressed. GSP elements include Greeting (an opening move), Address (defines addressee and their role), Approach (ice-breaking social topics to get the conversation going), Approach-Direct (introduction of topics concerning personal aspects of the interactants), Approach-Indirect (topics referring to the immediate situation, such as the weather), Centering (statements or questions that directly relate to the purpose of the interaction), Leave-taking (expressions indicating the desire to terminate the conversation), and Goodbye.

In their study, Togher and Hand (1999) analyzed the interactions of seven adults with TBI and seven spinal-injury matched controls, under two conditions. One condition was an information-giving interaction, where subjects were required to speak to teenage schoolboys as part of a community awareness driver education program. The second condition involved the subjects requesting information about the research project. Analysis involved calculating the mean percentage of moves made by both subject groups in each generic structural element. Results showed that with the removal of the data of one TBI subject, whose inappropriate interactions skewed the results, the mean percentage of moves produced by both groups in the information-giving interactions were similar for all structural elements.

Analysis of interactions of the information-requesting condition showed the TBI and control groups to produce similar amounts of Approach-Direct elements. In this condition, the TBI subjects produced a greater amount of moves to make up the Approach-Indirect element than the control subjects did. The mean percentage of moves making up the Centering element was higher in the control interactions than in the TBI interactions. Qualitative differences in the TBI and control subject interactions related to inappropriate, incomplete, or repeated structural elements produced by subjects with TBI. This study highlighted that the modification of the balance of power in interactional situations affected the ability of the TBI subjects to operate in a similar manner to normal subjects. When the TBI subjects were placed in a powerful information-giving role, they produced similar numbers of structural elements when compared with the control subjects.

The analyses described in the above studies revealed interesting patterns of interactional behaviors of TBI subjects, which were influenced by the power relationship and social distance between the interlocuters. Exchange structure analysis offers a comprehensive and systematic analysis of interpersonal exchanges, while GSP analysis provides a further means by which to examine the macrostructure of dynamic exchanges. Both methods of analysis offer insight into the characteristics of interpersonal communication that is so vulnerable to disruption in the TBI population. The subjects in the study, however, were included because they displayed impaired pragmatic behaviors. Further studies that examined the exchange structure with TBI subjects without marked pragmatic impairment would give valuable insight into the impact of TBI on pragmatic skill and provide further information to those working in the rehabilitation of communication of TBI individuals.

Limitations of Discourse Analyses in TBI

Discourse analysis has proven to be a fruitful means of delineating communication disorders in the TBI population. Collectively the analyses have the advantage of analyzing the micro- and macrolinguistic qualities of connected speech and the nature of interactional behaviors produced by subjects with TBI. All forms of discourse analysis have limitations in terms of their methodological soundness and social and ethnographic validity. Many studies of discourse production and behavior in the TBI population have been conducted under various methodological conditions on small subject numbers, and have involved broad interpretation of results. As a result, comparison across studies is difficult and the interpretation and clinical usefulness of results is limited. In particular, studies have varied in relation to the stimuli used to elicit discourse production, the nature of the control groups employed, and the analyses applied to the discourse samples. Comparison and extrapolation of results is further hampered by the inherent heterogeneity of the TBI population in terms of injury characteristics, time postinjury, sociolinguistic characteristics, and individual premorbid intellectual, personality, and psychosocial characteristics.

Another major factor that needs to be considered in the interpretation of findings into discourse production in TBI is the lack of available normative data relating to aspects of discourse produced. Many studies revealed high levels of variation in the discourse produced by normal control subjects on certain discourse variables. Such variations may represent differences in speaking style that occur across sociolinguistic sectors in the normal population. Interpretation of discourse quality and behaviors in the TBI population needs to be conducted with sensitivity to the sociolinguistic background of the individuals concerned. This highlights the need to use demographically matched control subjects when investigating discourse function in TBI. Snow et al. (1995) eloquently argue that the failure to use control subjects selected on the basis of demographic characteristics, exposes the results to the influence of artifact from educational and occupational status. In addition, when information regarding the normal discourse performance of people with a certain demographic profile is lacking, there is a risk that inappropriate sociolinguistic standards are applied to make arbitrary distinctions between normal and abnormal discourse function. There is a critical need, therefore, for improved information regarding the discourse abilities of non-brain-injured people across demographic sectors. Obtaining such information would involve broad-based studies that systematically describe the discourse skills of sectors of the normal population in tasks of differing discourse genres, elicited under various conditions, within various contexts and, where appropriate, with various communicative partners.

APPENDIX

The Businessman and the Tramp

A busy and hungry businessman arrived at the train station with his briefcase and sat down on the bench to wait for a train. He took some papers from his briefcase and then carefully placed the briefcase beside him. He busily read the papers as he waited for the train. Before too long, a dirty but good-natured tramp came along carrying a crumpled paper bag. He spied the smart briefcase and the distracted businessman. Carefully the tramp slid the briefcase off the bench and in its place he left his crumpled paper bag. After a while, the businessman looked up from his papers and was shocked to find a crumpled paper bag where his briefcase should have been. He looked inside the bag; "Someone has delivered my lunch!" he exclaimed.

References

Adamovich, B. (1990). Information processing, cognition, attention and communication following closed head injury. *Folia Phoniatre, 42,* 11–23.

Auerbach, S.H. (1986). Neuroanatomical correlates of attention and memory disorder in traumatic brain injury: An application of neurobehavioural subtypes. *Journal of Head Trauma Rehabilitation, 3,* 1–12.

Benjamin, L., Debinski, A., Fletcher, D., Hedger, C., Mealings, M., & Stewart-Scott, A. (1989). The use of the Bethesda Conversational Skills Profile in closed head injury. In V. Anderson & M. Bailey (Eds.), *Proceedings of the Fourteenth Annual Brain Impairment Conference: Theory and Function: Bridging the Gap* (pp. 57–64). Melbourne: Australian Society for the Study of Brain Impairment.

Biddle, K.R., McCabe, A., & Bliss, L.S. (1996). Narrative skills following traumatic brain injury in children and adults. *Journal of Communication Disorders, 29,* 447–469.

Bond, M.R. (1976). Assessment of the psychosocial outcome of severe head injury. *Acta Neurochirurgica, 34,* 57–70.

Braun, C.M. & Baribeau, J.M. (1987). Subclinical aphasia following closed head injury: A response to Sarno, Buonaguro and Levita. In R. Brookshire (Ed.), *Clinical Aphasiology, 17,* (pp. 326–333). Minneapolis: BRK Publishers.

Brooks, N., McKinlay, W., Symington, C., Beattie, A., & Campsie, L. (1987). Return to work within the first seven years after severe blunt head injury. *Brain Injury, 1,* 5–9.

Brown, P. & Levinson, S. (1987). *Politeness: Some Universals in Language Use.* Cambridge, England: Cambridge University Press.

Brown, M. & Vandergoot, D. (1998). Quality of life for individuals with traumatic brain injury: Comparison with others living in the community. *Journal of Head Trauma Rehabilitation, 13,* 1–23.

Cannito, M.P., Hayashi, M.M., & Ulatowska, H.K. (1988). Discourse in normal and pathological aging: Background and assessment strategies. *Seminars in Speech and Language, 9,* 117–134.

Chapman, S., Culhane, K., Levin, H., Harward, H., Mendelson, D., Ewing-Cobbs, L., Fletcher, J., & Bruee, D. (1992). Narrative discourse after closed head injury in children and adolescents. *Brain and Language, 43,* 2–62.

Clark, H.H. (1979). Responding to indirect speech acts. *Cognitive Psychology, 11,* 430–477.

Clark, H.H. & Clarke, E.V. (1977). *Psychology and Language: An Introduction to Psycholinguistics.* New York: Harcourt Brace Jovanovich.

Clark, H.H. & Schunk, D.H. (1980). Polite responses to polite requests. *Cognition, 8,* 111–143.

Coelho, C.A. (1995). Discourse production deficits following traumatic brain injury: A critical review of the recent literature. *Aphasiology, 9,* 409–429.

Coelho, C.A., Liles, B.Z., & Duffy, R.J. (1991a). Discourse analysis with closed head injured adults: Evidence for differing patterns of deficits. *Archives of Physical Medicine and Rehabilitation, 72,* 465–468.

Coppens, P. (1995). Subpopulations in closed head injury: Preliminary results. *Brain Injury, 9,* 195–208.

Ehrlich, J. (1988). Selective characteristics of narrative discourse in head-injured and normal adults. *Journal of Communication Disorders, 1,* 1–19.

Ehrlich, J. & Barry, P. (1989). Rating communication behaviors in head-injured adults. *Brain Injury, 3,* 193–198.

Fayol, M. & Lemaire, P. (1993). Levels of approach to discourse. In H.H. Brownell & Y. Joanette (Eds.), *Narrative Discourse in Neurologically Impaired and Normal Aging Adults* (pp. 3–20). San Diego: Singular Publishing Group Inc.

Friedland, D. & Miller, N. (1998). Conversation analysis of communication breakdown after closed head injury. *Brain Injury, 12,* 1–14.

Galski, T., Tompkins, C., & Johnston, M.V. (1998). Competence in discourse as a measure of social integration and quality of life in persons with traumatic brain injury. *Brain Injury, 12,* 769–782.

Garrison, J.W. (1986). Some principles of postpositivistic philosophy of science. *Educational Researcher, 15,* 12–15.

Glosser, G. & Deser, T. (1990). Patterns of discourse production among neurological patients with fluent language disorders. *Brain and Language, 40,* 67–88.

Grice, H.P. (1975). Logic and conversation. In F. Cole & J.L. Morgan (Eds.), *Syntax and Semantics 3: Speech Acts* (pp. 41–58). New York: Academic Press.

Hagen, C. (1984). Language disorders in head trauma. In A. Holland (Ed.), *Language Disorders in Adults: Recent Advances* (pp. 245–281). San Diego: College-Hill Press.

Halliday, M.A.K. (1985). *An Introduction to Functional Grammar.* London: Edward Arnold.

Halliday, M.A.K. (1994). *An Introduction to Functional Grammar,* Second Edition. London: Edward Arnold.

Halliday, M.A.K., & Hasan, R. (1976). *Cohesion in English.* London: Longman Group.

Hartley, L. (1995). *Cognitive-Communicative Abilities Following Brain Injury: A Functional Approach.* San Diego: Singular Publishing Group Inc.

Hartley, L. & Jensen, P.J. (1991). Narrative and procedural discourse after closed head injury. *Brain Injury, 6,* 271–281.

Hartley, L. & Jensen, P.J. (1992). Three discourse profiles of closed head injured speakers: Theoretical and clinical implications. *Brain Injury, 5,* 267–285.

Holland, A.L. (1982). When is aphasia aphasia? The problem of closed head injury. In R. Brookshire (Ed.), *Clinical Aphasiology, (Vol. 12)* (pp. 345–349). Minneapolis: BRK Publishers.

Jordan, F. & Murdoch, B. (1990). A comparison of the conversational skills of closed head injured children and normal adults. *Australian Journal of Communication Disorders, 18,* 69–82.

Kintsch, W. (1974). *The Representation of Meaning in Memory.* Hillsdale, NY: Lawrence Erlbaum.

Kintsch, W. & van Dijk, T.A. (1978). Toward a model of text comprehension and production. *Psychological Review, 5,* 363–394.

Labov, B.Z. (1972). *Language in the Inner City: Studies in the Black Vernacular.* Philadelphia: University of Pennsylvania Press.

Levin, H.S., Grossman, R.G., & Kelly, P.J. (1976). Aphasia disorder in patients with closed head injury. *Journal of Neurology, Neurosurgery, and Psychiatry, 39,* 1062–1070.

Levin, H.S., Grossman, R.G., Rose, S.E., & Teasdale, G. (1979). Long term neuropsychological outcome of closed head injury. *Journal of Neurosurgery, 50,* 412–422.

Lezak, M.D. (1978). Living with the characterologically altered brain-injured patient. *Journal of Clinical Psychology, 39,* 592–598.

Liles, B.Z., Coelho, C.A., Duffy, R.F., & Zalagens, M.R. (1989). Effects of elicitation procedures on the narratives of normal closed head-injured adults. *Journal of Speech and Hearing Disorders, 54,* 356–366.

Linscott, F.J., Knight, R.G., & Godfrey, H.P.D. (1996). The profile of functional impairment in communication (PFIC): A measure of communication impairment for clinical use. *Brain Injury, 10,* 397–412.

Mandler, J. & Johnson, N.S. (1977). Remembrance of things parsed: Story structure and recall. *Cognitive Psychology, 9,* 111–151.

Marsh, N. (1999). Social skill deficits following traumatic brain injury: Assessment and treatment. In S. McDonald, L. Togher, & C. Code (Eds.), *Communication Disorders Following Traumatic Brain Injury* (pp. 175–210). East Sussex: Psychology Press Ltd.

Marsh, N. & Knight, R.G. (1991). Relationship between cognitive deficits and social skill after head injury. *Neuropsychology, 5,* 107–117.

Marsh, N., Knight, R.G., & Godfrey, H.P.D. (1990). Long-term psychosocial adjustment following very severe head injury. *Psychological Medicine, 19,* 175–182.

McDonald, S. (1992). Differential pragmatic language loss following closed head injury: Ability to comprehend conversational implicature. *Applied Psycholinguistics, 13,* 295–312.

McDonald, S. (1993). Pragmatic language skills after closed head injury: Ability to meet the information needs of the listener. *Brain and Language, 44,* 28–46.

McDonald, S. & Pearce, S. (1995). "The Dice Game" a new test of pragmatic language skills after closed head injury. *Brain Injury, 9,* 255–271.

McDonald, S. & Pearce, S. (1998). Requests that overcome listener reluctance; impairment associated with executive dysfunction in brain injury. *Brain and Language, 61,* 88–104.

McDonald, S. & van Sommers, P. (1993). Pragmatic language skills after closed head injury: Ability to negotiate requests. *Cognitive Neuropsychology, 10,* 297–315.

Mentis, M. & Prutting, C. (1987). Cohesion in the discourse of normal and head injured adults. *Journal of Speech and Hearing Research, 30,* 88–89.

Milton, S., Prutting, C., & Binder, G. (1984). Appraisal of communication competence in head injured adults. In R. Brookshire (Ed.), *Clinical Aphasiology (Vol. 14)* (pp. 114–123). Minneapolis: BRK Publishers.

Mross, E.F. (1990). Text analysis: Macro- and microstructural aspects of discourse processing. In Y. Joanette and H.H. Brownell (Eds.), *Discourse Ability and Brain Damage* (pp. 50–68). New York: Springer-Verlag.

Newton, A. & Johnson, D.A. (1985). Social adjustment and interaction after severe head injury. *British Journal of Clinical Psychology, 24,* 225–234.

Pang, D. (1989). Physics and pathophysiology of closed head-injury. In I. Bodis-Wollner & E.A. Zimmerman (Series Eds.) & M.D. Lezak (Vol. Ed.), *Frontiers of Clinical Neuroscience: Vol.7 Assessment of the Behavioural Consequences of Head Trauma* (pp. 1–17). New York: Alna R. Liss.

Patry, R. & Nespoulous, J. (1990). Discourse analysis in linguistics: Historical and theoretical background. In Y. Joanette and H.H. Brownell (Eds.), *Discourse Ability and Brain Damage: Theoretical and Empirical Perspectives* (pp. 2–25). New York: Springer-Verlag.

Penn, C. & Cleary, J. (1988). Compensatory strategies in the language of closed head injured patients. *Brain Injury, 2,* 3–17.

Prigatano, G., Rouche, J., & Fordyce, D. (1986). Nonaphasic language disturbances after brain injury. In G.P. Prigatano (Ed.), *Neuropsychological Rehabilitation After Brain Injury* (pp. 18–28). Baltimore: John Hopkins University Press.

Prutting, C.A. & Kirchner, D.M. (1987). A clinical appraisal of the pragmatic aspects of language. *Journal of Speech and Hearing Disorders, 52,* 105–119.

Roth, F.P. & Spekman, N.J. (1986). Narrative discourse: Spontaneously generated stories of learning-disabled and normally achieving students. *Journal of Speech and Hearing Disorders, 51,* 8–23.

Searle, J. (1969). *Speech Acts.* Cambridge, England: Cambridge University Press.

Shadden, B.B., Burnette, R.F., Eikenberry, B.R., & DiBrezzo, R. (1991). All discourse tasks are not created equal. In T.E. Prescott (Ed.), *Clinical Aphasiology (Vol. 20)* (pp. 327–342). Austin, TX: Pro-Ed.

Snow, P., Douglas, J., & Ponsford, J. (1995). Discourse assessment following traumatic brain injury: A pilot study examining some demographic and methodological issues. *Brain Injury, 9,* 365–380.

Snow, P., Douglas, J., & Ponsford, J. (1997a). Procedural discourse following traumatic brain injury. *Aphasiology, 11,* 948–967.

Snow, P., Douglas, J., & Ponsford, J. (1997b). Conversation assessment following traumatic brain injury: A comparison of two groups. *Brain Injury, 11,* 409–429.

Snow, P., Lambier, J., Parsons, C., Mooney, L., Couch., & Russell, J. (1987). Conversation skills following closed head injury: Some preliminary findings. In C.D. Field, A.C. Kneebone, & M. Reid (Eds.), *Brain Impairment Proceedings of the Eleventh Annual Brain Impairment Conference* (pp. 87–97). Melbourne: AASBI.

Spence, S.E., Godfrey, H.P.D., Knight, R.G., & Bishara, S.N. (1993). First impressions count: A controlled investigation of social skill following closed head injury. *British Journal of Clinical Psychology, 32,* 309–318.

Stein, N. & Glenn, C. (1979). An analysis of story comprehension in elementary school children. In R. Freedle (Ed.) *New Directions in Discourse Processing* (pp. 53–120). Norwood NJ: Ablex.

Tate, R.L., Lulham, J.M., Broe, G.A., Strettles, B., & Pfaff, A. (1989). Psychosocial outcome for the survivors of severe blunt head injury: The results from a consecutive series of 100 patients. *Journal of Neurology, Neurosurgery and Psychiatry, 52,* 1128–1134.

Thompsen, I.V. (1975). Evaluation and outcome of aphasia in patients with severe closed head trauma. *Journal of Neurology, Neurosurgery and Psychiatry, 38,* 713–718.

Togher, L. & Hand, L. (1998). Use of politeness markers with different communication partners: An investigation of five subjects with traumatic brain injury. *Aphasiology, 12,* 755–770.

Togher, L. & Hand, L. (1999). The macrostructure of the interview: Are traumatic brain injury interactions structured differently to control interactions? *Aphasiology, 13,* 709–723.

Togher, L., Hand, L., & Code, C. (1996). Disability following head injury: A new perspective in the relationship between communication impairment and disempowerment. *Disability and Rehabilitation, 18,* 559–556.

Togher, L., Hand, L., & Code, C. (1997a). Analyzing discourse in the traumatic brain injury population: Telephone interactions with different communication partners. *Brain Injury, 11,* 169–189.

Togher, L., Hand, L., & Code, C. (1997b). Measuring service encounters in the traumatic brain injury population. *Aphasiology, 11,* 491–504.

Togher, L., Hand, L., & Code, C. (1999). Exchanges of information in the talk of people with traumatic brain injury. In S. McDonald, L. Togher, & C. Code (Eds.), *Communication Disorders Following Traumatic Brain Injury* (pp.113–145). East Sussex: Psychology Press Ltd.

Ulatowska, H.K., Allard, L., & Chapman, S.B. (1990). Narrative and procedural discourse in Aphasia. In Y. Joanette and H.H. Brownell (Eds.), *Discourse Ability and Brain Damage: Theoretical and Empirical Perspectives* (pp. 189–198). New York: Springer-Verlag.

Ulatowska, H.K. & Chapman, S.B. (1989). Discourse considerations for aphasia management. *Seminars in Speech and Language, 10,* 298–314.

Ulatowska, H.K., Weiss Doyel, A., Freedman Stern, R., & Macaluso Hayes, S. (1983) Production of procedural discourse in aphasia. *Brain & Language, 18,* 315–341.

van Dijk, T.A. & Kintsch, W. (1983). *Strategies of Discourse Comprehension.* New York: Academic Press.

Ventola, E. (1979). The structure of casual conversation in English. *Journal of Pragmatics, 3,* 267–298.

Westby, C.E., Van Dongen, R., & Maggart, Z. (1989). Assessing narrative competence. *Seminars in Speech and Language, 10,* 63–67. Merrill.

Willer, B., Rosenthal, M., Kreutzer, J.S. Gordon, W.A., Rempel, R. (1993). Assessment of community integration following rehabilitation for traumatic brain injury. *Journal of Head Trauma Rehabilitation, 8,* 75–87.

Wolfolk, W.B., Fucci, D., Dutka, F.E., Herberholz, L.M., & Latorre, T.M. (1992) Differences in narrative productions of closed head injured adults. *Bulletin of the Psychonomic Society, 30,* 226–228.

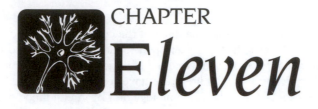

CHAPTER
Eleven

Language Disorders Following Traumatic Brain Injury in Childhood

Bruce E. Murdoch
and Deborah G. Theodoros

Introduction

Acquired childhood language disorders have been defined as those disturbances in language function resulting from some form of cerebral insult incurred after language acquisition has already commenced (Ozanne & Murdoch, 1990). The affected child has typically commenced learning language normally and has been acquiring developmental milestones at an appropriate rate prior to his/her injury. The cerebral insult causing acquired childhood language disorders can result from essentially the same range of neurological conditions that cause acquired language disorders in adults and include: traumatic brain injury (TBI), brain tumors, cerebrovascular accidents, infections, and convulsive disorders. However, the relative importance of each of the different etiologies to the occurrence of acquired language disorders in children differs from that seen in adults. In peacetime, cerebrovascular accidents are the most common cause of acquired language disorders in adults, whereas the most common cause of acquired childhood language disturbances is TBI (Lees, 1993; Ozanne & Murdoch,

1990). Although, as explained in Chapter 1 of the current book, head injuries associated with TBI can be classified as either open (penetrating) or closed (nonpenetrating), by far the majority of cases of acquired childhood language disorder associated with this etiology reported in the literature have resulted from closed head injuries. The mechanisms of TBI and the epidemiology of TBI in childhood are described in detail in Chapters 1 and 7, respectively, in this book and consequently will not be dealt with further in the present chapter.

Characteristics of the Language Disturbance in Childhood TBI

According to the traditional view, the prognosis for recovery from TBI in childhood is extremely good, the recovery often being considered to be rapid and complete. In particular, the recovery shown by children who have suffered mild head injuries has been reported to be excellent (Bijur, Haslum, & Gloning, 1990) while recovery from severe head injuries, although less certain, has been reported to be far better for children than for adults (Craft, 1972; Lenneberg, 1967). This difference between children and adults may result from three factors: First, it may be due to the different nature of the impacts causing TBI in children versus adults, childhood TBI generally being associated with lower-speed impacts (See Chapter 1); second, it may be related to differences in the basic mechanisms of brain damage following head injury in the two groups, which in turn are related to differences in the physical characteristics of children's heads and adult's heads (See Chapter 1); third, it may be the result of greater plasticity in the child's brain.

Contrary to the traditional view that children make a rapid and full recovery from TBI, over the past two decades a number of studies have documented the existence of persistent language deficits subsequent to severe TBI in children. Gilchrist and Wilkinson (1979) reported that almost two-thirds of young people with severe TBI exhibit aphasic-type disorders. Areas of language function reported to be deficient in children following TBI include: Verbal fluency (Chadwick, Rutter, Brown, Shaffer, & Traub, 1981a; Chadwick, Rutter, Shaffer, & Shrout, 1981b; Jordan, Ozanne, & Murdoch, 1990; Slater & Bassett, 1988), object naming (Jordan, Ozanne, & Murdoch, 1988, 1990; Levin & Eisenberg, 1979a, b), word and sentence repetition (Levin & Eisenberg, 1979a, b), and written output (Ewing-Cobbs, Fletcher, Levin, & Landry, 1985; Ewing-Cobbs, Levin, Eisenberg, & Fletcher, 1987). Unfortunately, the specific methodological approaches employed by different researchers to document the language abilities of children with TBI vary widely from study to study, making it difficult to determine the pattern of language impairment in this population. For instance, in some studies children with TBI have been included in larger groups of children with language difficulties arising from other neurological conditions (e.g., cerebrovascular accidents, brain tumors, etc.) making identification of specific areas of language impairment associated with TBI difficult (e.g., Alajouamine & Lhermitte, 1965; Hécaen, 1976). In addition, whereas some earlier researchers utilized aphasia batteries (e.g., Ewing-Cobbs et al., 1985, 1987; Levin & Eisenberg, 1979a,b) to assess the language abilities of children with TBI, others more recently have used tests more appropriate for use with pediatric subjects (e.g., Jordan et al., 1988).

The present chapter will provide a historical overview of research into the effects of childhood TBI on language abilities, in an attempt to establish the status of our understanding of the nature of language impairments in this population.

The language abilities of a group of 32 children with acquired aphasia associated with a variety of etiologies, including TBI, cerebrovascular malformation, aneurysm, and occlusion of the middle cerebral artery, among others, was evaluated by Alajouanine and Lhermitte (1965). They reported that the most obvious feature of the language disorder exhibited by the children in their group was a reduction in "expressive activities," with each child demonstrating a reduction in oral and written language and a reduction in the use of gestures.

Hécaen (1976) reported the language features of a group of 26 cases of acquired childhood aphasia of mixed etiology, which included 16 cases of head trauma. The associated aphasia was described by Hécaen as being characterized by a period of mutism followed by the recovery of language, marked by decreased initiation of speech, naming disorders, dyscalculia, and dysgraphia. Although less frequent, receptive language disorders were observed in one-third of the children with aphasia examined by Hécaen (1976). Due to the wide range of etiologies included in the subject groups examined by Alajouanine and Lhermitte (1965) and Hécaen (1976), however, any attempt to attribute the language features to any one etiological group, such as TBI, must out of necessity be guarded.

The early investigations of language in groups comprised only of children with TBI used standardized instruments such as aphasia batteries and tests of specific language behaviors to determine the profile of language impairment. For example, the Neurosensory Center Comprehensive Examination for Aphasia (NCCEA; Spreen & Benton, 1969) was used by Levin and Eisenberg (1979a) to examine the language abilities of a group of children and adolescents with closed head injury. Deficits in auditory comprehension were identified in 11% of the group, and verbal repetition was impaired in only 4%. Dysnomia for objects presented visually or tactually to the left hand were identified in about 12% of the group studied.

Ewing-Cobbs et al. (1985) also examined the language abilities of a group of children and adolescents with TBI, using the NCCEA. Their findings showed that during the early stages of recovery (less than 6 months posttrauma) a significant proportion of their subjects demonstrated linguistic impairments. In particular, naming disorders, dysgraphia, and reduced verbal productivity were prominent. These authors concluded that the language disorder identified was evidence of a "subclinical aphasia" rather than a frank aphasia disturbance. Ewing-Cobbs et al. (1985) speculated that, from a developmental perspective, the type of speech/language impairment incurred from a TBI is related to the language skills that are in primary ascendancy at the time of the injury. Further, comparison of recovery to the severity of injury indicated that children with moderate-severe TBI were more likely to demonstrate poorer performance on the naming and graphic subtests when compared to their mildly head-injured counterparts. In a further study of 23 children and 33 adolescents with TBI, Ewing-Cobbs et al.(1987) identified "clinically significant language impairment" in a large proportion of their subjects, with expressive and graphic functions most affected.

The most comprehensive series of studies to have documented the language abilities of children with TBI using tests developed for pediatric application is that reported by Jordan and colleagues (Jordan et al., 1988; Jordan, Cannon, & Murdoch, 1992, Jordan & Murdoch, 1990a, 1993, 1994). Jordan et al. (1988) assessed the language abilities of a group of 20 children with TBI, between 8 and 16 years of age, at least 12 months postinjury, using the Test of Language Development series and the NCCEA. They found the group with TBI to be mildly language-impaired when compared to a group of age- and sex-matched, non-neurologically-impaired controls. In particular, these investigators identified the presence of a specific deficit in naming in the group with TBI. The linguistic impairment exhibited by the children with TBI studied by Jordan et al. (1988), however, did not conform to any recognized developmental language disorder. Rather, it was noted by these researchers that the observed language disturbance was similar to that reported to occur following TBI in adults, in that the children with TBI also presented with a "subclinical aphasia" characterized by dysnomia. Jordan et al.(1988) concluded that, in contrast to the traditional view that the immature brain makes a rapid and full recovery following traumatic injury, TBI in children can produce long-term and persistent language deficits. In a follow-up study of the same group of children with TBI 12 months later, Jordan and Murdoch (1990a) observed that the naming deficit had persisted, while at the same time, verbal fluency abilities had deteriorated.

The high-level language functioning of a group of 11 children with severe TBI was assessed by Jordan, Cremona-Meteyard, and King (1996). Their findings indicated that the children with severe TBI had a lesser ability to create sentences with reference to social stimuli and a reduced ability to interpret ambiguous or figurative expressions than a group of matched controls. In contrast, Jordan et al. (1996) noted that the children with severe TBI were similar to the control children in their ability to make inferences.

Jordan et al. (1992) investigated the linguistic performance of a group of mildly head-injured children in adulthood but failed to identify any persistent linguistic deficits for this group, even in the very long term. In contrast, however, Jordan and Murdoch (1994) were able to identify late linguistic sequelae from 10 to 34 years following severe TBI sustained during childhood. Although overall scores achieved by these subjects fell within the average range on a standardized test of adolescent language development, scores were lower for the severely TBI individuals than for controls on measures of lexical recognition and retrieval as well as auditory comprehension of grammatically complex commands. Interestingly, a generalized reduction in linguistic skills across all areas of language competence assessed (syntax, semantics, pragmatics) was noted, suggesting a lack of specificity of linguistic impairment in their sample. It would appear, therefore, that children with mild TBI may be relatively spared in terms of persistent linguistic deficits when compared to their severely TBI counterparts, although marked variability in linguistic outcomes is evident within the severe TBI group.

In summary, contrary to the long-held view that children make a rapid and full recovery from TBI, a number of studies reported over the past 2 decades have documented the existence of persistent language deficits subsequent to severe TBI in childhood. In particular, studies of language function after pediatric TBI have shown that expressive oral language skills, including verbal fluency and naming to confrontation, are most consistently compromised, whereas receptive language is less impaired and tends to recovery earlier after injury. The observed language impairment is often characterized initially by reduced verbal output or, in its most severe form, mutism, which is followed in the longer term by subtle high-level language deficits. Subclinical language disturbance, as reflected in impoverished verbal fluency, dysnomia, and decreased word finding ability, is consistently reported in the literature. Frank aphasia, however, occurs in only a very small proportion of children suffering from TBI, if at all. The pattern of language impairment reported subsequent to childhood TBI is, therefore, similar in many ways to that reported in the literature relating to adult TBI (see Chapter 9).

Recovery of Language Function Following Childhood TBI

The traditionally held viewpoint that the child's brain exhibits a plasticity that enables rapid recovery of function following trauma had its origins in the work of Cotard (1868; cited in Levin, Benton, & Grossman, 1982). He reported that early or congenital damage to the left cerebral hemisphere did not lead to aphasia. This hypothesis was further supported by studies of a wide variety of brain injury cases, including children suffering congenital vascular disease and hemispherectomy for intractable seizures as well as traumatic head injury (Lenneberg, 1967; Smith, 1974). In more recent years, however, studies documenting the presence of persistent cognitive and behavioral as well as linguistic impairments subsequent to childhood TBI have cast some doubt on the traditional view of rapid and complete recovery in this population. Despite these doubts, few studies have documented the course of language recovery in children following TBI by way of a series of prospective evaluations.

Prospective Studies of Language Recovery in Childhood TBI

Jordan and Murdoch (1993) followed the course of speech and language recovery of a group of 11 children with TBI over an 18-month period postinjury. Although their findings confirmed that children with TBI have the potential for significant gains in speech and language skills subsequent to injury, Jordan and Murdoch (1993) noted that few of their subjects recovered to within normal limits on all language measures used, with 2 of the 11 subjects in particular experiencing severe, long-term speech and language deficits. Jordan and Murdoch (1993) commented that, although the patterns of language recovery demonstrated by their subjects were variable and very individual, naming and word-finding abilities, as measured on a test of confrontation naming, were particularly vulnerable to injury, with the majority of children with TBI experiencing persistent difficulties in this area of linguistic competence. Other authors have also reported dysnomia or word-finding difficulties to be a frequent persistent sequela to childhood TBI (Ewing-Cobbs et al., 1985; Levin & Eisenberg, 1979 a,b; Winogran, Knights, & Bawden, 1984).

Factors Affecting Language Recovery in Childhood TBI

A number of factors have been proposed as influencing the recovery of language following childhood TBI. These include the severity of the TBI (as measured by the Glasgow Coma Scale (GCS)—see Chapter 1), the site and size of lesion, and the age at injury. Severity of TBI has frequently been cited as one of the most important variables in determining the recovery of children with TBI, with more severe injuries tending to be associated with a poorer long-term prognosis for recovery (Chapman, 1995; Chapman, Levin, Wanek, Weyrauch, & Kufera, 1998; Fletcher & Levin, 1988; Jordan & Murdoch, 1993). Discourse measures have been reported to be lower in children who suffered a severe TBI, while children with mild TBI perform similarly to normal controls on discourse tasks (Chapman, 1995, Chapman et al., 1998). Similarly, severity of injury was found to affect the rate of recovery of the children with TBI investigated by Jordan and Murdoch (1993). They reported that it was in the first 6 months postinjury that the children with mild TBI tended to demonstrate most improvements in the language skills evaluated. In contrast, the children with severe TBI included in the group investigated by Jordan and Murdoch (1993) demonstrated more gradual improvement in language skills over the 18-month period of their prospective study. Jordan and Murdoch (1993) speculated that the observed differential rate of recovery is related to differences in the initial injury observed in children with severe TBI, compared to children with mild TBI. By definition, children with severe TBI are more likely to suffer extensive diffuse brain injury than their mild TBI counterparts. Indeed, Bruce, Alavi, Bilaniuk, Colinskas, Obrist, and Uzzell (1981) suggested that the degree of recovery subsequent to TBI is probably dependent on the extent of axonal injury. Jordan and Murdoch (1993) further speculated that, although children with mild TBI suffer less initial trauma in the form of diffuse axonal injury, they still experience the temporary secondary complication typical of TBI, that is, brain swelling (see Chapter 1). Rapid resolution of such brain swelling may well result in rapid restoration of function, provided there is no persistent local cerebral damage. In contrast, children with severe TBI, as well as experiencing these secondary effects of TBI, also experience more persistent primary axonal damage, leading to their poorer prognosis for recovery.

Despite the support in the literature for the notion that severity of TBI is an important factor influencing the degree of language recovery in children, it is evident that this factor alone does not fully account for degree of recovery in all cases. Examination of recovery patterns on an individual case basis often shows that the recovery patterns exhibited by individual children vary widely. In some cases children with severe TBI have been reported to show significant recovery of their language abilities while at the same time children with mild-to-moderate TBI may show poor recovery. For example, three of the children included in the prospective study of language recovery carried out by Jordan and Murdoch (1993) had very severe injuries (GCS = 3). Unexpectedly, only two of these three children experienced severe speech and language deficits in the long term. The third child demonstrated a "significant" recovery of his language skills, although he was reported to demonstrate a marked deficit in naming skills. Chapman, Watkins, Gustafson, Moore, Levin, & Kufera (1997) have likewise noted that severity of TBI does not always correspond to the degree of recovery of discourse abilities in children with TBI.

In addition to severity of injury, the site and size of the lesion has been identified as a possible factor influencing language recovery following childhood TBI. Although historically it was believed that children did not demonstrate the marked cerebral dominance for language observed in adults, more recent research has challenged this viewpoint, suggesting that significant language impairment is far more likely subsequent to dominant hemisphere damage than to nondominant hemisphere damage (Aram, Ekelman, Rose, & Whitaker, 1985; Aram, Ekelman, & Whitaker, 1986, 1987; Carter, Hohenegger, & Satz, 1982; Satz and Bullard-Bates, 1981). Aram et al. (1985, 1986, 1987) reported that the syntactic abilities of children who sustain early left hemisphere vascular lesions are compromised to a greater degree than children with early right hemisphere lesions. As further evidence of lateralization in childhood, Chapman (1997) noted that children with left hemisphere lesions as a consequence of TBI are more likely to show specific language disturbances on traditional language measures than children with an intact left hemisphere. Jordan and Murdoch (1993) suggested that the absence of significant localized damage to the dominant hemisphere may have been an important factor in the good recovery of linguistic competency observed in the majority of children with TBI included in their prospective study.

The size or volume of lesions incurred as a result of TBI has also been reported to be related to language abilities, with larger lesions being associated with greater levels of impairment (Levin, Ewing-Cobbs, & Eisenberg, 1995). In particular Levin et al. (1995) reported that the volume of left or right frontal lobe lesions in children increased the predictive value of performance on a verbal fluency task as well as on a response modulation task (i.e., respond to one stimulus and withhold response to another stimulus).

The relationship between age at injury and language outcome is somewhat controversial. It has been suggested that brain injury may have its greatest effect on the acquisition of new language skills rather than on the recovery of previously established abilities (Hebb, 1942). If true, this hypothesis may explain the noted relatively good recovery of lexical and grammatical aspects of language after brain injury, in that these abilities are often well established in children prior to injury. Consistent with this suggestion are the findings of recent studies that implicate a younger age at injury with a more deleterious impact on long-term language recovery (Chapman et al., 1998; Ewing-Cobbs et al., 1987; Ewing-Cobbs, Miner, Fletcher, & Levin, 1989). Chapman et al. (1998) reported poorer discourse abilities for children who suffered brain injuries prior to 5 years of age than for children injured at 5 years of age or older. Likewise, Ewing-Cobbs et al. (1989) identified that children with brain injuries incurred prior to 31 months of age performed more poorly on expressive language tasks than children with brain injuries sustained later than 31 months of age. Also consistent with this pattern, Ewing-Cobbs et al. (1987) noted that written language is more disrupted in children with TBI than in adolescents with TBI. Shaffer, Bijur, Chadwick, and Rutter (1980) reported that children who suffer brain injuries prior to 8 years of age have more significant reading problems than children who suffer TBI later in life.

Latent Behavioral Deficits Following TBI

Retrospective studies of the long-term consequences of TBI have provided evidence that TBI in childhood may lead to the manifestation of behavioral deficits at some later stage in the child's development, despite apparent recovery in the short term postinjury (Bates, Reilly, & Marchman, 1992; Chapman & Levin, 1994). According to Eslinger, Grattan, Damasio, and Damasio (1992), these latent deficits may not be evidenced until the child with TBI reaches maturity or even, in some cases, enters adult life. Although the mechanism underlying the manifestation of latent behavioral disturbances is not known, Chapman, Levin, and Lawyer (1999) outlined two possible explanations for their occurrence. First, brain injury may prevent the child from attaining the higher cognitive levels required to support later developmental processes. Second, that the latent deficits arise from damage to an immature brain region causing a delay of symptoms until that region reaches functional maturity. In fact, the latent deficits may result from an interaction between both of these mechanisms (Chapman et al., 1999).

Differential Recovery of Language Following Childhood TBI

As mentioned earlier in this chapter, the patterns of recovery of linguistic competency exhibited by children following TBI vary greatly from case to case. To illustrate the diversity of these recovery patterns, three cases seen in the current authors' research clinic are presented below. The first case demonstrates what would traditionally be described as a typical recovery pattern and serves to illustrate why children with TBI have, in the past, been renowned for making a rapid and full recovery. The second and third cases, however, show less typical courses of recovery, characterized by persistent significant language impairments.

Case 1 - Sara

Sara was a 9-year-old right-handed female who was admitted to hospital following a horse riding accident. Although she had not suffered any loss of consciousness immediately following the accident, Sara was unresponsive to commands. At the time of admission to hospital she was noted to be irritable and thrashing, and her eyes were deviated to the left. Her GCS score was 7, and she demonstrated focal fitting. A computerized tomographic (CT) scan performed shortly after admission revealed no abnormality except for a fracture of the skull in the region of the left occiput.

At 1 day posttrauma, Sara appeared able to recognize her mother but made no attempt to communicate. During the following 24 hours, rapid deterioration of her condition occurred to a point where she entered a state of deep coma. A repeat CT scan at this stage demonstrated the presence of right cerebral edema, with compressed ventricles and some midline shift. The child was electively ventilated and paralyzed for 1 week posttrauma, at which time she was weaned off the ventilator and the medication. Focal seizures continued; however, by 9 days postinjury Sara was able to open her eyes, and shortly after was able to follow simple commands. By 2 weeks postinjury, Sara was described as bright, and enjoyed watching television. However, she still failed to initiate communication and to respond socially. Response to yes/no questions at this time was demonstrated by the use of eye closing. Four weeks after the accident, Sara showed socially appropriate but simplified language, her speech at this time being described as labored. She was discharged from the hospital with regular medical and paramedical follow-up.

Sara's language abilities were then assessed at regular 6-month intervals over an 18-month period postinjury, using a battery of standardized language tests which included the NCCEA, the Test of Language Development-Intermediate (TOLD-I; Hammill & Newcomer, 1982), the Boston Naming Test (BNT; Kaplan, Goodglass, & Weintraub, 1983) and a selected subtests of the Clinical Evaluation of Language Functions (CELF; Semel-Mintz & Wiig, 1982). In addition to these standardized tests a conversation sample was also collected and analyzed for syntactic adequacy, using Prutting and Kirchner's (1987) Pragmatic Protocol.

Sara's performance on the NCCEA was essentially normal, even in the acute stage postinjury, and little variability in performance on this test occurred over the 18-month period. At initial assessment 1 month postinjury, Sara achieved a Spoken Language Quotient of 83 on the TOLD-I, which was just outside the normal range according to the test norms. Based on her performance on the TOLD-I, Sara made steady gains over the 18-month recovery period and at the final assessment was achieving scores within the normal range for all subtests. A raw score of 38 was achieved at the initial assessment with the BNT, Sara's performance at this time being marked by numerous semantic errors such as "dice" for dominoes and "penguin" for pelican. Sara did make continuous quantitative gains in her naming skills over the 18-month test period; however, performance on the BNT at final contact continued to be marked by semantic errors. At times during the course of the final assessment Sara requested the first sound of a word to cue her response. The accuracy score achieved by Sara for the confrontation naming subtest of the CELF, was well within normal limits at the initial assessment; however, speed of performance was markedly reduced. By 19 months postinjury, Sara had little difficulty on the confrontation naming test of the CELF, which requires rapid access of familiar names (for shapes and colors). Performance of the word association subtest of the CELF, which requires the naming of animals and food within a prescribed time period was within normal limits at each of the test intervals.

Sara demonstrated well-developed syntactic skills, and no deficit areas were identified. Although all communicative acts identified by the Pragmatic Protocol were found to be appropriate, it was noted in the acute stage postinjury that Sara's conversational fluency was often interrupted by repetitions and circumlocutory behavior as she appeared to search for the appropriate word. By 18 months postinjury, however, most evidence of word-searching behaviors had disappeared, with only the occasional linguistic dysfluency apparent. Based on Sara's initial conversational sample, it was evident that she had difficulty interpreting jokes in any more than a literal sense and also demonstrated some difficulty understanding complex instructions with frequent repetitions required. At the time of the final assessment, Sara was able to cope with complex verbal instructions; however, she continued to interpret according to literal meaning and demonstrated persistent difficulties with figurative language (e.g., Sara could only interpret proverbs in a purely literal sense).

In summary, Sara demonstrated a typical recovery from severe TBI characterized by significant language impairment during the acute stage of recovery, followed by a rapid return of functional communication skills during the first 6 months posttrauma. At the time of initial standardized testing (6 months postinjury), Sara demonstrated only minimal language impairment, which featured slightly reduced scores on tests of overall language abilities, and evidence of a mild word-finding difficulty. On the basis of the test results and

observation and analysis of Sara's conversational skills over the 18-month period postin-
jury, it was concluded that Sara presented with a high-level language deficit affecting both
verbal fluency and word retrieval and higher-level auditory comprehension abilities.

Case 2 - Jodie

Jodie, a 7-year-old, right-handed female, was admitted to hospital following a motor
vehicle-pedestrian accident. On admission to hospital she presented with a dilated right
pupil and left focal fitting involving the entire left arm. Jodie was assigned a GCS score of
3 on admission. A CT scan performed shortly after admission demonstrated the presence
of a small amount of blood in the right lateral ventricle, in the choroid plexus and fourth
ventricle. A small cerebral contusion was also identified in the right frontal region,
although no mass lesion was evident. A 5-cm long linear fracture was identified in the
outer table of the frontal bone. Jodie was intubated and hyperventilated. Intravenous val-
ium was prescribed for fitting.

At 1 day postinjury, Jodie presented with decerebrate rigidity with persisting bilateral
extensor spasms of both arms and legs. Pupils remained small and only reacted slightly. A
repeat CT scan at this time demonstrated scattered hemorrhagic contusions with sub-
arachnoid and intraventricular blood. There was diffuse brain swelling with small cis-
terns, but no evidence of hernification. Nine days after admission, Jodie remained in a
coma with quadriplegia and decerebrate rigidity. Brainstem function continued to be
unstable. An EEG performed 13 days posttrauma indicated a very abnormal pattern,
with diffuse slow wave activity; however, there were no frank epileptogenic features. At
this stage, the child remained unconscious, with eyes closed, and demonstrated no
response to speech. Jodie did, however, demonstrate suck and swallow reflexes. Two weeks
after the accident Jodie developed fitting, and there was a slight deterioration in her neu-
rological state. A CT scan taken 13 days postinjury demonstrated resolving cerebral con-
tusions, normal ventricular size, and generalized cerebral edema. No mass lesions,
however, were identified.

Three weeks postinjury Jodie spontaneously opened her eyes. It was reported, however,
that she demonstrated no comprehension at this time. Jodie continued in this state until
8 weeks postinjury, at which time medical charts continued to describe her as in a vegeta-
tive state. At 9 weeks following the accident, she was discharged from the hospital with reg-
ular medical and paramedical follow-up.

Evaluation of speech and language skills during the early stages of recovery proved
very difficult, since the child continued to remain unresponsive to formal evaluation.
Recovery of speech and language skills was, therefore, charted using observational tech-
niques. At 6 weeks postinjury, Jodie presented with periods of wakefulness. She was irri-
table and unresponsive. She demonstrated a severe spastic dysarthria, with extreme oral
hypersensitivity and the presence of the primitive oral reflexes (e.g., rooting, bite, suck-
swallow, and jaw thrust). Although Jodie had begun to take food orally, feeding was a
slow and tedious process.

Observation 12 weeks postinjury indicated that Jodie had increasing periods of wakeful-
ness and was inconsistently responsive to simple one-part commands (e.g., shut your eyes).
Responses were, however severely limited by her physical condition. Six months after the
accident Jodie remained in a severely impaired state. She was alert, could identify body
parts, and was responsive to simple commands, but demonstrated little expressive ability.

Vocalizations consisting of /g/ and /n/ plus a vowel were used in a noncommunicative manner. At this stage, Jodie could produce the reduplicated syllables of /nananana/.

At 10 months postinjury, Jodie began to spontaneously utter single words in appropriate contexts. Her first word was reported to be "daddy." The single-word stage lasted for only 3 days, at which time Jodie unexpectedly began to verbalize in well-structured and pragmatically appropriate sentences. Most of Jodie's expressions were in response to questions, with few spontaneous utterances, and speech was marked by slow and imprecise articulation. Informal assessment at this time indicated the presence of dysarthria, characterized by reduced speech rate, and fatigue with longer utterances. Jodie attempted "wh" type questions (What? Where? When? Why?) and functional questions (e.g., What do you do with a spoon?) with a high degree of accuracy. Tasks involving tactile naming resulted in naming errors characterized by errors within semantic class (e.g., Jodie substituted "glass" for "cup," and "pen" for "pencil.") At this time, Jodie was diagnosed as having bilateral optic atrophy, with no vision in the left eye and limited vision in the right eye.

Because of Jodie's limited concentration span and rapid fatigue, it was not until 12 months postinjury that formal assessment of her language skills could be carried out. During a 4-week period Jodie was administered a battery of tests designed to evaluate different aspects of language. As a result of Jodie's marked visual impairment, the test battery was somewhat limited but included selected subtests of the NCCEA, the TOLD-I, and selected subtests from CELF. A language analysis was performed using the Language Assessment and Remediation Screening Procedure (LARSP; Crystal, Fletcher, & Garman, 1976). Jodie was reassessed using the same test battery 6 months and 12 months after the initial assessment. At the final assessment (24 months postinjury) the BNT was also included in the test battery.

Subtests of the NCCEA administered at the time of initial testing (12 months postinjury) included: tactile naming (right hand and left hand), sentence repetition, repetition of digits, reversal of digits, word fluency, sentence construction, and articulation. Since Jodie was able to cooperate on more of the NCCEA subtests at the time of later assessments, further subtests, including visual naming, description of use, identification by name, and identification by sentence, were added to the test battery at these later times. Unfortunately Jodie's performance on all subtests of the NCCEA was indicative of severe impairment at all assessments. Likewise, Jodie's overall language quotient, as determined by the TOLD-I, remained more than two and one half standard deviations below the mean specified in the test manual for normals for the period of the study and was indicative of a severe persistent language impairment. Subtests for the CELF, that were administered included: processing relationships and ambiguities, processing spoken paragraphs, and producing word associations. At all occasions of testing, the percentiles achieved by Jodie on these subtests fell well below the prescribed range for normal. Jodie scored only 6 correct out of a possible 60 on the BNT when it was administered 24 months postinjury, her performance being marked by the presence of numerous semantic errors.

A syntactic analysis of conversational speech was carried out on a sample of 76 utterances from Jodi's initial language assessment (12 months postinjury) using LARSP. Analysis of the therapist-child interaction indicated that much of the sample was dominated by therapist questions, with only limited spontaneous speech on the part of the child (67 responses, 9 spontaneous). Results of the LARSP analysis at this stage placed Jodie at Stage III to Stage IV on the LARSP Profile (age equivalence of approximately 2; 6 to 3; 0). Jodie predominantly used utterances involving three clausal elements (subject-verb-object, subject-verb-complement, subject-verb-adverb) and three phrasal elements (determiner-adjective-noun, preposition-determiner-noun).

There was also some evidence of early coordination of sentences using the connective "and." Reevaluation 6 months later on a sample of 77 utterances indicated that Jodie had progressed to Stage V on the LARSP Profile, with some Stage VI structures appearing (age equivalence of approximately 3; 0 to 4; 6). At this time Jodie used predominantly 4 and 5 clausal element structures, with frequent use of coordination, subordination, and complex verb phrase structures. There was also an increase in the number of spontaneous utterances in the sample (58 responses, 19 spontaneous). Twenty-four months postinjury, Jodie demonstrated syntactic skills consistent with stages V and VI of the LARSP Profile. The sample at this time consisted of 94 utterances, with 81 classified as responses and 13 classified as spontaneous.

Overall, Jodie exhibited a range of symptoms consistent with those reported in cases of severe TBI (Levin, Madison, Bailey, Meyers, Eisenberg, & Guinto, 1983), including the presence of a persisting period of mutism, followed by a subsequent progression to syntactically intact, though limited verbalizations. Although Jodie could follow simple commands and interact with the environment soon after the return of consciousness, she failed to develop any systematic form of communication for a period of 10 months.

A number of researchers have identified the presence of a period of mutism following severe TBI in children (Levin et al., 1983; Hécaen, 1976, 1983), particularly in the presence of a diffuse increase in brain volume as evidenced in the present case. There has been only one reported case, however, of recovery subsequent to such a prolonged period of mutism as documented in the present case (Levin et al., 1983). Other researchers have reported that, of the cases who eventually regained verbal skills subsequent to severe TBI, 98.5% do so within 6 months postinjury (Levin et al., 1982). This would indicate the unlikelihood of the present case regaining verbal skills subsequent to such protracted mutism.

The TBI in the present case was associated with massive cerebral swelling, as evidenced by the early CT scans. Such a generalized increase in brain volume is reported to be common in young patients within 24 hours of a severe TBI (Levin et al., 1982; Levin et al., 1983). The resolution of such brain swelling is often thought to be associated with the recovery of function following severe TBI. Consequently, the rapid return of the brain to near normal proportions in the present case would seem to present a relatively positive prognosis for the rapid return of language function. Based on the CT scan evidence, the brain injury experienced by Jodie would seem insufficient to account for the prolonged period of mutism and subsequent language impairment characterized by generalized reduction in communication competency with an accompanying severe word-finding difficulty as documented in her case. Clearly, other factors must be sought to explain the presence of these features.

Snoek, Jennet, Adams, Graham, and Doyle (1979) reported that pathologic findings in the fatal cases of a series of severely TBI children demonstrating generalized cerebral swelling on CT scans identified the presence of diffuse white matter injury, hypoxic cortical damage, cerebral contusion, and signs of increased intracranial pressure. Importantly, the diffuse white matter injury in these cases was discernable only at a microscopic level. Bruce et al. (1981) concluded that the degree of recovery in children following TBI is dependent on the degree of primary axonal injury. It is possible, therefore, that in addition to transient swelling evident on the CT scans, Jodie may also have incurred permanent axonal damage at the microscopic level not evident in the CT scans. Although, if present, this permanent damage would serve to explain to some extent the prolonged period of mutism, it fails to explain the abrupt nature of the recovery of functional communication skills.

In summary, Jodie's case demonstrates the potential for recovery of at least functional communication skills after the seemingly critical 6-month recovery period following severe TBI in children. It also serves to demonstrate that, contrary to the traditional view that children make a full recovery from TBI, significant linguistic deficits may persist subsequent to severe TBI in some children.

Case 3 - John

John, a 13-year-old, right-handed male, was admitted to hospital subsequent to a cyclist-motor vehicle accident. He had been struck by a motor vehicle and was reportedly unconscious at the scene of the accident. On admission to hospital he presented with a fixed and dilated pupil and was assigned a GCS score of 3. A CT scan performed shortly after admission demonstrated marked generalized edema, with multiple small contusions. Small high-density areas indicative of hemorrhage were identified in the region of the right anterior lenticulate nucleus and deep in the left temporoparietal region. There was also a large left fracture in the temporal bone extending across the vertex. Parietal, frontal, and temporal trephine holes were drilled, revealing a small acute subdural hematoma, acute traumatic subarachnoid blood, and a tense, swollen brain. The subdural hematoma was evacuated and an intracranial pressure monitor inserted.

Ten days postinjury John began to demonstrate some purposeful movements and was reported to show recognition of some individuals. There was very little lower limb movement and very poor head control. Although cough and gag reflexes were reported to be intact, John had poor swallowing skills and was placed on nasogastric feeds. A repeat CT scan 14 days after admission demonstrated scattered intracerebral contusions, especially in the left temporal region, and widespread edema. A further CT scan performed 21 days postinjury indicated early cerebral atrophy with ventricular dilatation.

Assessment of oral-motor skills at 10 weeks postinjury indicated impaired oral-motor function due to increased tone in the facial muscles, minimal range of jaw movement, presence of primitive reflex patterns (biting, lip retraction), and marked oral and facial hypersensitivity. By 3 months postinjury John showed consistency in response to simple directions (e.g., open your eyes). A CT scan performed 5 months postinjury revealed dilation of both lateral ventricles as well as the third ventricle. There was also an increase in the subarachnoid space in the left temporal region where the left temporal horn of the left lateral ventricle was also more dilated, indicative of marked reduction in the volume of the cerebrum on the left.

At 6 months postinjury John demonstrated some consistent yes/no responses, and an informal assessment indicated that he could comprehend object names, match pictures, and make requests using an eye-pointing response. By 6 months postinjury, he was able to match words to pictures accurately 80% of the time. At this time, he presented as a spastic quadriplegic.

Formal assessment of language skills using a standardized test battery was not attempted until 12 months postinjury; however, even then due to John's severe physical impairments the use of these tests remained limited. Components of the Test of Adolescent Language-2 (TOAL-2; Hammill, Brown, Larson, & Weiderholt, 1987) and the NCCEA were administered. It must be noted that John's communication was entirely dependent on an augmentative communication system, either an adapted computer or a Cannon Communicator; hence, in all instances standard procedures for test administration was violated since John could not *respond in an oral manner. An informal oral-motor assessment was also completed. Testing was carried out at 12 months postinjury and then repeated at 24 months postinjury.*

At 12 months postinjury, John continued to exhibit severely impaired oral-motor skills. Oral-motor impairment was characterized by a minimal range of jaw movement, the persistence of primitive oral reflexes (jaw extension, bite reflex), extremely limited tongue mobility, reduced tone and mobility of facial muscles, and weakness of the pharyngeal and palatal muscles. Drooling was a constant problem, and his vocalizations were limited to three vowels. He could occasionally produce /m/ on command; however, coordination of lip closure and vocalization was extremely poor. The findings were consistent with the presence of a severe mixed spastic/flaccid dysarthria. Reassessment at 24 months postinjury indicated very minimal improvements in John's oral-motor skills.

Several subtests of the NCCEA were administered, using a "written" response mode or eye pointing in all instances. These subtests included: visual naming, description of use, tactile naming (right and left hand), sentence construction, identification by name, identification by sentence, reading for meaning, writing of names, writing to dictation, and writing (copying). At the time of initial testing, John's performance on the visual naming and the description of use subtests was considered to be severely impaired. In contrast, he achieved maximum scores on the subtests of identification by name, reading sentences for meaning, and reading words for meaning; hence his abilities in these areas were deemed to be intact. Performance on the NCCEA was, however, consistent with a marked word-finding difficulty. John's written responses were characterized by semantic paraphasic errors (e.g., "comb" became "brush"; "cup" became "bowl") at initial assessment. Marked improvement in scores in all subtests occurred over the 12-month period between initial and follow-up testing.

Because of the severe limitations in John's oral communication skills only the following subtests of the TOAL-2 were administered: listening/vocabulary, listening/grammar, reading/vocabulary, reading/grammar, writing/vocabulary, and writing/grammar. At both the initial and follow-up assessments, all scores achieved by John on these subtests fell below the range of average performance, with only very minimal improvement being evidenced over the 12-month period between tests. In particular, the skill areas most affected by John's injury appeared to be those involving a reading component (e.g., reading/grammar, writing/vocabulary, and writing/grammar all of which required John to read the stimulus material).

Overall, John demonstrated marked speech and language deficits subsequent to severe TBI. During the early stages of recovery, he remained semicomatose and any form of communication was severely limited for the first 6 months postinjury. Recovery of comprehension skills then proceeded rapidly, and John was able to demonstrate at least functional comprehension by 12 months postinjury. Severe oral-motor impairment persisted throughout the recovery stage, limiting any restoration of verbal communication. John continued to be reliant on an augmentative communication system for expressive function.

Performance on tests of overall language function demonstrated the presence of marked impairment in expressive and receptive syntax and expressive and receptive semantics, with a particular deficit in word-finding skills. The presence of a deficit in word-finding skills is consistent with much of the research on language recovery subsequent to pediatric TBI, which indicates the persistence of word-finding difficulties (Ewing-Cobbs et al., 1985, Levin & Eisenberg, 1979a). John's basic reading skills were preserved, as indicated by his performance on the NCCEA subtest of reading for meaning; however, more advanced reading abilities accessed by the reading/vocabulary and reading/grammar subtests of the TOAL-2 were found to be impaired. Although John demonstrated a number of language characteristics considered representative of typical recovery subsequent to pediatric TBI, the persistence of his language disorder is not consistent with the traditional view of recovery in this population.

Summary

The three cases of severe TBI presented above have served to highlight the heterogeneity that exists with regard to language recovery in the pediatric TBI population. Despite similar levels of severity (as demonstrated by the CGS scores) each case experienced a remarkably different pattern of recovery of linguistic skills in the long term. It is interesting to note, however, that a number of features were consistent despite the marked variability observed. It would appear that receptive language skills were least affected in each case, and although there were varying degrees of recovery, all three children progressed to a stage of at least functional communication skills. A special feature consistent across the three cases was the presence of a word-finding problem. Word-finding problems have frequently been reported in the literature as the most outstanding feature of language disorder subsequent to childhood TBI (Levin & Eisenberg, 1979b; Jordan et al., 1988; Winogran et al., 1984).

Based on the observations made in these three cases, it is obvious that children suffering TBI do not present as a homogeneous group with regard to language abilities, and consequently cannot be treated using a prescriptive approach. Rehabilitation programs for the child with TBI must, therefore, cater to the specific needs of the child in question. Communication management may require the use of an augmentative communication system, either in the acute stage or in the longer term, as demonstrated in Case 3, or may require the use of facilitative techniques that enable the child to manage his/her persistent communication deficits more effectively. The fact that all three cases presented above demonstrated some degree of word-finding deficit indicates that speech/language pathologists should provide the TBI child with strategies to overcome word-finding deficits from very early stages in recovery, in an attempt to prevent later breakdown of communication in response to this deficit. A number of authors in the past have addressed the issue of treatment of word-finding problems in the language-learning disabled population (McGregor & Leonard, 1989; Wallach & Butler, 1984), and it may be that strategies used with this latter group are appropriate for application to the child with TBI. Intervention strategies for children with language disorders subsequent to TBI are discussed more fully in Chapter 12.

Discourse Abilities Following Childhood TBI

As indicated earlier in the present chapter, traditional studies of the linguistic abilities of children who have suffered a TBI have focused primarily on the use of standard language assessment procedures to document the characteristics of the language impairment exhibited by this population. In particular, many studies have utilized aphasia batteries to describe the linguistic skills of children with TBI. Unfortunately, as many authors agree, traditional language measures may not adequately identify the range of language difficulties which manifest in persons with TBI

(Chapman, et al.,1992; Jordan et al., 1992; McDonald, 1992, 1993). In many instances, despite the existence of subtle, high-level linguistic deficits, people with TBI tend to score within normal limits on traditional aphasia tests (Chapman, et al., 1992; Jordan et al., 1992; Jordan & Murdoch, 1990a; Levin et al., 1982; McDonald, 1993). Further, despite apparent recovery of language function as identified by structured language measures, both children and adults have been shown to have persistent deficits at the discourse level of language following TBI (Chapman et al., 1998; Dennis & Barnes, 1990; McDonald, 1992, 1993; Mentis & Prutting, 1987). Consequently, in an attempt to better define the scope of communicative impairment in children with TBI, many researchers have recently advocated the use of discourse measures to identify those aspects of the language disorder that have proven elusive to traditional language batteries (Dennis & Barnes, 1990; Dennis & Lovett, 1990; Ewing-Cobbs et al., 1985; Jordan et al., 1988).

According to Dennis and Lovett (1990), discourse refers to the use of communicative language in context. Discourse reflects the complex interaction between cognition, linguistic, and information-processing abilities (Chapman et al., 1999). Given that children with severe TBI exhibit deficits in a variety of cognitive functions, including attention, memory, visuospatial function, and psychosocial function among others, in addition to linguistic impairments, discourse analysis may provide a better indication of communicative ability following childhood TBI than structured linguistic measures. Although a variety of different discourse types are recognized, including descriptive, conversational, narrative, procedural, and expository discourse, by far the majority of studies that have investigated the discourse abilities of children with TBI have used narrative discourse (Campbell & Dollaghan, 1990; Chapman, 1995; Chapman et al., 1992; Chapman et al., 1998; Dennis, Jacennik, & Barnes, 1994; Jordan, Murdoch, & Buttsworth, 1991).

Narrative tasks provide the opportunity to examine "complex language, sequencing of events, children's ability to make information explicit for the listener, and the knowledge of story structure" (Olley, 1989 p.44). In addition, Liles, Coelho, Duffy, and Zalagens (1989) suggested that story generation tasks are useful in rendering characterizations of language use in high-level TBI subjects. Consequently, the inclusion of narrative tasks in a test battery for children with TBI has been seen by several research groups as having the potential to provide valuable information for documenting further the linguistic characteristics of the TBI population. To that end, Jordan et al., (1991) used a story generation task to examine the story grammar skills and intersentential cohesion abilities of a group of 20 children with TBI, aged 8 to 16 years, at 1 to 4 years postinjury. Performance of the children with TBI was compared to that of a group of non-neurologically impaired accident victims matched for age, sex, and socio-economic status. No significant differences were found between the narrative skills of the children with TBI and the matched controls on any of the story grammar measures or in the use of cohesive devices. Jordan et al., (1991) inferred that the story generation task used in their study may not have yielded optimal narrative performance. In contrast, based on narratives collected during a story retelling task, Chapman, et al. (1992) reported deficits in the story grammar skills of 20 children and adolescents with TBI when tested at least 1 year postinjury. In particular, their findings indicated that the discourse of children with severe TBI differed from that of normal controls on both language and information structures, with the severe TBI cases producing less language and less information than the normal children in retelling a story. Further, the subjects with severe TBI differed from those with mild-moderate TBI on information structure measures of narratives. The disruption in story structure was reported by Chapman, et al. (1992) to be characterized primarily by omission of critical setting and action information.

Chapman et al. (1998) used a story retelling task to investigate the effects of severe TBI on discourse in children who were 6 to 8 years of age at the time of testing. In order to consider age-at-injury effects, these workers compared the narratives of children who sustained a TBI before the age of 5 years to those of children aged greater than 5 years at the time of injury. The results indicated that severe TBI has a deleterious effect on discourse in young children. In particular, Chapman et al. (1998) reported that their TBI cases exhibited marked reductions in the overall amount of information (propositions), in structural completeness, and in the expression of the central semantic meaning (gist) of the story. In contrast, measures of sentential length and complexity did not differ between the subjects with severe TBI and the control subjects. Consistent with the findings of Jordan et al., (1991), the ability of the children with severe TBI to manipulate certain cohesive devices (e.g., use of reference and connectors) was comparable to that of the control subjects. Although no significant differences were found by Chapman et al., (1998) according to age at injury, these researchers suggested that there was a consistent pattern of generally poorer discourse for the early injured group (i.e., less than 5 years of age at the time of injury).

Ewing-Cobbs, Brookshire, Scott, and Fletcher (1998) examined linguistic structure, cohesion, and thematic recall of the narrative discourse in two groups of children with TBI, selected on the basis of the presence or absence of acute language disturbance. A sibling comparison group was also included. Based on a story retelling task, the language-impaired TBI group produced fewer words and utterances than the sibling group, their stories being characterized by fewer complete referential and lexical ties and more referential errors, which Ewing-Cobbs et al. (1998) suggested were indicative of difficulty conjoining meaning across sentences. In addition, the language-impaired TBI group was reported as recalling only one-third of the propositions needed to maintain the story theme, and made more errors sequencing the propositions than did the other two groups. The language-impaired TBI group, however, did not differ from the other two groups on measures of rate and fluency of speech production, number or length of mazes, use of conjunctives, or naming errors. Overall, the majority of the findings reported by Ewing-Cobbs et al. (1998) are consistent with those of Chapman et al. (1992), who, as noted earlier, reported a reduction in the number of words, number of sentences, and amount of core information retained in the narratives of children and adolescents with severe TBI in conjunction with preservation of syntactic complexity and fluency.

To date, only two studies of the conversational discourse abilities of children with TBI have been reported (Campbell & Dollaghan, 1990; Jordan & Murdoch, 1990b). Campbell & Dollaghan (1990) collected a series of spontaneous conversation samples from nine children and adolescents with TBI over a period of approximately 13 months. At the time of initial assessment, 2 to 16 weeks postinjury, significant differences in all measures of expressive language were identified as compared to a normal control group. Significant improvement occurred, however, in the TBI group over the 13 months between the initial and final assessment. Although at the final follow-up the TBI group was reported to produce fewer utterances than the controls, their performance on other measures, including total number of words, total number of different words, mean length of utterance in morphemes, percentage of complex utterances, and percentage of utterances within mazes, was the same as the controls. Campbell and Dollaghan (1990) did note, however, that the patterns of deficit and recovery in the TBI group was heterogeneous, with five of the nine TBI cases continuing to exhibit marked deficits. Jordan and Murdoch (1990b) elicited conversations from a group of 20 children with TBI and examined their conversational skills using the Clinical Discourse Analysis (Damico, 1985). No significant differences were found between the performance of the children with TBI and a group of matched controls on this measure of conversational competency. Jordan & Murdoch (1990b) cautioned, however, that the children with TBI in their study were all between 1 and 5 years postinjury at the time of testing. They highlighted the need for further research of a prospective nature, examining the performance of children with TBI throughout the course of recovery on measures of conversational competency, to clarify the relationship between time postinjury and the occurrence of conversational error behaviors.

In summary, evidence is available to suggest that the discourse abilities of children with TBI are impaired in a number of ways, compared to normals. As yet, however, the relationship between factors such as age at injury, lesion site and size, severity of injury, etc., and the occurrence of deficits in discourse skills is unknown.

Assessment of Language Abilities Following Childhood TBI

Assessment of a child's language abilities subsequent to TBI should be carried out within the context of relevant medical and biographical information. This may include information such as the child's general physical and emotional condition, the presence of motor speech disorders, neurological status, radiological findings, cognitive status, and hearing abilities, among others. Within the confines determined by this essential background information, the speech-language pathologist should then proceed to draw up a profile of the child's language abilities based on a comprehensive evaluation of language, using a range of standardized and nonstandardized tests.

Test materials appropriate for use with children with acquired aphasia have been comprehensively reviewed by several authors (Cross & Ozanne, 1990; Lees & Urwin, 1991). Major factors to be kept in mind in selecting the particular language tests to be used include: the child's age, the presence of any concomitant disabilities such as motor or perceptual impairments, and the clinician's experience. Given that children with TBI have been reported to exhibit high-level language deficits, language evaluation for this population needs to include a wide range of formal and informal procedures capable of detecting subtle high-level language impairment. In addition, assessment of language skills subsequent to childhood TBI should cover both receptive and expressive language abilities and also include a developmental test as well as tests of specific skill areas, such as a visual naming test to determine the presence of dysnomia, which is a frequently documented sequela to TBI in childhood. The language evaluation should also include a collection of language samples which can be analyzed in terms of syntax, semantics, and pragmatics. A battery of language tests routinely used by the authors of the current chapter to assess the language abilities of children with TBI is outlined in Table 11-1.

The Preschool Language Scale–3 (PLS-3; Zimmerman, Steiner, & Pond, 1992) is an assessment commonly used in the clinical setting to examine language development and to identify the presence of language disorders in children aged from birth to 6 years. It includes both an auditory comprehension component and an expressive communication component, and includes tasks such as picture naming, repeating sentences, following directions (e.g., Point to the ———), and identifying concepts.

The language skills of infants can be assessed using the Receptive-Expressive Emergent Language Test-2nd Edition (REEL-2; Bzoch & League, 1991). The format of this test involves a checklist based on an interview with a significant caregiver of the child, in which observed behaviors of the child are explored with the interviewee. Each item is coded as "typical" of the child, "emergent," or "never observed." Several analyses of language development, including syntactic analyses, mean length of utterance, and type token ratio (vocabulary development) can also be carried out on samples of vocalization collected from children with TBI.

Table 11-1. Language tests suitable for use with children with TBI.

Test	Authors
Preschool Language Scale-3 (PLS-3)	Zimmerman et al. (1992)
Receptive-Expressive Emergent Language Test-Second Edition (REEL-2)	Bzoch & League (1991)
Clinical Evaluation of Language Fundamentals-Third Edition (CELF-3)	Semel, Wiig & Secord (1995)
Clinical Evaluation of Language Fundamentals-Preschool (CELF-P)	Wiig, Secord & Semel (1992)
Peabody Picture Vocabulary Test-Third Edition (PPVT-III)	Dunn et al. (1997)
Hundred Pictures Naming Test (HPNT)	Fisher & Glenister (1992)
Boston Naming Test (BNT)	Kaplan et al. (1983)
Test of Language Competence-Expanded Edition (TLC)	Wiig & Secord (1989)
Test of Word Knowledge (TOWK)	Wiig & Secord (1992)
Test of Problem Solving-Elementary (TOPS-Elementary)	Bowers et al. (1994)
Test of Problem Solving-Adolescent (TOPS-Adolescent)	Bowers et al. (1991)
Queensland University Inventory of Literacy (QUIL)	Dodd et al. (1996)
Test of Phonological Awareness (TOPA)	Torgesan & Bryant (1994)
School Age Oral Language Assessment (SAOLA)	Allen et al. (1993)

A general measure of the overall range of language skills exhibited by children with TBI can be determined using the Clinical Evaluation of Language Fundamentals-Preschool (CELF-P; Wiig, Secord, & Semel, 1992) and the Clinical Evaluation of Language Fundamentals–Third Edition (CELF-3; Semel, Wiig, & Secord, 1995). The CELF-P is suitable for children aged 3 years to 6 years, while the CELF-3 caters to ages 6 years to 15 years 11 months. Receptive and expressive vocabulary can be assessed in children with TBI, using the Peabody Picture Vocabulary Test-Third Edition (PPVT-III; Dunn, Dunn, & Williams, 1997) and the Hundred Pictures Naming Test (HPNT; Fisher & Glenister, 1992), respectively. The PPVT-III is a widely used test of receptive language and provides norms for children aged 2 years 6 months to 18 years 11 months. Each item within the test involves the child being presented with four pictures. He/she is then required to select the picture that best demonstrates the vocabulary item presented verbally by the examiner. The HPNT assesses expressive vocabulary and involves presenting the child 100 pictures of objects. He/she is then required to name each object while being timed.

Word-finding difficulties can be identified in children with TBI by using the BNT (Kaplan et al., 1983). This test is comprised of sixty pictures of common household objects that the child is asked to name. The assessment is standardized for children aged 5 years 5 months to 10 years 10 months as well as for normal and aphasic adults.

The Test of Language Competence-Expanded Edition (TLC; Wiig & Secord, 1989) assesses higher-level language abilities and was designed to be used in conjunction with other standardized measures of language performance, such as aphasia tests. The TLC is comprised of four subtests that include: understanding ambiguous sentences, making inferences, recreating sentences, and understanding metaphoric expressions.

Residual or recovered semantic knowledge following childhood TBI can be evaluated using the Test of Word Knowledge (TOWK; Wiig & Secord, 1992). It yields information regarding lexical knowledge, while accommodating two levels of age ranges. Each of the two levels consist of four core subtests and a number of supplementary subtests that target specific areas of difficulty. The subtests address aspects of receptive and expressive language such as vocabulary, definitions, opposites, multiple contexts, synonyms, and figurative usage.

The Test of Problem Solving-Elementary (TOPS—Elementary; Bowers, Huisingh, Barrett, Orman, & Lo Guidice, 1994) and the Test of Problem Solving-Adolescent (TOPS—Adolescent) (Bowers, Huisingh, Barrett, Orman, & LoGuidice, 1991) are standardized tests of language and problem solving that tap into higher-level language. The elementary version addresses problem solving, determining solutions, inference, empathizing, prediction, use of context, and thinking vocabulary, through the presentation of several pictures that show functional situations. The child is asked a series of open-ended questions about what is going on in each picture. The adolescent version of the test addresses aspects of language such as clarifying, evaluating, analyzing, effect, and fair-mindedness. Thirteen problem-solving passages are presented to the child, together with a series of open-ended questions.

Two tests that can be used to identify and describe phonological awareness skills of children in relation to literacy development are the Queensland University Inventory of Literacy (QUIL; Dodd, Holm, Oerlemans, & McCormack, 1996) and the Test of Phonological Awareness (TOPA; Torgenson & Bryant, 1994).

The QUIL includes several subtests that address various aspects of reading and writing skills, and it is standardized for school-aged children in grades 1–7. The TOPA measures young children's awareness of the individual sounds in words, a skill that occurs in readiness for literacy development. It is designed to be sensitive to the phonological structure of words in oral language and can be used to identify children of preschool age who are experiencing difficulty in this preliteracy area. The TOPA addresses a child's ability to hear or identify individual sounds in words, to blend individual sounds into words, as well as rhyming.

Finally, controlled narrative samples can be elicited from children with TBI by way of the School Age Oral Language Assessment (SAOLA; Allen, Leitão & Donovan, 1993). In this test, the child is told a story from a "wordless" book about "Peter and the Cat." The child is then required to retell the story using the pictures in the book.

Summary

Although traditionally, recovery of language abilities following TBI in childhood has been considered to be excellent, in recent years research utilizing specifically designed linguistic tasks has demonstrated the presence of significant, long-term language disorders in some children with severe TBI. In particular, expressive oral skills, including verbal fluency and naming to confrontation, have been reported to be consistently compromised, with receptive language abilities being less impaired and tending to recover earlier. Further, evidence is available to suggest that the discourse abilities of children with TBI are also impaired in a number of ways, compared to normal children.

The language abilities of children with TBI, however, are not homogeneous, with varying patterns of language recovery being described in the literature. Consequently, the language disorders demonstrated by children with TBI cannot be treated using a prescriptive approach. Rather rehabilitation programs need to be tailored to the specific needs of each child with TBI.

References

Alajouanine, T. & Lhermitte, F. (1965). Acquired aphasia in children. *Brain*, 88, 653–662.

Allen, L., Leitão, S., & Donovan, M. (1993). *School Age Oral Language Assessment.* South Fremantle, Western Australia: Language-Learning Materials, Research and Development.

Aram, D.M., Ekelman, B.L., Rose, D.F., & Whitaker, H.A. (1985). Verbal and cognitive sequelae following unilateral lesions acquired early in childhood. *Journal of Clinical and Experimental Neuropsychology, 7*, 55–78.

Aram, D.M., Ekelman, B.L., & Whitaker, H.A. (1986). Spoken syntax in children with acquired unilateral hemisphere lesions. *Brain and Language, 31*, 61–87.

Aram, D.M., Ekelman, B.L., & Whitaker, H.A. (1987). Lexical retrieval in left and right brain lesioned children. *Brain and Language, 27*, 75–100.

Bates, E., Reilly, J., & Marchman, E. (1992). Discourse and grammar after early focal brain injury. Abstract from Academy of Aphasia Meeting, Toronto, Canada.

Bijur, P.E., Haslum, M., & Gloning, J. (1990). Cognitive and behavioral sequelae of mild head injury in children. *Pediatrics, 86*, 337–344.

Bowers, L., Huisingh, R., Barrett, M., Orman, J., & LoGuidice, C. (1991). *Test of Problem Solving — Adolescent.* Queensland: Pro-Ed.

Bowers, L., Huisingh, R., Barrett, M., Orman, J., & LoGuidice, C. (1994). *Test of Problem Solving — Elementary.* Queensland: Pro-Ed.

Bruce, D.A., Alavi, A., Bilaniuk, K., Colinskas, C., Obrist, W., & Uzzell, B. (1981). Diffuse cerebral swelling following head injuries in children: The syndrome of malignant brain edema. *Journal of Neurosurgery, 54*, 170–178.

Bzoch, K.R. & League, R. (1991). *Receptive-Expressive Emergent Language Test Second Edition.* Austin, TX: Pro-ed.

Campbell, T.F. & Dollaghan, C.A. (1990). Expressive language recovery in severely brain-injured children and adolescents. *Journal of Speech and Hearing Disorders, 55*, 567-581.

Carter, R.L., & Hohenegger, M.K., & Satz, P. (1982). Aphasia and speech organization in children. *Science, 219*, 797–799.

Chadwick, O., Rutter, M., Brown, G., Shaffer, D., & Traub, M. (1981a.) A prospective study of children with head injuries: II Cognitive sequelae. *Psychological Medicine, 11*, 49–61.

Chadwick, O., Rutter, M., Shaffer, D., & Shrout, P.E. (1981b). A prospective study of children with head injuries: IV. Specific cognitive deficits. *Journal of Clinical Neuropsychology, 3*, 101–120.

Chapman, S.B. (1995). Discourse as an outcome measure in pediatric head-injured populations. In S.H. Broman & M.E. Michel (Eds.), *Traumatic Brain Injury in Children* (pp. 95–116). New York: Oxford University Press.

Chapman, S.B. (1997). Cognitive-communication abilities in children with closed head injury. *American Journal of Speech-Language Pathology, 6*, 50–58.

Chapman, S.B., Culhane, K.A., Levin, H.S.., Harward, H., Mendelsohn, D., Ewing-Cobbs, L., Fletcher, J.M., & Bruce, D. (1992). Narrative discourse after closed head injury in children and adolescents. *Brain and Language, 43*, 42–65.

Chapman, S.B. & Levin, H.S. (1994). Discourse abilities and executive function in head-injured children. Paper presented at the American Speech-Language and Hearing Association Convention, New Orleans, USA.

Chapman, S.B., Levin, H.S. & Lawyer, S.L. (1999). Communication problems resulting from brain injury in children: Special issues of assessment and management. In S. McDonald, L. Togher, & C. Code (Eds.), *Communication Disorders Following Traumatic Brain Injury* (pp. 235–269). Hove, Sussex: Psychology Press.

Chapman, S.B., Levin, H.S., Wanek, A., Weyrauch, J., & Kufera, J. (1998). Discourse after closed head injury in young children: Relation of age to outcome. *Brain and Language, 61*, 420–449.

Chapman, S.B., Watkins, R., Gustafson, C., Moore, S., Levin, H.S., & Kufera, J.A. (1997). Narrative discourse in children with closed head injury, children with language impairment and typically developing children. *American Journal of Speech-Language Pathology, 6*, 66–75.

Craft, A.W. (1972). Head injury in children. In P.J. Vinken & G.W. Bruyn (Eds.), *Handbook of Clinical Neurology* Vol. 23 (pp. 445–458) Holland: Elsevier.

Cross, J.A. & Ozanne, A.E. (1990). Acquired childhood aphasia: Assessment and treatment. In B.E. Murdoch (Ed.), *Acquired Neurological Speech/Language Disorders In Childhood* (pp. 66–123). London: Taylor & Francis.

Crystal, D., Fletcher, P., & Garman, M. (1976). *The Grammatical Analysis of Language Disability.* London: Edward Arnold.

Damico, J. (1985). Clinical discourse analysis: A functional approach to language assessment. In C.S. Simon (Ed.), *Communication Skills and Classroom Success* (pp.165–203). London: Taylor & Francis.

Dennis, M. & Barnes, M.A. (1990). Knowing the meaning, getting the point, bridging the gap, and carrying the message: Aspects of discourse following closed head injury in childhood and adolescence. *Brain and Language, 39*, 428–446.

Dennis, M. Jacennik, B., & Barnes, M.A. (1994). The content of narrative discourse in children and adolescents after early-onset hydrocephalus and in normally developing age peers. *Brain and Language, 46,* 129–165.

Dennis, M. & Lovett, M.W. (1990). Discourse ability in children after brain damage. In Y. Joanette & H.H. Brownell (Eds.), *Discourse Ability and Brain Damage: Theoretical and Empirical Perspectives* (pp. 199–223). New York: Springer-Verlag.

Dodd, B., Holm, A., Oerlemans, M., & McCormack, M. (1996). *Queensland University Inventory of Literacy.* Queensland, Australia: The University of Queensland.

Dunn, L.M., Dunn, L.M., & Williams, K.T. (1997). *Peabody Picture Vocabulary Test–Third Edition.* Minnesota: American Guidance Service.

Eslinger, P., Grattan, L.M., Damasio, H., & Damasio, A.R. (1992). Developmental consequences of childhood frontal lobe damage. *Archives of Neurology, 49,* 764–769.

Ewing-Cobbs, L., Brookshire, B., Scott, M.A., & Fletcher, J.M. (1998). Children's narratives following traumatic brain injury: Linguistic structure, cohesion and thematic recall. *Brain and Language, 61,* 395–419.

Ewing-Cobbs, L., Fletcher, J.M., Levin, H.S., & Landry, S.H. (1985). Language disorders after pediatric head injury. In J.K. Darby (Ed.) *Speech and Language Evaluation in Neurology: Childhood Disorders* (pp. 97–112). Orlando, FL: Grune & Stratton.

Ewing-Cobbs, L., Levin, H.S., Eisenberg, H.M., & Fletcher, J.M. (1987). Language functions following closed head injury in children and adolescents. *Journal of Clinical and Experimental Neuropsychology, 9,* 575–592.

Ewing-Cobbs, L., Miner, M.E., Fletcher, J.M., & Levin, H.S. (1989). Intellectual motor and language sequelae following closed head injury in children and adolescents. *Journal of Pediatric Psychology, 9,* 575–592.

Fisher, J.P. & Glenister, J.M. (1992). *The Hundred Pictures Naming Test.* Victoria: ACER.

Fletcher, J.M. & Levin, H.S. (1988). Neurobehavioural effects of brain injury in children. In D.K. Routh (Ed.), *Handbook of Pediatric Psychology.* New York: Guilford Press.

Gilchrist, E. & Wilkinson, M. (1979). Some factors determining prognosis in young people with severe head injuries. *Archives of Neurology, 36,* 355–359.

Hammill, D.D. Brown, V.L., Larsen, S.C., & Weiderholt, J.L. (1987). *Test of Adolescent Language–2.* Austin, TX: Pro-Ed.

Hammill, D.D. & Newcomer, P.L. (1982). *Test of Language Development–Intermediate.* Austin, TX: Pro-ed.

Hebb, D.O. (1942). The effect of early and late brain injury upon test scores and the nature of abnormal adult intelligence. *Proceedings of the American Philosophical Society, 1,* 265–292.

Hécaen, H. (1976). Acquired aphasia in children and the ontogenesis of hemispheric functional specialization. *Brain and Language, 3,* 114–134.

Hécaen, H. (1983). Acquired aphasia in children: Revisited. *Neuropsychologia, 21,* 581–587.

Jordan, F.M. Cannon, A., & Murdoch, B.E. (1992). Language abilities of mildly closed head injured children 10 years postinjury. *Brain Injury, 6,* 39–44.

Jordan, F.M. Cremona-Meteyard, S., & King, A. (1996). High-level linguistic disturbances subsequent to childhood closed head injury. *Brain Injury, 10,* 729–738.

Jordan, F.M. & Murdoch, B.E. (1990a). Linguistic status following closed head injury: A follow-up study. *Brain Injury, 4,* 147–154.

Jordan, F.M. & Murdoch, B.E. (1990b). A comparison of the conversational skills of closed head injured children and normal children. *Australian Journal of Human Communication Disorders, 18,* 69–82.

Jordan, F.M. & Murdoch, B.E. (1993). A prospective study of the linguistic skills of children with closed head injuries. *Aphasiology, 7,* 503–512.

Jordan, F.M. & Murdoch, B.E., (1994). Severe closed head injury in childhood: Linguistic outcomes into adulthood. *Brain Injury, 8,* 501–508.

Jordan, F.M., Murdoch, B.E., & Buttsworth, D.L. (1991). Closed head injured children's performance on narrative tasks. *Journal of Speech and Hearing Research, 34,* 572–582.

Jordan, F.M., Ozanne, A.E., & Murdoch, B.E. (1988). Long-term speech and language disorders subsequent to closed head injury in children. *Brain Injury, 2,* 179–185.

Jordan, F.M., Ozanne, A.E., & Murdoch, B.E. (1990). Performance of closed head-injured children on a naming task. *Brain Injury, 4,* 27–32.

Kaplan, E., Goodglass, H., & Weintraub, S. (1983). *Boston Naming Test.* Philadelphia: Lea & Febiger.

Lees, J.A. (1993). *Children with Acquired Aphasias.* London: Whurr Publishers.

Lees, J.A. & Urwin, S. (1991). *Children with Language Disorders.* London: Whurr Publishers.

Lenneberg, E.H. (1967). *Biological Foundations of Language.* New York: John Wiley & Sons.

Levin, H.S. Benton, A., & Grossman, R.G. (1982). *Neurobehavioural Consequences of Closed Head Injury.* Oxford: Oxford University Press.

Levin, H.S. & Eisenberg, H.M. (1979a). Neuropsychological impairment after closed head injury in children and adolescents. *Journal of Pediatric Psychology, 4,* 389–402.

Levin, H.S. & Eisenberg, H.M. (1979b). Neuropsychological outcome of closed head injury in children and adolescents. *Child's Brain, 5,* 281–292.

Levin, H.S., Ewing-Cobbs, L., & Eisenberg, H.M. (1995). Neurobehavioral outcome of pediatric closed head injury. In S.H. Broman & M.E. Michel (Eds.), *Traumatic Head Injury in Children* (pp.70–94). New York: Oxford University Press.

Levin, H.S., Madison, C.F., Bailey, C.B., Meyers, C.A., Eisenberg, H.M., & Guinto, F.C. (1983). Mutism after closed head injury. *Archives of Neurology, 40,* 601–607.

Liles, B.Z., Coelho, C.A., Duffy, R.J., & Zalagens, M.R. (1989). Effects of elicitation procedures on the narratives of normal and closed head-injured adults. *Journal of Speech & Hearing Disorders, 54,* 356–366.

McDonald, S. (1992). Communication disorders following closed head injury: New approaches to assessment and rehabilitation. *Brain Injury, 6,* 283–292.

McDonald, S. (1993). Pragmatic language skills after closed head injury: Ability to meet the informational needs of the listener. *Brain and Language, 44,* 28–46.

McGregor, K.K. & Leonard, L.B. (1989). Facilitating word-finding skills in language impaired children. *Journal of Speech and Hearing Disorders, 54,* 141–147.

Mentis, M. & Prutting, C.A. (1987). Cohesion in the discourse of normal and head injured adults. *Journal of Speech and Hearing Research, 30,* 88–98.

Olley, L. (1989). Oral narrative performance of normal and language impaired school aged children. *Australian Journal of Human Communication Disorders, 17,* 43–65.

Ozanne, A.E. & Murdoch, B.E. (1990). Acquired childhood aphasia: Neuropathology, linguistic characteristics and prognosis. In B.E. Murdoch (Ed.), *Acquired Neurological Speech/Language Disorders in Childhood* (pp. 1–65). London: Taylor & Francis.

Prutting, C.A. & Kirchner, D.N. (1987). A clinical appraisal of the pragmatic aspects of language. *Journal of Speech & Hearing Disorders, 52,* 105–119.

Satz, P. & Bullard-Bates, C. (1981). Acquired aphasia in children. In M.T. Sarno (Ed.), *Acquired Aphasia* (pp. 398–426). New York: Academic Press.

Semel, E.,. Wiig, E.H., & Secord, W.A. (1995). *Clinical Evaluation of Language Fundamentals–Third Edition.* San Antonio, TX: The Psychological Corporation.

Semel-Mintz, E. & Wiig, E.H. (1982). *Clinical Evaluation of Language Functions.* Columbus, OH: Charles E. Merrill.

Shaffer, D., Bijur, P., Chadwick, D.F., & Rutter, M.L. (1980). Head injury and later reading disability. *Journal of the American Academy of Child Psychiatry, 19,* 592–610.

Slater, E.J. & Bassett, S.S. (1988). Adolescents with closed head injuries. *American Journal of Diseases of Children, 142,* 1048–1051.

Smith, E. (1974). Influence of site of impact upon cognitive performance persisting long after closed head injury. *Journal of Neurology, Neurosurgery and Psychiatry, 37*, 719–726.

Snoek, J., Jennett, B., Adams, J.H., Graham, D.I., & Doyle, D. (1979). Computerized tomography after recent severe head injury in patients without acute intracranial hematoma. *Journal of Neurology, Neurosurgery & Psychiatry, 42*, 215–225.

Spreen, O. & Benton, A.L. (1969). *Neurosensory Centre Comprehensive Examination for Aphasia.* Victoria: University of Victoria.

Torgenson, J.K. & Bryant, B.R. (1994). *Test of Phonological Awareness.* Queensland: Pro-Ed.

Wallach, G.P. & Butler, K.G. (1984). *Language Learning Disabilities in School-Age Children.* Baltimore: Williams & Wilkins.

Wiig, E.H. & Secord, W. (1989). *Test of Language Competence–Expanded Edition.* San Antonio: The Psychological Corporation.

Wiig, E.H. & Secord, W. (1992). *Test of Word Knowledge.* San Antonio, TX: The Psychological Corporation.

Wiig, E.H. Secord, W., & Semel, E. (1992). *Clinical Evaluation of Language Fundamentals–Preschool.* San Antonio: The Psychological Corporation.

Winogran, H.W., Knights, R.M., & Bawden, H.N. (1984). Neuropsychological deficits following head injury in children. *Journal of Clinical Neuropsychology, 6*, 269–286.

Zimmerman, I.L., Steiner, V.G., & Pond, R.E. (1992). *Preschool Language Scale–3.* San Antonio, TX: The Psychological Corporation.

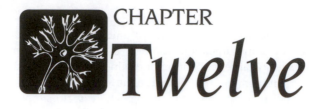

CHAPTER

Twelve

Treatment of Cognitive-Linguistic Communication Disorders Following Traumatic Brain Injury

Fiona J. Hinchliffe, Bruce E. Murdoch, and Deborah G. Theodoros

Introduction to Cognitive-Linguistic Communication Rehabilitation in Adults Following TBI

Communication is fundamental to all levels of daily activity, and effective communication is necessary for the maintenance of a positive quality of life and psychosocial well-being. Even the most subtle communication impairments can seriously influence the success with which an individual achieves his or her occupational, personal, and interpersonal goals. In the adult population, traumatic brain injury (TBI) typically occurs in young males, with the highest incidence befalling those in the 15–24-year-old age group (Australian Bureau of Statistics [ABS], 1990; Kraus et al., 1984). Consequently many individuals who sustain a TBI must cope with communicative difficulties for the greater part of their adult lives. Intervention by the speech-language pathologist that aims to ameliorate the social and personal handicap imposed by communication disorders is an essential component in the functional and psychosocial rehabilitation of the individual with TBI.

The planning and implementation of treatment for language and communication deficits following TBI is invariably challenging. There is no simple prescription of therapy for this population, which is characteristically heterogenous. The communicative ability of each person who has sustained a TBI is likely to be the product of their premorbid personality, sociolinguistic, and behavioral characteristics, combined with the neurobehavioral sequelae of diffuse brain trauma and the acquired manifestations of cognitive and linguistic impairment. Further diversity is also present in the extent and nature of the impact that a communication impairment can have on an individual. That is, the functional effects of an acquired communication deficit may vary from person to person, depending on the individual's educational, vocational, social, and cultural situation and needs.

While the treatment plan for each TBI case will necessarily be unique, there are several general principles of treatment, which are theoretically driven and are integral to the design of a comprehensive, effective, and socially valid program that is directed toward meaningful real-world outcomes that promote personal and communal linkages. This chapter addresses current general principles for designing and implementing treatment programs for individuals with language and communication disorders following TBI, as well as outlines some therapy strategies for specific language and communication deficits.

A Framework for Assessing and Treating Communication Impairment

The World Health Organization (WHO, 1997) produced a revision of the most widely recognized conceptual framework for describing consequential aspects of illness, the International Classification of Impairments, Activities and Participation (ICIDH-2). This classification provides a framework by which to assess the consequential phenomena of an illness and systematically structure an intervention program and measure its outcome. The ICIDH-2 presents a social model of human functioning and disablement that classifies disturbances of function associated with health conditions at the body (impairment), person (activity and activity limitation), and society (participation) levels. According to this framework, impairment refers to any abnormality of function of the body's structure or function. "Activity and activity limitation" is concerned with the nature and extent of functioning at the level of the person, referring to the individual's integrated activities associated with everyday life. "Participation and participation restriction" addresses the societal consequences of disability, referring to the nature and extent of a person's involvement in life situations in relation to impairments, activities, health conditions, and contextual factors. To illustrate, according to the WHO framework (1997), the consequences of TBI could be represented on a continuum of deficits in auditory processing, verbal memory, word finding, attention, and verbal organization (impairments); limited ability to converse fluently and observe normal interactive behaviors (activity limitation); and inability to fulfill a normal life role with respect to vocational and family status (participation restriction).

Table 12-1 summarizes the application of the ICIDH-2 framework to the assessment and treatment of language-based communication disorders following TBI. Each component of this approach will be discussed in subsequent sections of this chapter.

Table 12-1. Framework for assessment and treatment of cognitive-communication disorders of traumatic brain injury, using the IDICH-2 model of human functioning and disablement (WHO,1997).

Level of Disablement	Example	Assessment Approach	Treatment Approach
Impairment	Auditory processing deficit	Standardized diagnostic assessments	Restorative and compensatory approach using modality-specific or component process exercises
Activity Limitation	Limitations in maintaining a conversation in contexts requiring rapid exchanges of information	Tests of pragmatic ability Investigation of features of discourse production and comprehension	Compensatory approach aimed at altering the behavior of the individual
		Tests of skill on specific functional tasks	Behavioral Approach Specific functional skills training
Participation Restriction	Restricted involvement in social relationships. Denied participation in particular employment activities.	Quality-of-life scales Handicap inventories	Compensatory approach aimed at manipulating the environment—physical, contextual, personal

The Nature of the Cognitive-Linguistic Communication Disorders

As discussed in earlier chapters, communication difficulty in the TBI population often occurs in the presence of minimal or no primary language impairment. Deficits in language skills requiring higher-level and integrated cognitive-linguistic components are, however, consistently apparent. Deficits in lexical-semantic and sentential-semantic manipulations, complex comprehension, oral fluency, and attention have been identified as cardinal cognitive-linguistic impairments following severe TBI (Hinchliffe, Murdoch, Chenery, Baglioni, & Harding-Clark, 1998).

In addition to, and as a consequence of, impairment in these components of cognitive-linguistic function, individuals with TBI experience a complex range of difficulties both in daily communicative activities and in wider social contexts (e.g., Coelho, 1995; Hartley, 1995; Hartley & Jensen, 1991; McDonald 1993; Mentis & Prutting, 1987; Penn & Cleary, 1988). These include, but are not limited to, the use of excessive or inappropriate language for the situation, poor word-finding skills, inappropriate lexical selection, difficulty structuring discourse, difficulty maintaining a topic or sustaining a conversation, reduced understanding of subtle meaning or abstract language, difficulty processing language in demanding situations, reduced sensitivity to nonverbal or situational cues, and poor use of vocal intonation, gesture, and facial expression in conversation (Braun, Lussier, Baribeau, & Malmus, 1989; Hagen, 1984; Holland, 1982; McDonald & van Sommers, 1993; Prigatano, Roueche, & Fordyce, 1985). Such difficulties in communication are termed "cognitive-communication" disorders, and are considered to arise from the above-described impairments in linguistic and metalinguistic skill as well as impairments in nonlinguistic cognitive functions such as perception discrimination, organization, reasoning, attention, and memory (ASHA, 1991).

Along with impairments in linguistic and cognitive processes, communication skills are potentially disrupted by disorders of executive function. Executive functions mediate and regulate all other cognitive activities and are necessary for the formation and execution of goal-directed behavior (Lezak, 1995). Executive disruption is common in TBI and is considered to be the result of damage to the frontal lobes (Stuss & Benson, 1986). Several dimensions of executive function that are necessary for functional communication skill have been identified (Ylvisaker & Szekeres, 1989). These include self-awareness and goal setting, planning, self-directing, self-inhibiting, self-monitoring, self-evaluation, and flexible problem solving. Deficits in executive functioning, particularly reduced self-awareness and self-monitoring, may contribute to disruptions in functional communicative activity as well as being detrimental to successful communication rehabilitation.

A cognitive-communication disorder is thought to underlie the ability to effectively use language, in terms of lexical choice and adherence to the social rules of language-based interactions (Hartley, 1995; Watt, Penn, and Jones, 1996). Such a disorder can, therefore, underpin reduced pragmatic abilities and associated deficits in social skills. Indeed, cognitive-communication disorders following TBI have been shown to be associated with unsatisfactory interpersonal communication experiences and poor social integration (Galski, Tompkins, & Johnston, 1998; O'Flaherty & Douglas, 1997), as well as contributing to poor quality of life, psychosocial handicap, and failure to achieve work reentry (Brown & Vandergoot, 1998; Galski et al., 1998; Isaki & Turkstra, 2000; Snow, Douglas, & Ponsford, 1998). Thus, cognitive-communication disorders can be said to manifest as limitations in communicative activity and participation within society.

The Issue of Candidacy for Treatment

In contemporary health care settings, where the emphasis on measuring outcomes and the cost-benefit relationship of rehabilitation have become critical, the selection of candidates for rehabilitation is a sensitive and challenging first step in the rehabilitation process. Often those with very severe injuries are not considered candidates for therapy if the neurobehavioral consequences of the trauma are deemed unlikely to respond to intervention. At the other end of the spectrum are those with relatively minor brain injury, who are often discharged from acute hospital settings and denied access to rehabilitation services. In both cases, decisions as to the selection of candidacy for therapy have traditionally been driven by medically-orientated consideration of the assessable impairment, rather than the activity limitation or participation restriction that may potentially be experienced by the individual.

In some cases, those with mild impairments who are discharged without follow-up can experience significant functional difficulties and fail to return in an effective manner to their valued life roles (Hinnant, 1999; Wrightson, 1989), and have been shown to judge themselves as having reduced quality of life postinjury (Brown & Vandergoot, 1998). In contrast, Burke et al. (2000) described an extended rehabilitation program offered to a 15-year-old girl who had sustained a very severe traumatic brain injury. With an integrated, intense, and comprehensive rehabilitation program, the young girl made significant functional gains in mobility, swallowing, communication, personal care, and psychological adjustment, eventually being reintegrated into the home and school environments.

As long as financial and practical resources for rehabilitation are universally limited, parsimonious judgment needs to be applied to selection of rehabilitation candidates and the design of their therapy (Donabedian, 1980). Speech-language pathologists, along with other rehabilitation specialists, however, must endeavor to educate funding bodies and administrators as to the importance of rehabilitation at the level of participation in society (Burke et al., 2000; Snow & Douglas, 1999). All individuals who have suffered a TBI should be considered "at risk" of social handicap. It is this risk and the attitude of the individual with TBI towards this risk, that should drive the decision to offer therapy beyond the acute phase of recovery.

Establishing the Stakeholders in Communication Therapy

The aims and outcomes of communication therapy are, of necessity, individually determined entities. Before the process of assessment, therapy design, and administration commences, it is important for the speech-language pathologist to identify the "stakeholders" in the therapy process (Rosenthal, 1995). The stakeholders are those who have a vested interest in the outcome of treatment and may include the individual with TBI, his/her family, service providers, friends, and work associates. The stakeholders in the therapy will help affect an ecologically valid assessment of communication problems and assist in the design of a therapeutic program that achieves socially meaningful outcomes for the individual with TBI.

Assessment of Cognitive-Linguistic Communication Functioning

Traditionally, speech-language pathology assessments, and the subsequent treatment regimes, have been principally concerned with standardized test batteries designed to evaluate impairments in isolated linguistic skills. While such tests, when carefully selected, can reliably determine the presence of any deficits in linguistic components that underpin social communication, they fall short of providing a sensitive measure of interactional communicative function or communicative ability beyond the confined context of the clinical room. Indeed, the highly structured nature of clinical language tests may only serve to obscure the functional communication difficulties encountered by the TBI individual within more demanding communication contexts. As a consequence, when designing treatment for TBI individuals, researchers and clinicians alike have come to rely less on tests of discrete language function and more on determining the impact of linguistic deficits on interactive and noninteractive discourse skills (e.g., Chapman et al., 1992; Coelho, Liles, & Duffy, 1991; Ehrlich & Barry, 1989; Liles, Coelho, Duffy, & Zalagens, 1989; Hartley & Jensen, 1991, 1992; Mentis & Prutting, 1987; McDonald, 1993; McDonald & Pearce, 1995; Snow, Douglas & Ponsford, 1995, 1997a, 1997b, 1998, 1999; Togher, Hand, & Code, 1997a), social skills (Marsh & Knight, 1991), and quality-of-life perceptions (Brown & Vandergoot, 1998).

The first step in the management of communication disorders following TBI should involve a comprehensive assessment of communication skills at the levels of impairment, activity, and participation. In this way, clinicians may be alerted to the presence of a deficit in language skills necessary for communication, as well as gain insight into the ability of the individual with TBI to use verbal and nonverbal cues and behaviors in order to interact successfully within his/her relevant communicative environments.

Assessment of Language Impairment Following TBI

There are few well-designed, standardized language assessments that are sensitive and broad ranging enough to reliably delineate the linguistic deficits in the TBI population. As a result, clinicians must adopt a collection of assessments, often designed for language-impaired populations other than TBI. A comprehensive assessment should aim to sample all modalities of language processing in a hierarchical manner and should include evaluation of auditory and reading comprehension, lexical selection and retrieval, verbal and written expression, verbal memory and learning, verbal integration and semantic organization, abstract language use such as comprehension of humor, proverbs, and idiomatic expressions, and ability to use language for problem solving and reasoning (Hartley, 1995). Table 12-2 lists suggested standardized assessments batteries that include tests of primary language function as well as those that have been found to be sensitive to deficits of higher-order linguistic and metalinguistic ability (Lethlean & Murdoch, 1997; Hinchliffe, Murdoch, & Chenery, 1998). For example, The Test of Language Competence—Expanded, Level II (Wiig & Secord, 1989) and The Word Test—Revised (Huisingh, Barrett, Bachman, Bagcen, & Orman, 1990), which examine the integrity of linguistic skill on complex and linguistically demanding tasks, have been found to discriminate between TBI and control subjects (Hinchliffe, Murdoch, & Chenery, 1998) and contain subtests that are associated with deficits in discourse production (Wiig, Alexander, & Secord, 1988).

***Table* 12-2.** Assessments of language impairment (component processes).

	Component Process	Suggested Test/Subtest
Primary Language Processes	Auditory Comprehension—word level	• Boston Diagnostic Aphasia Examination (BDAE) (Goodglass & Kaplan, 1983) • Western Aphasia Battery (WAB; Kertesz, 1982)
	Auditory Comprehension—sentence level/commands	• BDAE (Goodglass & Kaplan, 1983)—Following Commands • WAB (Kertesz, 1982) • Revised Token Test (McNeil & Prescott, 1978)
	Auditory Comprehension—paragraph level	• BDAE (Goodglass & Kaplan, 1983)—Paragraph Comprehension
	Oral Expression—naming	• Boston Naming Test (Kaplan et al., 1983) • WAB (Kertesz, 1982)—Object Naming • BDAE (Goodglass & Kaplan, 1983)—Picture Naming; Responsive Naming
	Oral Expression—verbal fluency	• BDAE (Goodglass & Kaplan, 1983) and WAB (Kertesz, 1982)—Animal Naming • Neurosensory Centre Comprehensive Examination of Aphasia (NCCEA; Spreen & Benton, 1969)—Word Fluency • Controlled Oral Word Association Test (COWAT) (Benton & Hamsher, 1983)
	Oral Expression—sentence generation	• NCCEA (Spreen & Benton, 1969)—Sentence Construction
	Oral Expression—picture description	• BDAE (Goodglass & Kaplan, 1983)—Cookie Theft • WAB (Kertesz, 1982)—Spontaneous Speech Content and Fluency Scales
	Reading Comprehension—word level	• BDAE (Goodglass & Kaplan, 1983) • WAB (Kertesz, 1982)
	Reading Comprehension—sentence to paragraph level	• BDAE (Goodglass & Kaplan, 1983) • WAB (Kertesz, 1982)

(continues)

Table 12-2. (*continued*)

	Component Process	Suggested Test/Subtest
Primary Language Processes	Written Expression	• BDAE (Goodglass & Kaplan,1983 • WAB (Kertesz, 1982)
Higher-Order Language Processes	Auditory Comprehension and Reasoning	• Test of Language Competence—Extended (TLC-E; Wiig & Secord, 1989)—Listening Comprehension • Wiig-Semel Test of Linguistic Concepts (Wiig & Semel, 1974)
	Semantic Knowledge and Expressive Vocabulary	• The Word Test—Revised (TWT-R; Huisingh et al., 1990)
	Comprehension of Ambiguity	• TLC-E—Ambiguous Sentences
	Comprehension of inferred meaning	• TLC-E—Listening Comprehension: Making Inferences • Right Hemisphere Language Battery (RHLB; Bryan, 1989)—Comprehension of Inferred Meaning
	Comprehension of Absurdities	• TWT-R—Semantic Absurdities
	Comprehension of Humor	• RHLB—Appreciation of Humor
	Comprehension of Figurative and Idiomatic Expression	• RHLB—Metaphor Picture Test, Written Metaphor Test • TLC-E—Figurative Language
	Verbal Reasoning and Problem Solving	

Several commentators have questioned the ecological validity of standardized tests and warned against the sole reliance on, or unguarded interpretation of, clinical testing of cognitive-linguistic processes in the TBI population (Hartley, 1995; Snow & Douglas, 1999; Snow & Ponsford, 1995). When used in combination with other methods of evaluation, such as pragmatic assessments, functional communication assessments, and ethnographic observations, the standardized assessment battery can provide useable objective information. While clinical offline tasks are not designed to fully describe communication problems following TBI, information from these standardized assessments can serve to highlight the cognitive-linguistic strengths of the individual, as well as alert the clinician to the presence of a communication disorder. In addition, information from such tests can help explain the underlying nature of deficits in communicative ability. Such information would affect the design of treatment, whether it be choosing to focus on improving a cognitive-linguistic function, or adapting the communicative environment in order to compensate for the anticipated difficulties caused by the cognitive-linguistic deficit.

Assessment of Limitations in Communication Activity Following TBI

Assessment of the consequences of TBI on communicative activity involves the evaluation of how the speaker effectively plans and delivers or understands message content in different interactive contexts. Such an examination requires the use of both pragmatic and functional techniques of assessment. The boundaries of these approaches have been blurred by theoretical and terminological confusions, resulting in the terms "pragmatic assessment" and "functional assessment," often being used synonymously (e.g., Snow & Ponsford, 1995). It has been argued, however, that each approach is theoretically discreet, and that therapy that is driven by a theoretical structure should consider the notions of pragmatic competence and functional skill as related rather than interchangeable entities (Penn, 1999).

Pragmatics is essentially concerned with the way language is used in natural contexts (Levinson, 1983). Pragmatic competence requires the possession of three types of knowledge (knowledge of language and its structure, knowledge of the world and of objects, knowledge of the rules of social behavior), as well as the ability to adapt to the environment, and the ability to use multiple cognitive processes in real-time processing (Penn, 1999). Dissociation of these abilities leads to diminished pragmatic competence in certain environments. Pragmatic assessment, therefore, focuses on exploring the component pragmatic processes and behaviors required to achieve communication in various contexts.

A variety of pragmatic assessments have been used in the TBI population that have their basis in differing theoretical frameworks, such as the Speech Act Theory (Searle, 1969) and Grice's Cooperative Principle (Grice, 1975). Some measures have examined splinter components of pragmatic competence such as comprehension of conversational implicature (McDonald, 1992), detection of sarcasm (McDonald & Pearce, 1996), the ability to negotiate requests (McDonald & van Sommers, 1993), and specific measures of discourse production—for example, cohesion and information content (e.g., Hartley & Jensen, 1991; Mentis & Prutting, 1987). Other assessments have been more inclusive and incorporate a wide range of communicative behaviors (Benjamin, Debinski, Fletcher, Hedger, Mealings, & Stewart-Scott, 1989; Jordon & Murdoch, 1990; Milton, Prutting, & Binder, 1984; Snow, Douglas, & Ponsford 1995; 1997b; 1998). Table 12-3 lists a number of pragmatic assessments that measure broad components of pragmatic function.

In contrast to measures of pragmatic ability, the goal of functional assessments is not to identify deficits in components of pragmatic skill, but rather to determine the quality of the "endproduct" of the attempts to communicate (Manochiopining, Sheard, & Reed, 1992). Some measures of functional skill determine the impact of cognitive-linguistic and pragmatic disorders on social and vocational domains, and hence tap into measuring the social handicap or participation restriction resulting from disorders in communication. Table 12-3 includes a list of direct and indirect measures of functional communication that can be used in the TBI population. Indirect methods involve interviews, surveys, self-reports, or ratings by familiar communicative partners. Direct methods entail quantitative measures of discourse comprehension and production, observation, and rating of communicative ability in clinical and/or natural environments (Hartley, 1995).

Table 12-3. Assessments of communication activity and participation restriction.

	Assessments	Authors
Pragmatic Assessments	Pragmatic Protocol	Prutting & Kirchner, 1987
	The Profile of Communicative Appropriateness (PCA)	Penn, 1985
	The Discourse Abilities Profile	Terrell & Ripich, 1989
	The Edinburgh Functional Communication Profile (revised)	Wirz, Skinner, & Dean, 1990
	Communicative Abilites in Daily Living (CADL)—Revised	Holland, Frattali, & Fromm, 1998
	Conversational Rating Scale	Ehrlich & Barry, 1989
	Conversational Skills Rating Scale (CSRS)	Spitzburg & Hurt, 1987
	Checklist of Listening Behaviors	Hartley, 1995
	Analysis of Topic	Hartley, 1995
	Conversational Analysis Profile for People with Cognitive Impairments	Perkins, Whitworth, & Lesser, 1998
	Discourse Comprehension Test (DCD)	Brookshire & Nicholas, 1993
	Analysis of Monologic Discourse: Clinical elicitation and analysis of narrative, procedural, expository, or persuasive discourse along the dimensions of sentential structure productivity, information, content, cohesion, and coherence	See Hartley, 1995 for a summary of quantitative measures
Functional Assessments	Functional Communication Profile	Sarno, 1975
	The Rating of Functional Performance	Wertz, Collins, Weiss, Kurtzke et al., 1981
	The Everyday Communication Needs Assessment (ECNA)	Worrall, 1999
	The Functional Linguistic Communication Inventory (FLCI)	Bayles & Tomoeda, 1995
	The Functional Assessment of Communication Skills for Adults (ASHA FACS)	Frattali, Thompson, Holland, Wohl, & Ferketic, 1995
Functional Assessments— Participation Restriction	Communicative Effectiveness Index (CETI)	Lomas, Pickard, Betser, Elbard, Finlayson, & Zoghaib, 1989
	Checklist of Adaptive Listening Skills	Morreau & Bruinks, 1991
	Communicative Adequacy in Daily Situations	Clark & Witte, 1995
	The Communication Profile	Payne, 1994
	Environmental Needs Assessment	Hartley, 1995

Tests of pragmatic skill, including specific discourse analyses and functional communication assessments, provide opportunity to examine real-time communication function beyond the boundaries of sentence-level offline clinical tasks. Clinicians should be cautious, however, in the interpretation of the TBI person's performance on such tasks, and should carefully examine the variables that may diminish the sensitivity of the assessment and threaten its validity and reliability. Kearns (1990) has cautioned clinicians on assessing pragmatic skills by using rating scales which are vulnerable to changes in observer expectancy and feedback and gradual changes in observer coding behaviors. In addition, Snow and Douglas (1999) have highlighted some of the limitations of discourse assessment and analysis in clinical practice. These include the time-consuming nature of the analyses and the lack of normative data that is sensitive to demographic and sociolinguistic variations, by which to compare the features of discourse produced by the individual with TBI.

Through assessment and guarded interpretation of interactive and discourse skills, the clinician can establish how the linguistic deficits may impede the ability of the individual with TBI to perform activities that constitute his/her routines and participate meaningfully in society. The clinician should discuss with the TBI individual, and other stakeholders, the functional consequences of the language, discourse, and pragmatic impairments, and in doing so, commence the process of establishing ecologically valid intervention goals.

Assessment of Restriction in Participation Resulting from Cognitive Linguistic Communication Disorders Following TBI

In the establishment of treatment goals and priorities, it is necessary to determine the impact of cognitive-linguistic impairment and reduced pragmatic competence on the communicative activity and societal participation of the individual with TBI. That is, the speech-language pathologist must gain an understanding of the personal significance of the injury by examining the individual's past communicative style, activities, and roles in society in relation to his/her present and proposed future communicative activities.

First, the speech-language pathologist should obtain an understanding of aspects of the individual's premorbid communication style and experiences. This involves interviews with the TBI individual and the significant people in his/her life in order to gain insight into the individual's sociocultural background, educational history, psychosocial functioning, employment history, leisure interests, and personal communicative style. It is also necessary to determine the nature of the present communicative environments that are unique to the individual and to identify the significant communicative partners within that environment. Finally, long-term goal planning requires the contemplation of the future communication needs in terms of social relationships, independent living, vocational aspirations, and community participation. Thus, in treatment planning, it is necessary to identify what regular activities the individual is involved in, or wishes to become involved in, establish the communicative demands of each one and the possible environmental supports available. With this knowledge, the degree to which the person encounters limitations in communication activity or participation can be determined and compensatory intervention can be planned.

An environmental needs assessment or ecological inventory, such as the one proposed by Hartley (1995), would provide the clinician with a systematic method for identifying the present and future communicative environments of the individual and the activities, roles, and communicative partners within those environments. Another structured approach for determining how important certain everyday communication skills are to individuals with TBI, is The Communication Profile (Payne, 1994). This assessment lists 26 everyday functional communicative skills and requires the individual to rate, on a five-point scale, the importance of these skills in their daily lives. For example, the respondent is asked to rate how important activities such as reading a prescription label or talking on the telephone to family are to them. Other methods of assessing the level of participation in communication based activities are listed in Table 12-3.

Ethnographic techniques have recently been promoted as useful methods by which to collect qualitative data regarding an individual's communicative behavior in multiple life situations (Hartley,1995; McGann & Werven, 1995; Rees & Gerber, 1992; Snow & Douglas, 1999).Ethnography involves obtaining information from multiple direct observations of behaviors or interviews and the subsequent evaluation of the interview and observational data in order to determine communicative strengths and difficulties (Ripich & Spinelli, 1985).

An ecologically valid assessment of cognitive-communication deficits following TBI is a dynamic process that uses multiple inputs to develop a complete picture of an individual's communicative competence in terms of impairment, activity limitation, and participation restriction. Given that clinical assessment forms the basis of decisions regarding treatment goals and priorities, it is imperative that the assessment provides the therapist with valid information that is sensitive to the communicative history, style, contexts, and needs of the individual concerned. Such information can then be used to develop a treatment plan that is socially valid and personally meaningful.

Principles of Goal Setting

In consultation with the TBI individual and other stakeholders, the clinician needs to establish a set of realistic, specific, and structured goals of treatment that are objective and measurable. These goals will depend on the stage of recovery, the identified impairments and limitations of communication, the accessibility of resources and support, the time frame available, as well as the motivation of the individual with TBI and the other stakeholders in the rehabilitation process. Well-managed goal setting paves the way for therapy to be continuously motivating, socially valid, and meaningful for the individual and, therefore, most likely to ultimately promote participation in the life domains most valued by the individual.

There are several principles that can be applied to goal setting in the design of a communication rehabilitation program for the brain-injured person. Some of these principles are summarized in Table 12-4 and discussed here briefly. Goal setting should be a natural progression from the assessment and data-gathering phase of therapy. Having completed an ecologically valid assessment, the therapist should discuss the identified communication-related problems with the injured person and the other stakeholders. Care must be taken to ensure that the injured person possesses a metacognitive awareness of the impact of the injury on his/her communicative function, so that he/she can participate in the goal setting and design of treatment strategies. It is important that the

***Table* 12-4.** Principles of goal setting.

- Goals should be based on assessment results.
- The person with TBI should contribute to decision making regarding the targets of therapy.
- Goals should be realistic with respect to the targets chosen and the time line available.
- Goals should be clearly defined and measurable.
- Goals should be easily communicated to all stakeholders.
- Goals should be constantly monitored and modified.

---

goal setting context provides an environment that encourages freedom of expression, mutual respect, and cooperation. This not only establishes a positive environment for treatment, but also ensures that the individual with TBI is identified as an equal contributor to the design of therapy. Such an environment promotes a positive attitude and a sense of ownership and shared responsibility for the treatment goals, which in turn enhances motivation and commitment.

Intervention will not be effective if the treatment goals are not realistic or do not relate well to the identified communicative impairments and functional needs of the individual. In some cases it is difficult to determine the likelihood of a person achieving a seemingly ambitious long-term goal. In order to promote success and the motivation to attain such a goal, the clinician should structure a number of achievable goals that will effect a more immediate functional change. The realistic setting of goals must also be completed with the availability of time and resources in mind. In cases where the TBI individual has less than ideal access to regular therapy or little support for therapeutic regimes outside of the clinic, the nature of the goals and the time frame for achievement must be modified.

Each goal should be clearly defined and measurable, so that success can be easily communicated and understood. The goals should be simply expressed in language that is meaningful to the individual with TBI (Snow & Douglas, 1999), and success should be easily and reliably measured. Snow & Douglas (1999) suggest that the injured person should be encouraged to take responsibility for recording the success of performance within a therapy session, thereby increasing motivation to accomplish the goals.

Goals that are well defined and measurable are easily communicated to all stakeholders in therapy and to other members of the rehabilitation team. They also ensure monitoring of progress and accountability of service delivery. When goals are not being achieved, it is necessary for the clinician, the injured person, and the other stakeholders to determine the reason for limited success. It is possible that the goal may no longer be realistic or relevant, or that the methods being used to achieve the goal are ineffective. Accordingly, the therapeutic strategy may need to be changed or the goal itself amended.

Goal setting, therefore, is not simply an "outset" stage of therapy. Goal setting is a dynamic and evolving process that is pivotal to each therapy session and to each effort the individual makes in communication outside the therapy session.

The Structure of Therapeutic Goals

The determination of therapeutic goals is driven by the findings of the assessment procedures. Consistent with the approach for assessment of communication problems following TBI, therapy goals may be constructed within the ICIDH-2 framework (WHO, 1997). This framework allows for the establishment of treatment goals at three levels of function. The *long-term* goal concerns the desired global outcome of treatment. This holistic goal addresses, in functional terms, the overall expected living outcome for the individual and specifies how the person aims to participate in society. For example, the long-term outcome for an injured individual with minimal physical difficulties may be to return to living with his wife and child and resuming his occupation on a part-time basis. Thus, his long-term goal is to successfully participate in society as a husband, father, and employee, and for the community to accept the individual within these roles.

After establishing the societal goal of therapy, it is necessary to identify the intermediate goals aimed at achieving success in the personal communicative activities that shape an individual's role. These *intermediate* goals relate to the information gained during assessment, especially the environmental needs assessment, and aim to promote functional communication skills. For example, one goal may be for the TBI individual to be able to deliver a verbal report at monthly staff meetings. Hartley (1995) has summarized an extensive list of functional communication goals across different life domains such as the home, community, and work environments.

The third level of goal formation identifies the short-term or *immediate* objectives of treatment. Typically these goals target the modality-specific or component process skills that are required to attain the intermediate goals of functional activity. These goals therefore, target the impairment level of disablement. For example, some immediate goals for the TBI individual who hopes to return to work and deliver monthly verbal reports, might be to be able to organize verbal content in a logical order and to be able to express content without excessive verbal dysfluencies.

General Methods and Principles for Treating Communication Disorders Following TBI

Several approaches to rehabilitation of cognitive disorders following TBI have been described. Essentially these approaches can be considered restorative, compensatory, or behavioral (Gross and Schultz, 1986; Diller, 1987; Gordon, 1990; Coelho, DeRuyter, & Stein, 1996; Mazaux & Richer, 1998). The restorative approach assumes that repetitive exercise of neuronal circuits will facilitate neuronal growth and hence, improve function. Thus it aims to restore cognitive function within the context of its premorbid organization. In contrast, the compensatory approach assumes that certain functions cannot be restored and is therefore aimed at developing skills and strategies to circumvent impaired function and achieve functional competence (Mazaux & Richer, 1998). It has been argued, however, that it is artificial to separate restoration from compensation within a rehabilitation program and that both approaches should occur simultaneously (Coelho et al., 1996). Similarly, the behavioral approach to therapy can be integral to treatment that targets deficits in component processes or compensatory strategies. This approach involves the use of behavior modification techniques to reinforce or discourage discrete behaviors, or to promote the speed and accuracy of learning a task or skill (Gross & Schultz, 1986; Jacobs, 1993).

Regardless of the type of intervention strategy used, or the nature of the goals being targeted, there are some general treatment principles that should be applied to the delivery of therapy for individuals with TBI (Hartley, 1995; Prigatano, 1987; Snow & Ponsford, 1995; Snow & Douglas, 1999). These principles, which are based on behavioral learning techniques, are summarized in Table 12-5 and serve to maximize the learning potential of the individual, promote motivation, and facilitate goal achievement.

Table 12-5. General treatment principles for communication disorders following TBI.

Create a positive learning environment	• Display a positive regard and unconditional support for the injured person.
	• Avoid applying personal "value judgments" to behavior or goals.
	• Establish a role of mentor, adviser, or coach rather than autocratic instructor.
	• Instill a sense of ownership of therapy:
	   - Allow participation in goal setting.
	   - Allow input into scheduling time and place of treatment.
	   - Allow decision making when trying out skills.
	• Use effective reinforcement:
	   - Ensure that reinforcement is meaningful for the individual.
	   - Ensure that reinforcement is consistent across environments.
	   - Ensure that reinforcement is immediate and clear.
	   - Ensure that reinforcement is used at every opportunity.
	• Select an environment conducive to success:
	   - Minimize distractions/embarrassment.
	   - Add variety to minimize boredom.

Ensure positive therapy organization	• Therapy should be hierarchical, moving from the simple to the complex, within and between sessions. • Goals should be clearly defined/reiterated at the beginning of each session. • Closure should occur at the end of each session, with success/goal achievement reviewed and planning for next session discussed.
Implement general therapy strategies	• Problem Solving • Verbal Mediation or "Self-Talk"

(continues)

***Table* 12-5.** (*continued*)

Implement general therapy strategies	• Task Analysis
	• Behavioral Learning:
	    - Direct instructions/scripting
	    - Modeling and imitation
	    - Shaping
	    - Fading of cues/structure

Provide opportunities for practice and generalization	• Role-Playing • Behavioral Rehearsal • Group Therapy • Task Relocation
Develop skills of self-evaluation and self-monitoring	• Video feedback • Promote Self-Instruction. • Promote Self-Reinforcement. • Promote Environmental Feedback.

Treatment of Cognitive-Linguistic Communication Difficulties at the Impairment Level of Dysfunction

From the perspective of the impairment-activity limitation-participation restriction hierarchy, traditional therapy aimed at restoration of specific, defective linguistic skills targets the impairment level of disablement. This approach involves the psychometric assessment of component processes of cognitive and linguistic function, followed by repetitive practice on structured clinical tasks such as drills and computer-based or worksheet activities (Mateer, Sohlberg, & Youngman, 1990; Sohlberg & Mateer, 1989). Examples of such activities in the speech pathology clinic may include lexical-semantic tasks of word-finding, categorizing and sequencing and verbal organization tasks. These exercises aim to train or improve function in areas that are found to be defective on testing and that are thought to underpin the difficulties in functional communicative activities.

In the move toward functionalism in speech pathology, intervention using component process retraining has been widely criticized. The nature of such intervention is essentially domain-specific whereby, in their effort to ameliorate deficits in the component processes of cognition following TBI, the various professionals involved each assess and treat the TBI individual according to their specialty. The tasks for treatment are determined by the performance on test scores. The outcome of treatment is evaluated by the amount of gain on retesting, and it is hoped that any decrease in impairment would have a spontaneous effect on associated functional activity. There is little evidence, however, that can fuel such a hope. It has been demonstrated that individuals with TBI have difficulty generalizing the use of skills on structured, clinical tasks to activities performed in real time and in real-life situations (Ben-Yishay & Prigatano, 1990; Ponsford & Kinsella, 1988; Prigatano, 1997; Szekers, 1994), and improvement on structured tasks does not necessarily manifest as improved skill in everyday performance (Ponsford & Kinsella, 1988; Mateer & Sohlberg, 1988). Thus, an inherent shortcoming of the restorative approach to therapy stems from the limited understanding of the relationship between the training task used and the cognitive deficit being targeted (Snow & Ponsford, 1995).

Thus, in a component process restoration program, the TBI individual receives a splintered approach to dealing with the difficulties of daily life, with each professional concerned with improvement in specific processes. The functional consequences of TBI, however, are not discreet, and rehabilitation necessarily involves the blurring of professional boundaries in order to attain a common long-term goal. It is not surprising that therapy programs that are aimed purely at restoration of cognitive-linguistic processes are often unsuccessful. In such programs, it is unlikely that a thorough understanding of the communicative needs of the TBI individual has been established. It is also unlikely that the injured person has actively participated in the goal formation, and the tasks may have little or no functional relevance to the individual concerned. In addition, the relationship between the immediate, intermediate, and long term goals is likely to be non-specific. Unfortunately, it has not been uncommon to hear a young person with TBI undergoing such therapy to remark "I can't do these exercises . . . I couldn't do them at school . . . I hated them then too." If, however, the therapeutic process is approached using the goal-setting structure and process described above, the goals of therapy will be salient, and hence motivating, for the individual with TBI.

Well-thought-out goal-setting procedures will identify the communicative activities the individual needs to perform. These activities can then be analyzed in terms of their component features. In this way, the component processes, be they cognitive-linguistic operations or components of pragmatic skill, that are necessary to achieve a meaningful real-life goal, can form the immediate goals of therapy. Component process retraining combined with compensatory strategies can then be applied at this level. For example, instead of administering multiple nonspecific word-finding tasks to a person with a word retrieval deficit, it would be more relevant and motivating to choose tasks that facilitate retrieval of the names of food and household items so that a grocery order can be successfully placed. With this approach, component process retraining is used in a purposeful, functional goal-driven manner and is not merely "cookbook" therapy. Table 12-6 presents a list of common cognitive-linguistic impairments following TBI, along with some examples of component process retraining activities.

Table 12-6. Suggested therapy exercises for common linguistic impairments following TBI.

Impairment	Suggested Therapy Activity
Lexical-Semantic Processing	
Difficulty with identifying word meanings Difficulty identifying salient semantic features Difficulty with semantic categorization	Identifying synonyms and antonyms; semantic choice questions; defining words by class; defining words by attribute; defining using negation; matching words with definitions; defining words; producing multiple definitions; identifying correct meanings of homonyms and homophones; naming semantic categories; identifying semantic features of categories and category members; naming category members

(continues)

Table 12-6. (*continued*)

Impairment	Suggested Therapy Activity
Comprehension of Spoken Instructions	
Difficulty following instructions with multiple critical elements	Following instructions that increase in number of critical semantic elements
Comprehension of Lengthy or Complex Auditory Information	
Difficulty detecting and remembering main ideas Difficulty making inferences and drawing conclusions Difficulty interpreting abstract ideas Difficulty discriminating between relevant and irrelevant information Difficulty recognizing incongruency Difficulty resolving ambiguity	Summarizing tasks; story retelling; answering specific questions; deriving punch lines; anticipating next episode; interpreting abstract expressions; defining abstract expressions; recognizing correct interpretations of proverbs and/or metaphorical statements; distinguishing fact from opinion in isolated statements and in connected argument; providing definitions for multiple-meaning words; identifying phrases with multiple meanings arising from surface- or deep-structure characteristics; using semantic, syntactic and pragmatic cues to accurately interpret embedded multiple-meaning sentences in narratives; produce nonliteral meaning of words
Comprehension of Complex Written Information	
Difficulty recognizing and retaining main points Difficulty interpreting information Difficulty integrating information and drawing conclusions Difficulty detecting and comprehending inference	Explain stimuli by theme or gist; demonstrate appreciation of a character's motives, an implied outcome, or the moral of the story; identify essential, optional, and irrelevant information; identify and explain absurdities that arise from contextual incongruence; recognize alternate interpretations of information
Word Retrieval	
Reduced word association skills	Word association tasks; interpreting definitions; providing category names; comparing semantic items according to attributes; providing synonyms and antonyms

(*continues*)

***Table* 12-6.** (*continued*)

Organization of Verbal Expression	
Difficulty with efficient production of organized, meaningful verbal expression	Sequencing tasks; summarizing tasks; providing instructions to blind listener; syntactic judgment tasks; story retelling; story generation; analysis and self-correction of recorded verbal expression.

Organization of Written Expression	
Difficulty with efficient production of written expression	Sequencing tasks; summarizing tasks; providing step-by-step written instructions; short narrative production using narrative schema; self-correction of written information

Intervention at the Activity Level of Communicative Function

To attain the intermediate goals that target certain functional behaviors, compensatory strategies and functional skills training, along with behavioral techniques can be used. Compensatory strategy training aims to teach the individual methods by which to overcome their deficits through the use of self-initiated procedures. Compensatory strategies may be overt and involve the use of physical aids (e.g., a notebook to assist memory) or external behaviors (e.g., requests for repetition of information). Alternately, a compensatory strategy may be covert or internal, such as the use of self-cuing instruction, mental associations, or visual imagery (Ylvisaker & Holland, 1985).

For a compensatory strategy to be successful, it must eventually be able to be accessed at an automatic level. To promote efficient learning of a compensation, the strategy must be carefully selected. During the assessment stage of therapy, the clinician should observe strategies spontaneously used by the injured person to facilitate language functions such as word retrieval, verbal organization, or verbal memory. In addition, the therapist should interview the person about the strategies used (Ylvisaker & Holland, 1985). This process will help identify the type of compensatory strategies that are most naturally used by the injured person, as well as those that are inefficient or maladaptive. Selection of compensatory strategies should also be guided by the person's particular strengths and weakness. For example, a person who is verbose and tangential, but possesses little self-awareness and poor self-monitoring, would be a candidate for an external aid (e.g., significant other) to assist him/her to monitor the relevance of output. Alternately, a person who displays some insight into his/her tendency to be verbose may be taught to read the nonverbal signs conveyed by the listener and to employ a verbal checking strategy, such as "Do you follow me?"

Compensatory strategies can be used to improve efficiency with particular cognitive or linguistic operations, or can be used to facilitate the execution of functional communication. For example, an injured person who has been identified as having a word retrieval impairment may be encouraged to use circumlocution to successfully convey the message. If functional assessments and needs analysis have also revealed that this person has anxiety and difficulty organizing verbal expression to make appointments over the telephone. He/she may be encouraged to write a "script" prior to making the phone call and learn to make requests such as "Could you repeat that time and date please?" Behavioral learning strategies (see Table 12-5) would be utilized to promote successful learning of these compensatory strategies.

Functional skills training aims to improve the ability to perform a specific function through learning and repetition (Szekeres, Ylvisaker, & Holland, 1985). Treatment is conducted within the functional communicative environment and is, by nature, activity-based. For example, a functional skills task may involve specific training in the way to answer the telephone, convey feelings to a doctor, or operate a communication device. Functional skills training involves the use of behavioral learning principles outlined in Table 12-5 and summarized by Hartley (1995). These include direct instructions and scripting, behavioral rehearsal and role-playing, behavior shaping, and fading of cues. For example, the process of talking to a doctor about symptoms can be discussed and a general script for the situation practiced internally or subvocally, or in a role-play situation. If an injured person has difficulty initiating information-giving in the doctor-patient situation, behavior-shaping techniques may initially aim for the person to attend and respond appropriately to the doctor's questioning. A subsequent goal may be for the injured person to be able to initiate discussion of information regarding the major symptom. The eventual goal would be for the injured person to engage more equally in the communicative exchange.

Functional skills training can be adapted to address the common discourse sequelae in TBI. Some difficulties are specific to the genre (e.g., narrative or procedural discourse) being produced, while others, such as problems with information transfer and topic maintenance, occur in both interactive and monologic discourse (McDonald, 1993; McDonald & Pearce, 1995). The first step in discourse therapy is to outline the nature and rules of the genre being targeted. To improve the organization of content in narrative discourse, the TBI individual should be made aware of the sequential structure (the story grammar) required for a complete and organized narrative. The therapist can then illustrate the importance of the organizational components by omitting them from a text and discussing the effect of the deconstruction with the TBI individual (Snow & Douglas, 1999). The individual with TBI must also be aware of the need to establish clear and logical links between events in the story. Without the establishment of such links, the narrative may be disjointed or ambiguous. With increased awareness of the need for specific structure and logical connection of information, the individual can then practice and evaluate the production of narratives in terms of structure, clarity, and success of information transfer.

Disorders of conversational discourse are pervasive and persistent sequelae of TBI (Snow, Douglas, & Ponsford, 1998). Conversational skills are central to the establishment and maintenance of personal, social, and vocational relationships, and are therefore, inextricably related to psychosocial well-being. Therapy for conversational skill difficulties should commence with discussions about the features of good conversational skills and the rules of conversation behavior (e.g., the need to take turns, the need to be relevant, the need to make eye contact). A theoretical framework relevant for therapy targeting conversational function in TBI can be found in the theory of systemic functional grammar (SFG) (Togher, Hand, & Code, 1996, 1997a, 1997b). This theory holds that the language used in each communicative interaction is differentially influenced by the context of the exchange. The context has three major components: field, tenor, and mode. The field describes the nature of the interaction (e.g., a patient-doctor exchange, a conversation with a familiar person, asking for directions); the tenor identifies the people who are involved in the exchange (e.g., doctor-patient; girlfriend-boyfriend); the mode is the role that the language is playing (e.g., spoken or written).

Often conversational deficits following TBI are characterized by the selection of language that is inappropriate to the tenor and field of the context (Hartley, 1992). Therapy for conversational disorders may involve selecting a communicative context, identifying the field, tenor, and mode of the exchange, and discussing the appropriate language and interactive behaviors expected within the context. Several of the strategies discussed above, such as scripting, behavioral rehearsal, and role-playing, can then be used to practice the appropriate interactive language and behaviors. Therapy sessions, however, typically fail to vary the tenor of interaction. To promote the effectiveness of therapy and foster generalization of skills, efforts should be made to provide the TBI individuals with experiences of different fields, modes, and tenor relationships.

Environmental manipulation directly targets the achievement of functional activity as well as being integral to attaining long-term goals. This method endeavors to modify the physical and communicative environment so as to facilitate communicative success for the individual with TBI. Environmental intervention may include advising potential communicative partners as to strategies to facilitate interaction with the TBI individual, or altering the physical layout of a work office so that the person with TBI is able to operate with limited distractions and extraneous noise. As with personal behavioral techniques, compensations within the environment can be shaped and faded. Initially, a person may require overt cues from significant others to assist the communicative exchange. With time, these cues may be modified and eventually withdrawn and replaced with internal strategies to ensure effective communication.

Intervention at the Participation Level of Function

Intervention at the Participation level of the ICIDH-2 (WHO, 1987) framework involves the strategies used to facilitate achievement of the long-term and life outcome goals. Intervention at this level is generally concerned with two areas: the maintenance, transfer, and generalization of functional communicative skills to real-life situations; adaptation, reform, and education of the personal, physical, and social environments that are relevant to the brain-injured individual.

The ultimate goal of therapy for communication disorders is for the brain-injured person to use the skills they have learned in therapy to participate in real-world roles. Transfer of learning and generalization of skills should not, however, be something addressed only at the end stage of therapy. Techniques that promote generalization of communicative skill should be an integral component of the intervention program from assessment and goal setting through to discharge. Table 12-7 summarizes strategies that can be used throughout therapy in order to foster generalization of communicative skills. It can be noted that some of these strategies are restatements of some of the general treatment principles outlined in Table 12-5.

Table 12-7. Strategies that promote generalization of communicative skills.

- Where possible, attempt communication activities in the natural environment or gradually relocate the task to a more normal environment.
- Increase the number of environments that a communication activity is practiced in.
- Gradually fade cues and external reinforcement.
- Practice and promote self-instruction—systematically replace external cues with overt self-instruction, then gradually encourage the instructions to become covert (Ylvisaker & Holland, 1985).
- Practice and promote self-monitoring by training the individual to recognize and record the occurrence of target behavior (Hartley, 1995).
- Encourage self-reinforcement by teaching the use of positive self-statements (Hartley, 1995).
- Use group therapy to provide opportunity for practicing skills, obtaining feedback from peers, and boosting confidence before attempting real-world activities.
- Train the other stakeholders in therapy in providing cues and giving appropriate reinforcement.
- Teach organized problem solving and practical reasoning strategies (Ylvisaker & Holland, 1985) so that the individual may be able to generate alternate solutions to deal with unexpected social challenges.

Environmental manipulation or compensation can increase the opportunity the individual has to participate in meaningful roles in society. Environmental manipulation may involve structural modifications of a work environment or household alterations to allow the person with TBI to function independently. Environmental compensation may involve educating those people who are significant communication partners, to provide communication support to the brain-injured person. Communicative support may include making allowances for communication inefficiencies. For example, an employer may be encouraged to allow more time for the person to convey their message verbally or to complete written tasks. In addition, significant communicative partners may be taught to provide external cues and appropriate reinforcement in order to promote ongoing positive communicative experiences for the individual with TBI.

Reducing the restrictions on participation within society for the individual with TBI also requires society to accommodate the activity limitations following TBI. Speech-language pathologists, along with all the professionals involved in the rehabilitation process, have a responsibility to become advocates for brain-injured individuals and educate government funding bodies and the general public as to the social and vocational needs of TBI individuals. Through the provision of adequate and sustainable funding, and the reduction of social prejudice and ignorance, the goal of community reentry for individuals with TBI may be more easily attained.

The following case study, "Kylie," illustrates the design of a treatment program for a young woman with a cognitive communication disorder following TBI. The assessment, goal setting, and a therapy plan were developed according to the ICIDH-2 (WHO, 1997) framework of impairment, activity limitation, and participation restriction. The case report illustrates how the long-term, participation level goal can be achieved through deriving intermediate goals, which aim to accomplish the activities involved in the participation goal. Similarly, the intermediate goals can be analyzed and broken down into component processes, which form the short-term, immediate goals.

Case Report - Kylie

Kylie was a 23-year-old teacher who was involved in a single vehicle accident outside a small rural town. At the time of retrieval from the accident, she was unconscious, but her Glasgow Coma Score was not recorded. Following hospital admission, Kylie was diagnosed with a closed-head injury, although neuroradiological investigations failed to reveal any abnormalities.

Kylie had successfully completed a 3-year course in Early Childhood Education. At the time of her accident, she was employed as a preschool teacher in a small rural school and was enrolled in a part-time Bachelor of Education course. Kylie had no premorbid history of neurological impairment, learning disability, drug abuse, or psychiatric disturbance.

At the time of commencing rehabilitation, Kylie was 3 months postinjury, was alert and cooperative, and had reached a score of VIII on the Level of Cognitive Functioning Scale (Hagen, 1984). To achieve this score, patients must be purposeful and appropriate in their response to the environment and must be able to recall and integrate past and recent events and display carry-over for new learning. On standardized language batteries, Kylie had little difficulty completing tests of primary language function. There was some evidence of inefficiency on word retrieval tasks. Kylie displayed a natural tendency to use circumlocution to facilitate verbal retrieval or achieve information transfer. On more complex and linguistically demanding tasks, Kylie showed some difficulty with lexical-semantic manipulations. For example, she had difficulty retrieving semantically associated words and displayed some impairment in the ability to recognize alternate meanings of words. There was also evidence on sentence construction tasks of reduced efficiency with verbal planning and monitoring.

Investigation of monologic discourse (narrative) production indicated that Kylie's discourse was marked by a high level of verbal disruption (mazes and fillers), high verbal output, decreased amount of propositions and decreased propositional production in relation to the amount of output. This tendency to be verbose was reflected in conversational discourse, which was characterized by the propensity to deliver intricate detail in explanations so that the main message was either forgotten or difficult to determine. In terms of interactional behaviors, Kylie was able to take turns, and was sensitive to the nonverbal cues of the listener. She often became aware of her verbosity and would acknowledge this by saying something to the effect of "Oh I'm going on and on and on . . . . I always do that . . . my mother always said I could talk . . . ." Case history notes indicated that Kylie was extroverted, with an easy-going nature. Postinjury, Kylie was a friendly and pleasant conversationalist, but could often be "overfamiliar" and inappropriately casual in her interactions. Kylie had no difficulty conversing with her peers, but displayed inappropriate conversational behaviors when talking with hospital staff, elderly people, and her employer. Thus, she appeared to have little sensitivity to the demands of field and tenor of the context and had difficulty altering her choice of topic and style of interaction accordingly. Unlike her awareness of her tendency to be verbose, Kylie did not always appear aware of the impact of her inappropriate conversation in certain contexts.

An ecological inventory indicated that Kylie possessed most of the skills to regain independent function in the home and within the community. Returning to work posed more difficulty. Participating in work necessitated planning daily activities and completing a written record of the plan. It also required the real-time formulation of clear instructions and explanations. Kylie's position also required her to meet with parents and other staff on formal and informal bases. Assessment of the functional communication activities revealed that Kylie had difficulty formulating well-organized explanations that were fluent and not overinclusive. In addition, the speech pathologist was concerned about Kylie's ability to converse at a professional level with other staff and parents.

After consultation with Kylie and her employer and coworker, a functional cognitive-linguistic communication therapy plan was devised and is displayed in Table 12-8. Kylie's global "lifetime" goal was to return to work as a preschool teacher. Given her minimal disruption of primary language and cognitive processes and her capacity for self-evaluation, along with her motivation and emerging insight, it was decided that this goal was a realistic long-term aim. The intermediate goals selected for targeting were to improve efficiency of formulation of instructions to children, to reduce verbosity when talking to friends, and to increase sensitivity to the context of discourse and adapt conversational behaviors accordingly. Several immediate goals were agreed upon. These goals targeted the component processes needed to achieve the intermediate goals. A variety of strategies involving compensation and behavioral learning techniques were used (see Table 12-8).

After 3 months of inpatient therapy, Kylie was discharged to her parents' home. From there, she attended weekly outpatient therapy, and an increasing emphasis was put on homework exercises. This encouraged Kylie to practice her communication skills in different settings and helped to develop self-monitoring and self-evaluation skills. Kylie made progress in all areas, particularly in her ability to reduce her verbosity in conversational speech and alter her communicative style to suit the conversational context. After a further 6 months, Kylie returned to her hometown and began to work two mornings a week. By this time, Kylie had developed reliable internal strategies to prevent or curtail verbosity, but occasionally needed addition external cues. Therapy included telephone discussions with Kylie's supervisor and coworker. These discussions served to educate and encourage Kylie's colleagues in their understanding of her communicative difficulties and the importance of their participation in her rehabilitation. Weekly phone calls were made to monitor Kylie's progress and discuss any issues within the program requiring modification.

In her part-time capacity, Kylie was able to interact well with the children and had little problem in conversing with peers and parents. Her supervisor reported favorably on her appropriateness and efficiency of interactions. After 4 months, Kylie was able to increase her work to four mornings a week and was considering resuming her studies in education.

Introduction to Treatment of Cognitive-Linguistic Communication Deficits in Children Following Traumatic Brain Injury

Cognitive-linguistic communication difficulties are frequent, but highly variable sequelae of TBI in childhood (Blosser & DePompeii, 1994). Many of the issues that complicate the investigation and management of communication difficulties in adults with TBI also affect the rehabilitation of pediatric brain injury. Other issues, such as the age at the time of injury and the possible coexistence of developmental learning problems, are peculiar to the pediatric population and further influence the long-term outcome profile of the child with TBI.

Table 12–8. Example of a communication therapy plan targeting levels of impairment, activity limitation, and participation restriction.

Communication Therapy Plan

Name: *Kylie*

Communication Environment:
Home: *Living alone, independently*
Work: *Preschool—interactions with children, staff, and parents.*

Date:
Communication Partners:
Home: *Lives alone, but socializes with friends regularly; Often calls parents on the phone.*
Work: *Children, senior staff, parents*

Motor Speech: NAD
Vision: NAD

Long-term goal: *To return to work as a preschool teacher—ability to complete all tasks associated with the job.*

Motor Control: NAD
Mobility: NAD

Suggested Strategy: *Compensatory strategies, functional retraining, environmental modification*

Intermediate Goals	Immediate Goals	Suggested Strategy	Suggested Intervention
1. To be able to formulate instructions to children	1a. Improve word retrieval	Workout and practice scripts Role-play Rehearsal	Encourage circumlocution. Verbal association tasks relevant to work context
	1b. Improve verbal planning		Plan one-sentence explanations, increasing to more complex explanations
2. To reduce verbosity in conversations with friends	2a. Identify the salient information in the narrative	Production of familiar to unfamiliar narratives Video feedback Rehearsal	Discuss/teach differentiation of content into: essential, embellishment, irrelevant
	2b. Identify the organizational structure of the narrative	Group therapy Stakeholder feedback	Discuss the concept of narrative structure and the necessary components of a story. Practice identifying the presence or absence of components Story retelling and story generation tasks

(continues)

Table 12-8. (*continued*)

Intermediate Goals	Suggested Strategy	Immediate Goals	Suggested Intervention
2. To reduce verbosity in conversations with friends		2c. Produce narratives that contain essential information and adhere to structure	Decide on a less obvious verbal cue
			Learn to subvocalize the cue
		2d. Internalize self-initiated cues to reduce verbosity	Eventually fade the cue out
3. To improve appropriateness of conversational style with senior staff and parents	Role-play Task relocation Education of stakeholder (staff)	3a. To increase awareness of the effects of contexts	Discuss the need to vary the type of language and the manner of speaking with different people. Have Kylie evaluate appropriateness of various interactions and identify the aspects contributing to inappropriateness.
		3b. To be able to alter communicative style in different contexts	Role-play interactions. Move interactions into different environments. Increase practice opportunities with multiple partners.
		3c. To be able to self-monitor	Use video feedback. Increase awareness of listener cues.

Treatment Schedule: 2 *individual/wk and* 1 *group/wk*

Maintenance Schedule:

Neurobehavioral deficits in children with TBI must be viewed within the context of a dynamic developmental process (Ponsford, 1995). The sequelae of TBI in children influence not only their ability to perform former functions, but also their capacity to acquire and refine skills as they progress through childhood and adolescence.

Thus, the essential difference between TBI in children and adults is that the impairments encountered by children are unstable. Areas of deficit in language and components of cognition may appear or increase after a period of time. The instability of the impairment level of function will influence the child's ability to perform the range of communicative activities that are appropriate for his/her age and sociocultural environment.

The Nature of the Language and Communication Disorders Following Pediatric TBI

Earlier research has described language problems following pediatric TBI as subtle (Sarno, 1980), with many TBI children encountering minimal residual impairments in the recovery and acquisition of formal components of the language system (Chapman, Levin, Matejka, Harwar, & Kufera, 1995; Klonoff, Low, & Clark, 1977; Ylvisaker, 1993). Nevertheless, not all children with TBI escape specific language deficits. The most common residual deficits in language function that have been noted following severe TBI in children and adolescents include reduced verbal fluency and confrontation naming skills (Ewing-Cobbs, Levin, Eisenberg, & Fletcher, 1987; Ewing-Cobbs, Miner, Fletcher, & Levin, 1989; Jordan, Ozanne, & Murdoch, 1988; Jordan & Murdoch, 1993), as well as generalized reduction in developmental verbal and cognitive abilities (Jordan & Murdoch, 1990).

Increasingly, researchers have noted that impairments in communication following TBI in children may not be well delineated by highly structured standardized testing and that there exists significant communication deficits in this population that are more apparent at higher-level aspects of language representation (Chapman, Levin, & Lawyer, 1999; Dennis & Barnes, 1990; Ewing-Cobbs, Brookshire, Scott, & Fletcher, 1998). The diffuse brain damage associated with TBI in children results in impairments in cognitive functions, including memory, attention, visuospatial skills, and executive functions (Fletcher, Ewing-Cobbs, Miner, Levin, & Eisenberg, 1990; Levin et al., 1993; Perrott, Taylor, & Montes, 1991). To a greater extent, assessment of language and communication skills using methods that rely on integrated functioning of cognitive-linguistic processes, such as discourse measures, are complementing the use of traditional language batteries (Chapman et al., 1999). Investigations of discourse are considered to be more sensitive to the sequelae of pediatric TBI and are able to better highlight limitations in functional communicative abilities experienced by children with TBI.

Some aspects of discourse production by children do not appear to be vulnerable to the effects of TBI, while problems with other aspects of discourse production have been found to be more prevalent than specific language problems (Chapman et al., 1992) and more persistent (Chapman, 1997; Dennis &

Barnes, 1990). Surface structure measures, such as sentential length and complexity, and measures of intersentential cohesion have failed to discriminate between normal children and TBI children on narrative tasks (Chapman, Levin, Wenek, Weyrauch, & Kufera, 1998; Jordan, Murdoch, & Buttsworth, 1991). Other investigations of narrative discourse in this population have revealed that spoken narrative production is marked by a reduction in the amount of overall information produced, as well as in the amount of core propositional, or most salient, information contained in the output (Chapman et al., 1992; Chapman, Watkins, Gustafson, Moore, Levin, & Kufera, 1997). Children with TBI also display difficulty in completing macrostructure tasks, such as paraphrasing story content or synthesizing and retaining the central meaning of a story (Chapman et al., 1992; Chapman et al., 1997).

The information content of written discourse may be even more vulnerable to the effects of severe TBI than oral discourse production is (Ewing-Cobbs et al., 1997). Written narratives of children have been found to contain less information and greater disruptions of episodic structure. Given the importance of written skills for all aspects of academic education, it is necessary that the assessment of written, as well as spoken, discourse be incorporated into the management of communication problems in children with TBI (Chapman et al., 1999).

Establishing the Stakeholders in Cognitive-Linguistic Communication Therapy

The assessment and treatment of communication deficits in a child with TBI cannot be properly achieved without the input of the significant people in that child's life. Parents or guardians are vital members of the rehabilitation team and are essential to the provision of relevant information concerning the premorbid development and characteristics of the child (e.g., birth history, medical history, developmental history, learning style, academic status, and social behavior). In addition, those involved with the education of the child would have an integral role in the development and generalization of therapy strategies. In essence, the involvement of stakeholders will facilitate an ecologically valid assessment of function and promote the design of a meaningful and motivating therapy program.

Assessment of Language and Communication Disorders in Pediatric TBI

Assessment procedures should commence with the identification of stakeholders and the gathering of case history information. Important information regarding the factors that influence outcome, such as the mechanism of injury, site and extent of lesion, age at injury, premorbid personality and developmental and academic history should be considered.

Although formal tests of language impairment are generally considered insensitive to the effects of pediatric TBI, their inclusion in the assessment process is critical. It is vital that deficits in primary linguistic operations be identified, so that their effect on social communication and academic achievement can be minimized. Follow-up use of formal assessment is also necessary to ensure that impairments in developmental language operations do not go undetected. The formal language tests selected for administration will depend on the age of the individual and his/her stage of metalinguistic and metacognitive development. The language measures should be comprehensive, covering all modalities of language function and should include tasks that rely on integrated cognitive-linguistic operations (e.g., verbal fluency, resolution of semantic ambiguity, sentential-semantic manipulation). In addition, it is important that the test battery include tests of the specific skills (e.g., confrontation naming) that are frequently documented as being vulnerable to TBI.

Assessment of oral and written discourse should complement the formal tests so that the limitations in communicative function can be more clearly realized. Along with specific discourse measures, tests of pragmatic function are a vital component of the comprehensive assessment of communication problems following TBI, since they provide an opportunity to examine real-time communication function beyond the boundaries of clinical tasks. Some tests of formal language function and pragmatic skill that are suitable for assessing function in children and adolescence, are listed in Table 12-9.

Table 12-9. Some tests of language and communicative function for children, following TBI.

General Tests of Developmental Language

Clinical Evaluation of Language Fundamentals—Revised (CELF-R)	Semel, Wiig & Secord, 1987
Test of Language Development-2 (TOLD-P)	Newcomer & Hammill, 1988
Test of Language Development-2 Intermediate (TOLD-2I)	Hammill & Newcomer, 1988
Test of Adolescent Language (TOAL)	Hammill, Brown, Larsen, & Weiderholt, 1987
Test of Language Competence—Expanded	Wiig & Secord, 1989
The Token Test for Children	Di Simone, 1978
Test of Problem Solving	Zachman, Jorgensen, Huisingh, & Barrett, 1984

Semantics

Peabody Picture Vocabulary Test—Revised	Dunn & Dunn, 1981
Test of Word Knowledge	Wiig & Secord, 1992
The Word Test	Jorgensen, Barrett, Huisingh, & Zachman 1981
Double Administration Naming Technique	Fired-Oken, 1987

Pragmatics

The Bus Story: A Test of Continuous Speech, 2nd Edition	Renfrew, 1991
Let's Talk Inventory for Adolescents	Wiig, 1982
Clinical Discourse Analysis	Damico, 1985
Pragmatic Protocol	Prutting & Kirchner, 1987

Nonstandardized and informal testing should also be incorporated into the diagnostic protocol. Informal testing is valuable in the early stages of recovery from TBI, when rapid daily improvement can render the results of standardized assessments invalid. Informal methods of assessment may include observation of isolated play behavior, conversation interaction, and classroom and playground behavior. Informal methods involving observation techniques are also valuable throughout the treatment program, providing insight into the efficacy or generalization of a treatment strategy.

Treatment of Language and Communication Deficits in Pediatric TBI

Intervention for children with language and communicative disorders following TBI is by necessity individually designed. General principles of therapy design (see Table 12-5) should, however, apply. The goals of therapy should be derived from the comprehensive assessment and reflect not only the identified areas of impairment, but also the functional communicative needs of the individual. Therapy goals will also be influenced by the occurrence of concomitant disorders, such as behavioral disturbances and physical limitations, and the amount of environmental support available. At all times, the stakeholders should be involved in the therapy process. In addition, therapy should be conducted in a positive learning environment that fosters participation on behalf of the child in goal setting and task design. The quality of reinforcement is particularly important for continued motivation and generalization of skills.

In the adult TBI population, rehabilitation specialists generally concede that methods of compensation are more valuable than methods aimed at restitution of impaired function. The issue of compensation versus restoration is not so clear in pediatric rehabilitation, where certain component cognitive and linguistic processes are still developing or have not yet been acquired. It has been suggested that skills in a rapid stage of development may be more vulnerable to disruption by TBI than skills that are well consolidated or overlearned (Ewing-Cobbs et al., 1987; Ewing-Cobbs et al., 1998). With this in mind, clinicians should consider techniques to promote restoration of function and maximize developmental potential. It is expected however, that compensatory strategies, either personal or environmental, will also be integral to a therapy program that aims to achieve an increase in functional communicative activity.

While many children with TBI do not display deficits in specific language function, therapy aimed at linguistic operations may be required. For example, a child with a specific confrontation naming impairment may benefit from exercises aimed at increasing semantic awareness and organization. Such tasks include activities involving sentence completion, categorization and association of lexical items, semantic judgment, and convergent and divergent naming. Compensatory strategies might include teaching the use of circumlocution or synonyms, or subvocal closure cues (e.g., I write with a ____).

Therapy for oral and written discourse production and comprehension may be aimed at the common discourse sequelae in pediatric TBI, including difficulty retaining and conveying the most essential information, poor organization of verbal and written discourse, understanding inference and comprehending meaning across the text, as well as reduced ability to paraphrase and synthesize information (Chapman et al., 1999). The content of discourse treatment should be related to situations that are relevant to the child's recreational life or academic focus. Discourse therapy should move beyond the clinic room to be conducted in a variety of natural contexts and with a number of significant communicative partners.

Treatment for pragmatic disturbances will depend on the age and expected social-interactive behaviors of the child. Therapy should include many of the strategies used in the adult population, such as increasing self-awareness and self-monitoring, behavioral rehearsal, direct instruction and scripting, behavior shaping, and fading of cues. Group therapy is a valuable strategy because of its ability to provide children with the opportunity to practice pragmatic skills and receive feedback in a nonthreatening environment.

Follow-up Assessment Treatment for Language and Communication Disorders in Pediatric TBI

The effects of brain injury on the language, cognitive, and communication abilities of children are not always apparent immediately after the brain insult. Even those children who fail to exhibit deficits in specific language function and possess minimal disturbances of discourse behavior should be monitored throughout their academic years so that latent disturbances in communication ability can be detected. Communicative function in brain-injured children should, therefore, be monitored as they move through adolescence and into adulthood.

Communication is fundamental to the social skill and psychosocial well-being of people of all ages. Ongoing evaluation of the communicative activities of children with TBI is critical, in order to prevent these children from experiencing restricted participation and social isolation in adulthood.

Summary

The management of cognitive-linguistic communication disorders following TBI is critical to the success with which a person resumes valued roles in the community. The model presented in this chapter provided a framework for assessment and treatment of communication across a continuum from impairments in cognitive-linguistic and pragmatic components to the ability to achieve functional communicative activities and societal participation. Regardless of age, sensitive assessments, involving both standardized and ethnographic techniques, must be used to illuminate the extent of the communication impairments and the impact they have on the person's functional activities and societal participation. With the knowledge gained from the assessment, relevant, real-life goals may be derived in collaboration with the injured person and other stakeholders. Throughout the program, it is necessary that the injured person remain an active participant in goal setting, treatment regime, and target monitoring. Therapy is by nature dynamic and evolving and should monitored and modified according to its effectiveness.

Given that communication is central to participation in society, the ultimate goal of communication therapy can only be measured by the success with which an individual is able to gain reentry into their community and the quality of life they experience within that community.

References

ASHA (American Speech-Language-Hearing Association). (1991). Guidelines for speech-language pathologists serving persons with language, socio-communicative and/or cognitive-communication impairments. *Asha, 3* (Suppl. 5), 21–28.

Australian Bureau of Statistics (ABS). (1990). *Hospital Morbidity in Queensland (Cat. No. 4303.3)*. Canberra, Australian Capital Territory.

Bayles, K. & Tomeoda, C. (1995). *Functional Linguistic Communication Inventory (FLCI)*. Oxcon, UK: Winslow Press.

Benjamin, L., Debinski, A., Fletcher, D., Hedger, C., Mealings, M., & Stewart-Scott, A. (1989). The use of the Bethesda Conversational Skills Profile in closed head injury. In V. Anderson & M. Bailey (Eds.), *Proceedings of the Fourteenth Annual Brain Impairment Conference: Theory and Function: Bridging the Gap* (pp. 57–64). Melbourne: Australian Society for the Study of Brain Impairment.

Benton, A.L. & Hamsher, K. (1983). *Multilingual Aphasia Examination* (Rev. ed.). Iowa City: AJA Associates.

Ben-Yishay, Y. & Prigatano, G.P. (1990). Cognitive remediation. In M. Rosenthal, E.R. Griffith, M. Bond, & J.D. Miller (Eds.), *Rehabilitation of the Adult and Child with Traumatic Brain Injury* Second edition. (pp. 393–409). Philadelphia, PA: F.A. Davis Co.

Blosser, J.L. & DePompeii, R. (1994). *Pediatric Traumatic Brain Injury Proactive Intervention*. San Diego, CA: Singular Publishing Group, Inc.

Brookshire, R.H. & Nicholas, L.E. (1993). *Discourse Comprehension Test*. Tucson, AZ: Communication Skill Builders.

Brown, M. & Vandergoot, D. (1998). Quality of life for individuals with traumatic brain injury: Comparison with others living in the community. *Journal of Head Trauma Rehabilitation, 13*, 1–23.

Bryan, K. (1988). Assessment of language disorders after right hemisphere damage. *British Journal of Disorders of Communication, 23*, 111–125.

Burke, D., Kirrily, A., Baxter, M., Baker, F., Connell, K., Diggles, S., Feldman, K., Horny, A., Kokinos, M., Moloney, D., & Withers, J. (2000). Rehabilitation of a person with severe traumatic brain injury. *Brain Injury, 14*, 463–471.

Chapman, S.B., Levin, H.S., Matejka, J., Harward, H.N., & Kufera, J. (1995). Discourse ability in head-injured children: Considerations of linguistic, psychosocial, and cognitive factors. *Journal of Head Trauma Rehabilitation, 10*, 36–54.

Chapman, S., Culhane, K., Levin, H., Harward, H., Mendelson, D., Ewing-Cobbs, L., Fletcher, J., & Bruee, D. (1992). Narrative discourse after closed head injury in children and adolescents. *Brain and Language, 43*, 2–62.

Chapman, S.B. (1997). Cognitive-communication abilities in children with closed head injury. *American Journal of Speech and Language Pathology, 6*, 50–58.

Chapman, S.B., Levin, H.S., & Lawyer, S.L. (1999). Communication problems resulting from brain injury in children: Special issues of assessment and management. In S. McDonald, L. Togher & C. Code (Eds.), *Communication disorders following traumatic brain injury*. East Sussex: Psychology Press.

Chapman, S.B., Levin, H.S., Wanek, A., Weyrauch, J., & Kufera, J. (1998). Discourse after closed head injury in young children: Relation of age to outcome. *Brain and Language, 61*, 420–449.

Chapman, S.B., Watkins, R., Gustafson, C., Moore, S., Levin, H.S., & Kufera, J.A.(1997). Narrative discourse in children with closed head injury, children with language impairment, and typically developing children. *American Journal of Speech-Language Pathology, 6*, 66–75.

Clark, L.W. & White, K. (1995). Nature and efficacy of communication management in Alzheimer's disease. In R. Lubinski (Ed.), *Dementia and Communication* (pp. 238–256). San Diego: Singular.

Coelho, C.A. (1995). Discourse production deficits following traumatic brain injury: A critical review of the recent literature. *Aphasiology, 9*, 409–429.

Coelho, C.A., DeRuyter, F., & Stein, M. (1996). Treatment efficacy: cognitive-communicative disorders resulting from traumatic brain injury in adults. *Journal of Speech and Hearing Research, 39*: S5–S17.

Coelho, C.A., Liles, B.Z., & Duffy, R.J. (1991). Discourse analysis with closed head-injured adults: Evidence for differing patterns of deficits. *Archives of Physical Medicine and Rehabilitation, 72,* 465–468.

Damico, J.S. (1985). Clinical discourse analysis. A functional language assessment technique. In C.S. Simon (Ed.), *Communication Skills and Classroom Success: Assessment of Language-Learning Disabled Students.* San Diego: College Hill Press.

Dennis, M. & Barnes, M.A. (1990). Knowing the meaning, getting the point, bridging the gap, and carrying the message: Aspects of discourse following closed head injury in childhood and adolescence. *Brain and Language, 39,* 428–446.

Diller, L. (1987). Neuropsychological rehabilitation. In M.J. Meier, A.L. Benton, & Diller, L. (Eds.), *Neuropsychological Rehabilitation.* London: Churchill-Livingstone, 1–17.

Di Simone, F. (1978). *The Token Test for Children.* Hingham, MA: Teaching Resources.

Donabedian, A. (1980). *Explorations in Quality Assessment and Monitoring. Volume 1: The Definition of Quality and Approaches to Its Assessment.* Ann Arbor, MI: Health Administration Press.

Dunn, L.M. & Dunn, L.M. (1981). *Peabody Picture Vocabulary Test-Revised.* Minnesota: American Guidance Service.

Ehrlich, J. & Barry, P. (1989). Rating communication behaviors in head-injured adults. *Brain Injury, 3,* 193–198.

Ewing-Cobbs, L., Brookshire, B., Scott, M.A., & Fletcher, J.M. (1998). Children's narratives following traumatic brain injury: Linguistic structure, cohesion, and thematic recall. *Brain and Language, 61,* 395–419.

Ewing-Cobbs, L., Levin, H.S., Eisenberg, H.M., & Fletcher, J.M. (1987). Language functions following closed head injury in children and adolescents. *Journal of Clinical and Experimental Neuropsychology, 9(5),* 575–592.

Ewing-Cobbs, L., Miner, M.E., Fletcher, J.M., & Levin, H.S. (1989). Intellectual, motor, and language sequelae following closed head injury in infants and preschoolers. *Journal of Pediatric Psychology, 14,* 531–547.

Fletcher, J.M., Ewing-Cobbs, L., Miner, M.E., Levin, H.S., & Eisenberg, H.M.(1990). Behavioral changes after closed head injury. *Journal of Consulting Clinical Psychology, 58,* 93–98.

Frattali, C.M., Thompson, D., Holland, A., Wohl, C., Ferketic, M. (1995). *American Speech-Language Hearing Association Functional Assessment of Communication Skills for Adults.* Rockville, MD: ASHA.

Fried-Oken, M. (1987). Qualitative examination of children's naming skills through test adaptations. *Language, Speech and Hearing Services in Schools, 18,* 206–216.

Galski, T., Tompkins, C., & Johnston, M.V. (1998). Competence in discourse as a measure of social integration and quality of life in persons with traumatic brain injury. *Brain Injury, 12,* 769–782.

Goodglass, H. & Kaplan, E. (1983). Boston Diagnostic Aphasia Examination. In H. Goodglass & E. Kaplan (Eds.), *The Assessment of Aphasia and Related Disorders* Second edition. Philadelphia: Lei and Febiger.

Gordon, W.A. (1990). Approaches to cognitive rehabilitation. In R.L.I. Wood (Ed.), *Management of Behavioral Sequelae of Traumatic Brain Injury.* Baltimore: Brookes.

Grice, H.P. (1975). Logic and conversation. In F. Cole & J.L. Morgan (Eds.), *Syntax and Semantics 3: Speech Acts* (pp. 41–58). New York: Academic Press.

Gross, Y. & Schultz, L.E. (1986). Intervention models in neuropsychology. In B. Uzzell & Y. Gross (Eds.), *Clincial Neuropsychology of Intervention.* New York: Guilford.

Hagen, C. (1984). Language disorders in head trauma. In A. Holland (Ed.), *Language Disorders in Adults: Recent Advances* (pp. 245–281). San Diego: College-Hill Press.

Hammill, D.D., Brown, V.L., Larsen, S.C., & Wiederholt, J.L. (1987). *Test of Adolescent Language*. Austin, TX: Pro-Ed.

Hammill, D.D. & Newcomer, P.L. (1988). *Test of Language Development-2 Intermediate*. Austin, TX: Pro-Ed.

Hartley, L. (1992). Assessment of functional communication. *Seminars in Speech and Language, 13*, 264–279.

Hartley, L. (1995). *Cognitive-Communicative Abilities Following Brain Injury: A Functional Approach*. San Diego: Singular Publishing Group, Inc.

Hartley, L. & Jensen, P.J. (1991). Narrative and procedural discourse after closed head injury. *Brain Injury, 6*, 271–281.

Hartley, L. & Jensen, P.J. (1992). Three discourse profiles of closed-head-injured speakers: Theoretical and clinical implications. *Brain Injury, 5*, 267–285.

Hinchliffe, F.J., Murdoch, B.E., & Chenery, H.J. (1998). Towards a conceptualization of language and cognitive impairment in closed head injury: use of clinical measures. *Brain Injury, 12*, 109–132.

Hinchliffe, F.J., Murdoch, B.E., Chenery, H.J., Baglioni, A.J., & Harding-Clark, J. (1998). Cognitive-linguistic subgroups in closed head injury. *Brain Injury, 12*, 369–398.

Hinnant, D.W. (1999). Neurobehavioral consequences: Assessment, treatment and outcome. In D.W. Marion (Ed.), *Traumatic Brain Injury*. New York: Thieme.

Holland, A.L. (1982). When is aphasia aphasia? The problem of closed head injury. In R. Brookshire (Ed.), *Clinical Aphasiology, Vol. 12*. (pp. 345–349). Minneapolis: BRK Publishers.

Holland, A.L., Frattali, C., & Fromm, D. (1998). *Communication Activities of Daily Living (CADL-2)*. Austin, TX: Pro-Ed.

Huisingh, R., Barrett, M., Bagcen, C., & Orman, O. (1990). *The Word Test-Revised*. Ilinois: Lingui Systems.

Isaki, E. & Turkstra, L. (2000). Communication abilities and work reentry following traumatic brain injury. *Brain Injury, 14*, 441–453.

Jacobs, H.E. (1993). *Behavior Analysis Guidelines and Brain Injury Rehabilitation: People, Principles and Programs*. Gaithersburg, MD: Apsen Publishers.

Jordan, F.M. & Murdoch, B.E. (1990). A comparison of the conversational skills of closed-head-injured children and normal adults. *Australian Journal of Communication Disorders, 18*, 69–82.

Jordan, F.M. & Murdoch, B.E. (1993). A prospective study of the linguistic skills of children with closed head injuries. *Aphasiology, 7*, 503–512.

Jordan, F.M, Murdoch, B.E., & Buttsworth, D.L. (1991). Closed head injured children's performance on narrative tasks. *Journal of Speech and Hearing Research, 34*, 572–582.

Jordan, F.M., Ozanne, A.E., & Murdoch, B.E., (1988). Long-term speech and language disorders subsequent to closed head injury in children. *Brain Injury, 2*, 179–185.

Jorgensen, C., Barrett, M., Huisingh, R., & Zachman, L. (1981). *The Word Test: A Test of Expressive Vocabulary and Semantics*. Illinois: Lingui Systems, Inc.

Kearns, K.J. (1990). Procedures and measures. In L.B. Olswang, C.K. Thompson, S.F. Warren, & N.J. Minghetti (Eds.), *Treatment Efficacy Research in Communication Disorders* (pp. 79–90). Rockville, MD: American Speech-Language-Hearing Foundation.

Kertesz, A. (1982). *The Western Aphasia Battery*. New York: Grune and Stratton.

Klonoff, H., Low, M.D., & Clark, C. (1977). Head injuries in children: A prospective five-year follow-up of children with head injuries. *Journal of Neurology, Neurosurgery and Psychiatry, 40*, 1211–1219.

Kraus, J.F., Black, M.A., Hessol, N., Ley, P., Rokaw, W., Sullivan, C., Bowers, S., Knowlton, S., & Marshall, L. (1984). The incidence of acute brain injury and serious impairment in a defined population. *American Journal of Epidemiology, 119*, 186–201.

Lethlean, J.B. & Murdoch, B.E. (1997). Performance of subjects with multiple sclerosis on tests of high level language. *Aphasiology, 11* 39–57.

Levin, H.S., Culhane, K.A., Mendelsohn, D., Lilly, M.A., Bruce, D., Fletcher, J., Chapman, S., Harward, H., & Eisenberg, H.M. (1993). Cognition in relation to magnetic resonance imaging in head-injured children and adolescents. *Archives of Neurology, 50*, 897–905.

Levinson, S.C. (1983). *Pragmatics.* Sydney: Cambridge University Press.

Lezak, M. (1995). *Neuropsychological Assessment* Third edition. New York: Oxford University Press.

Liles, B.Z., Coelho, C.A., Duffy, R.F., & Zalagens, M.R. (1989). Effects of elicitation procedures on the narratives of normal closed head-injured adults. *Journal of Speech and Hearing Disorders, 54,* 356–366.

Lomas, J., Pickard, L., Betser, S., Elbard, H., Finlayson, A., & Zoghaib, C. (1989). The communicative effectiveness index: development and psychometric evaluation of a functional communication measure for adult aphasia. *Journal of Speech and Hearing Disorders, 54,*113–224.

Manochiopining, S., Sheard, C., & Reed, V.A. (1992). Pragmatic assessment in adult aphasia: A clinical review. *Aphasiology, 6,* 519–534.

Marsh, N. & Knight, R.G. (1991). Relationship between cognitive deficits and social skill after head injury. *Neuropsychology, 5,* 107–117.

Mateer, C.A. & Sohlberg, M.M. (1988). A paradigm shift in memory rehabilitation. In H.A. Whitaker (Ed.), *Neuropsychological Studies of Nonfocal Brain Damage* (pp. 202–225). New York: Springer-Verlag.

Mateer, C.A., Sohlberg, M.M., & Youngman, P.K. (1990). The management of acquired attention and memory deficits. In R.L. Wood & I. Fussey (Eds.), *Cognitive Rehabilitation in Perspective* (pp. 68-95). London: Taylor & Francis.

Mazaux, J.M. & Richer, E. (1998). Rehabilitation after traumatic brain injury in adults. *Disability and Rehabilitation 20,* 435–447.

McDonald, S. (1992). Differential pragmatic language loss following closed head injury: Ability to comprehend conversational implicature. *Applied Psycholinguistics, 13,* 295–312.

McDonald, S. (1993). Pragmatic language skills after closed head injury: Ability to meet the information needs of the listener. *Brain and Language, 44,* 28–46.

McDonald, S. & Pearce, S. (1995). "The Dice Game" a new test of pragmatic language skills after closed head injury. *Brain Injury, 9,* 255–271.

McDonald, S. & Pearce, S. (1996). Clinical insights into pragmatic theory: Frontal lobe deficits and sarcasm. *Brain and Language, 53,* 81–104.

McDonald, S. & Pearce, S. (1998). Requests that overcome listener reluctance:impairment associated with executive dysfunction in brain injury. *Brain and Language, 61,* 88–104.

McDonald, S. & van Sommers, P. (1993). Pragmatic language skills after closed head injury: Ability to negotiate requests. *Cognitive Neuropsychology, 10,* 297–315.

McGann, W. & Werven, G. (1995). Social competence and head injury: A new emphasis. *Brain Injury, 9,* 93–102.

McNeil, M.R. & Prescott, T.E. (1978). *Revised Token Test.* Baltimore: University Park Press.

Mentis, M. & Prutting, C. (1987). Cohesion in the discourse of normal and head-injured adults. *Journal of Speech and Hearing Research, 30,* 88–89.

Milton, S., Prutting, C., & Binder, G. (1984). Appraisal of communication competence in head-injured adults. In R. Brookshire (Ed.), *Clinical Aphasiology (Vol. 14)* (pp.114–123). Minneapolis: BRK Publishers.

Morreau, L.E. & Bruininks, R.H. (1991). *Checklist of Adaptive Listening Skills.* Allen,TX: DLM.

Newcomer, P.L. & Hammill, D.D. (1988). *Test of Language Development-2 Primary.* Austin, TX: Pro-Ed.

O'Flaherty, C. & Douglas, J. (1997). Living with cognitive-communication difficulties following traumatic brain injury: using a model of interpersonal communication to characterize the subjective experience. *Brain Injury, 11,* 889–1011.

Payne, J.C. (1994). Communication Profile: A Functional Skills Survey. Arizona: Communication Skill Builders.

Penn, C. (1985). The profile of communicative appropriateness: A clinical tool for the assessment of pragmatics. *The South African Journal of Communication Disorders, 32,* 18–23.

Penn, C. (1999). Pragmatic assessment and therapy for persons with brain damage: What have clinicians gleaned in two decades? *Brain and Language, 68,* 535–552.

Penn, C. & Cleary, J. (1988). Compensatory strategies in the language of closed-head-injured patients. *Brain Injury, 2,* 3–17.

Perkins, L., Whitworth, A., & Lesser, R. (1998). Conversing in dementia: A conversational analytic approach. *Journal of Neurolinguistics, 11,* 33–54.

Perrott, S.B, Taylor, H.G., & Montes, J.F. (1991). Neuropsychological sequelae, familial stress, and environmental adaptation following pediatric head injury. *Developmental Neuropsychology, 7,* 69–86.

Ponsford, J.L. (1995). Traumatic brain injury in children. In J. Ponsford, S. Sloan, & P. Snow (Eds.), *Traumatic Brain Injury: Rehabilitation for Everyday Adaptive Living.* Hillsdale: Lawrence Erlbaum Associates.

Ponsford, J.L. & Kinsella, G. (1988). Evaluation of a remedial program for attentional deficits following closed head injury. *Journal of Clinical and Experimental Neuropsychology, 10,* 693–708.

Prigatano, G.P. (1997). Recovery and cognitive retraining after craniocerebral trauma. *Journal of Learning Disabilities, 20 (10),* 603–613.

Prigatano, G., Roueche, J., & Fordyce, D. (1986). Nonaphasic language disturbances after brain injury. In G.P. Prigatano (Ed.), *Neuropsychological Rehabilitation After Brain Injury* (pp. 18–28). Baltimore: John Hopkins University Press.

Prutting, C.A. & Kirchner, D. (1987). A clinical appraisal of the pragmatic aspects of language. *Journal of Speech and Hearing Disorders, 52,* 105–109.

Rees, N.S. & Gerber, S. (1992). Ethnography and communication: Social-role relations. *Topics in Language Disorders, 12(3),* 15–27.

Renfrew, C. (1991). *The Bus Story: A Test of Continuous Speech* Second edition. Oxford: C. Renfrew.

Ripich, D.N. & Spinelli, F.M. (1985). An ethnographic approach to assessment and intervention. In D.N. Ripich & F.M. Spinelli (Eds.), *School Discourse Problems* (pp. 199–216). San Diego: Singular Publishing Group.

Rosenthal, M. (1995) Sheldon Berrol, MD Senior Lectureship: The ethics and efficacy of brain injury rehabilitation—myths, measurements and meaning. *Journal of Head Trauma Rehabilitation, 11,* 88–95.

Sarno, M.T. (1975). *The Functional Communication Profile.* New York: NYU Medical Center, Institute of Rehabilitation Medicine.

Sarno, M.T. (1980). The nature of verbal impairment after closed head injury. *Journal of Nervous and Mental Disorders, 168(11),* 685–692.

Searle, J. (1969). *Speech Acts.* Cambridge: Cambridge University Press.

Semel, E., Wiig, E.H., & Secord, W. (1987). *Clinical Evaluation of Language Fundamentals—Revised.* Orlando: Harcourt Brace Jovanovich, Inc.

Snow, P. & Douglas, J. (1999). Discourse rehabilitation following traumatic brain injury. In S. McDonald, L. Togher, & C. Code (Eds), *Communication Disorders Following Traumatic Brain Injury.* East Sussex: Psychology Press.

Snow, P., Douglas, J., & Ponsford, J. (1995). Discourse assessment following traumatic brain injury: A pilot study examining some demographic and methodological issues. *Brain Injury, 9,* 365–380.

Snow, P., Douglas, J., & Ponsford, J. (1997a). Procedural discourse following traumatic brain injury. *Aphasiology, 11,* 948–967.

Snow, P., Douglas, J., & Ponsford, J. (1997b). Conversation assessment following traumatic brain injury: A comparison of two groups. *Brain Injury, 11,* 409–429.

Snow, P., Douglas, J., & Ponsford, J. (1998). Conversational discourse abilities following severe traumatic brain injury: a follow-up study. *Brain Injury, 12,* 911–935.

Snow, P. & Ponsford, J. (1995). Assessing and managing changes in communication and interpersonal skills following TBI. In J. Ponsford, S. Sloan, & P. Snow (Eds.), *Traumatic Brain Injury Rehabilitation for Everyday Adaptive Living.* Hillsdale: Lawrence Erlbaum Associates.

Sohlberg, M.M. & Mateer, C.A. (1989). Introduction to Cognitive Rehabilitation: Theory and Practice. New York: Guilford.

Spitzberg, B.H. & Hurt, H.T. (1987). The measurement of interpersonal skills in instructional contexts. *Communication Education, 36,* 28–45.

Spreen, O. & Benton, A.L. (1969). *Neurosensory Centre Comprehensive Examination for Aphasia: Manual for Directions.* Victoria, BC: University of Victoria.

Sohlberg, M.M. & Mateer, C.A. (1989). Training use of compensatory memory books: A three stage behavioral approach. *Journal of Clinical and Experimental Neuropsychology, 11,* 871–891.

Stuss, D. & Benson, F. (1986). *The Frontal Lobes.* New York: Raven Press.

Szekers, S., Ylvisaker, M., & Holland, A. (1985). Cognitive rehabilitation therapy: A framework for intervention. In M. Ylvisaker (Ed.), *Head Injury Rehabilitation: Children and Adolescents* (pp. 219–246). Austin, TX: Pro-Ed.

Terrell, B.Y. & Ripich, D.N. (1989). Discourse competence as a variable in intervention. *Seminars in Speech and Language, 10,* 282–297.

Togher, L., Hand, L., & Code, C. (1996). Disability following head injury: A new perspective in the relationship between communicative impairment and disempowerment. *Disability and Rehabilitation,* 18(11), 169-189.

Togher, L., Hand, L., & Code, C. (1997a). Analyzing discourse in the traumatic brain injury population: Telephone interactions with different communication partners. *Brain Injury, 11,* 169–189.

Togher, L., Hand, L., & Code, C. (1997b). Measuring service encounters in the traumatic brain injury population. *Aphasiology, 11,* 491–504.

Watt, N., Penn, C., & Jones, D. (1996). Speech-language evaluation of closed head injured subjects in South Africa: Cultural applicability and ecological validity of a test battery. *South African Journal of Communication Disorders, 43,* 85–92.

Wertz, R.T., Collins, M., Weiss, D., Kurtzke, J.F., Friden, T., Brookshire, R.H., Pierce, J., Holzapple, P., Hubbars, D., Porch, B., West, J., Davis, L., Matovich, V., Orley, G., & Resurrection, E. (1981). Veterans Administration cooperative study on aphasia: A comparison of individual and group treatment. *Journal of Speech and Hearing Disorders, 24,* 580–594.

WHO (World Health Organization). (1997). *ICIDH-2: International Classification of Impairments, Activities and Participation.* Geneva, Switzerland: WHO.

Wiig, E. (1982). *Let's Talk Inventory for Adolescents.* Ohio: Charles E. Merrill Publishing Company.

Wiig, E., Alexander, E., & Secord, W. (1988). Linguistic competence and level of cognitive functioning in adults with traumatic closed head injury. In H. Whitaker (Ed.), *Neuropsychological Studies of Nonfocal Brain Injury: Trauma and Dementia* (pp. 186–199). New York: Springer-Verlag.

Wiig, E. & Secord, E. (1989) *Test of Language Competence—Expanded.* Ohio: Charles E. Merrill.

Wiig, E. & Secord, E. (1992). *Test of Word Knowledge.* Ohio: Charles E. Merrill.

Wirz, S. L., Skinner, C., & Dean, E. (1990). *Revised Edinburgh Functional Communication Profile.* Tucson, AZ: Communication Skill Builders.

Worrall, L. (1999). *The Everyday Communication Needs Assessment (ECNA).* London: Winslow Press.

Wrightson, P. (1989). Management of disability and rehabilitation services after mild head injury. In H. Levin, H. Isenberg, & A. Benton (Eds.), *Mild Head Injury.* New York: Oxford University Press.

Ylvisaker, M. (1993). Communication outcome in children and adolescents with traumatic brain injury. *Neuropsychological Rehabilitation, 3,* 367–387.

Ylvisaker, M. & Holland. A. (1985). Coaching, self-coaching, and rehabilitation of head injury. In D. Johns (Ed.), *Clinical Management of Neurogenic Communicative Disorders* Second edition. Boston: Little Brown and Company.

Ylvisaker, M. & Szekeres, S.F. (1989). Metacognitive and executive impairments in head-injured children and adults. *Topics in Language Disorders, 9,* 34–42.

Zachman, L. Jorgensen, C., Huisingh, R., & Barrett, M. (1984). *Test of Problem Solving.* Illinois: Lingui Systems.

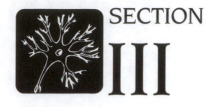

SECTION

III

Swallowing Disorders Following Traumatic Brain Injury

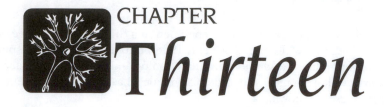

CHAPTER
Thirteen

Swallowing: Neuroanatomical and Physiological Framework

Angela T. Morgan and Elizabeth C. Ward

Introduction

Swallowing, or deglutition, has been recognized as one of the most basic biological functions. Although it is referred to as a "basic" or "fundamental" function, the act of swallowing is by no means a simple process. The oropharyngeal phase of swallowing lasts under 1.5 seconds and requires highly coordinated neurological control in order to modulate the movements of the 31 paired muscles involved in the swallowing process (Dodds, Stewart, & Logemann, 1990; Donner, Bosma, & Robertson, 1985; Nelson & Castell, 1988). The normal swallowing process occurs so effortlessly that the complexity of the neurocontrol orchestrating this complex sequence is often overlooked (Dodds, 1989). However, impairment to the neurological control of swallowing results in dysphagia, and may lead to potential deleterious effects on respiratory status, nutrition, and quality of life.

The mechanisms of traumatic brain injury (TBI) have been recognized in the literature as predisposing factors to dysphagia. With severe head injury in particular, there is a possibility of combined focal, multifocal, and diffuse cortical and brainstem damage, which may affect the neurological control of swallowing. Essential to the understanding of swallowing impairment is a thorough knowledge of the normal deglutitive process (Kennedy & Kent, 1988). Subsequently, it is the purpose of this chapter to outline the physiological functioning and neuroanatomical control of the normal swallowing process in order to provide a basis for the comprehension of dysphagia present following TBI.

The Swallowing Process

The swallowing process has generally been referred to as involving a number of sequences or phases. Traditionally swallowing has been discussed in four phases, consisting of the: (a) oral preparatory phase, (b) oral phase, (c) pharyngeal phase, and (d) esophageal phase. In addition to these four stages, Leopold and Kagel (1983, 1997) proposed an additional fifth stage, the preoral anticipatory stage, which is highly relevant for individuals with TBI.

Preoral Anticipatory Stage

Leopold and Kagel (1983, 1997) have been the pioneers in advocating a new approach to the current classification of dysphagia. The authors highlighted the fact that the traditional swallowing paradigm, comprising of four stages, is constrained, with dysphagia being grounded in the analysis of the anatomical structure and physiological functioning of the oral preparatory, oral, pharyngeal, and esophageal phases. A more inclusive approach to the classification of dysphagia has been proposed, involving consideration of a preoral, or anticipatory, stage of swallowing. Leopold and Kagel (1997) suggested that this stage encompasses the interaction of preoral motor, cognitive, psychosocial, and somatoesthetic elements involved during mealtimes. Siebens et al. (1986) have also proposed a paradigm that recognizes the cognitive, affective, motor, and sensory stimuli seen as important preoral characteristics to be considered in relation to the ability to induce or exacerbate dysphagia.

Groher (1997) referred to oral movements as being the beginning of the continuum of coordinated oral-pharyngeal movements during swallowing. The majority of speech pathologists view the swallowing mechanism in this way in relation to clinical management of a patient. As with any bodily function, however, it is known that the swallowing process actually begins at the neurological level, hence the proposal to change the view to consider an initial swallowing phase, which actually commences prior to the contact of food with the oral cavity. Speech pathologists already give "special consideration" to the effects of cognitive, psychosocial, and somatoesthetic elements on swallowing when managing a patient with dysphagia, particularly one with a swallowing impairment of neurogenic origin, e.g., TBI. However, it is proposed that these elements deserve classification as a distinct anticipatory stage, rather than their current status of "special considerations." Indeed, for the head-injured population, in which cognitive deficits are recognized as a substantial factor influencing feeding and swallowing (Cherney & Halper, 1989; Logemann, 1989; Mackay, Morgan, & Bernstein, 1999), this preoral anticipatory stage has particular significance. Until these elements are recognized by clinicians as representing a distinct stage in the swallowing process, their role in the presentation of dysphagia will continue to be undermined by the more widely recognized clinical pathology of the lingual, pharyngeal, and esophageal phases. Leopold and Kagel (1997) stressed the importance of adopting this additional stage into the swallowing paradigm, in particular for patients with neurological impairment.

Oral Preparatory Phase

The oral preparatory phase is a voluntary process, involving the manipulation of food or liquid in order to form a cohesive bolus ready for swallowing. This phase consists of: tasting the food; mastication, if necessary; combination of the food with saliva; and finally, formation of the food or fluid into a bolus of appropriate size and consistency for movement into the pharynx and esophagus (Derkay & Schechter, 1998). Extremely complex neuromuscular control is required to achieve this phase. Logemann (1983, 1988) summarized the work of Flowers and Morris (1973) to classify the fine-graded movements of the oro-facial musculature that are required. These include: (a) lip closure; (b) rotary and lateral motion of the jaw; (c) buccal or facial tone; (d) rotary, lateral motion of the tongue, and (e) the anterior bulging of the soft palate to widen the nasal airway and narrow the oropharyngeal inlet.

During the oral phase, once the food has been placed in the mouth, the mouth is closed, the lips are compressed together and pressed against the incisors, and the anterior tongue is raised and pressed against the hard palate in order to hold the bolus (Arvedson, Rogers & Brodsky, 1993; Derkay & Schechter, 1998; Logemann, 1988; Zemlin, 1988). If the substance is a liquid, oral manipulation and avoidance of anterior spillage of liquid from the oral cavity is heavily dependent on lip seal (Arvedson et al., 1993).

Elevation of the tongue is achieved via the combined actions of the digastric, genioglossus, geniohyoid, and mylohyoid muscles (Derkay & Schechter, 1998). As Derkay and Schechter (1998) stated, if the food is a solid bolus, then the tongue will also spread it out in the oral cavity in order to expose the food to mastication by the teeth. Mastication involves extremely fine neuromuscular control necessary not only to prevent injury to the tongue, but also to hold a cohesive bolus and prevent premature spillage of the bolus into the pharynx (Logemann, 1988; Derkay & Schechter, 1998).

Of the aforementioned neuromuscular actions of normal oral preparation, Logemann (1988) reported that the rotary, lateral motion of the tongue is the most crucial for controlling the bolus in the mouth and for positioning it superiorly on the teeth to be mixed with saliva. During this phase the soft palate is lowered by contraction of the palatoglossus muscles to help prevent a bolus of food or liquid from entering the pharynx before a swallow is triggered (Arvedson et al., 1993; Derkay & Schechter, 1998). Logemann (1988) explained that at the end of oral preparation, the tongue gathers food particles in the oral cavity together to form a cohesive bolus ready for initiation of the swallow. The tongue generally surrounds the bolus during this collection process, and just before initiating the swallow, the tongue holds the bolus near the front or center of the palate (Logemann, 1988). The tongue surrounding the bolus forms a shape similar to that seen during the production of /sh/ (Logemann, 1983).

A number of authors have provided a clear summary of the neurocontrol of the oral preparatory phase of deglutition (Kennedy & Kent, 1985; Larson, 1985). The cranial nerves involved include: trigeminal (lip closure), facial (facial tone), facial (rotary lateral jaw movement), vagus (palatoglossus—soft palate), and hypoglossal (rotary lateral tongue movement).

Oral Phase

Like the oral preparatory phase, the oral phase is a voluntary stage of the eating process. This phase begins with the posterior propulsion of the food bolus by the tongue and ends with the trigger or production of a "reflex" swallow. The oral phase begins with elevation of the tongue (holding the bolus), which allows for contact with both the hard and soft palate, and a sequential stripping action that is produced largely by the action of the styloglossus muscles (Arvedson et al., 1993; Derkay & Schecter, 1998; Logemann, 1988; Ramsey, Watson, Gramiak, & Weinberg, 1955). This action creates posterior propulsion of the bolus past the anterior tonsillar pillars into the pharynx to trigger the "reflex" swallow (Derkay & Schechter, 1998). As the bolus is propelled posteriorly into the pharynx, the soft palate elevates against the posterior pharyngeal wall (Arvedson et al., 1993). The nasopharynx is sealed off to prevent nasopharyngeal reflux and the pharyngeal phase of swallowing begins.

There has been significant debate over the placement of the receptors for the swallowing reflex initiated at the end of the oral phase (Linden, Tippett, Johnston, Siebens, & French, 1989; Miller, 1982, 1986; Pommerencke, 1928). The majority of receptors have been reported to be placed at the base of the anterior pillars, with further receptors being located in the tongue base, epiglottis, and pyriform fossae (Derkay & Schechter, 1998). Thus it appears that the receptors for swallowing overlap the oral and pharyngeal areas. However, a significant proportion of the debate is concerned with the role of the tongue, or more specifically the posterior tongue, in initiating the swallow reflex. Due to the anatomical placement of the tongue in the oral cavity, and due to the trigger of the "reflex" swallow signaling the end of the oral phase, discussion of the debate regarding receptor placement will be covered in this section on the oral phase of swallowing.

Storey (1968) has suggested that, since the posterior tongue covers the anterior faucial arches at initiation of the oral phase, small amounts of the bolus escape through the fauces into the pharyngeal region of the epiglottis. This region then becomes the area for initiation of a swallow. Shedd, Kirchner, and Scatliff (1961) documented contractions of the faucial isthmus in oral preparation of the bolus, providing evidence that the tongue plays some part in eliciting the pharyngeal swallow. Seminal research by Miller (1982) found that swallowing initiation is reliant upon sensory feedback from a number of areas, with the faucial arches being the primary area of input. Miller (1982) discovered that the uvula, soft palate, posterior tongue, and pharynx are also important areas for feedback.

Disagreement also exists regarding the exact nature of the trigger of the reflexive swallow. A number of authors have suggested that the presence of a bolus itself does not automatically trigger the swallowing process. Miller (1982) found that the threshold for triggering the reflex swallow can be changed by input from higher cortical and hypothalamic regions (areas involved in integrating swallowing with visceral and somatic sensations). Logemann (1988) also suggested that the presence of a bolus may alert the brain that there is food, liquid, or saliva to be swallowed. Logemann (1988) believed that the posterior propulsion of the bolus is more likely to trigger the pharyngeal swallow, through the base of the tongue contacting the faucial arch area and the oropharynx, stimulating the oropharyngeal receptors or the tongue-base receptors, and triggering the reflexive swallow. Another area of research has concentrated on the effects of temperature on the swallowing reflex. Lazarra, Lazarus, and Logemann (1986) found that the peripheral stimulus of coldness alters the swallowing trigger threshold. Further research is needed, however, to fully understand the exact mechanisms of the swallowing reflex. Thus, the oral preparatory phase of swallowing is a complex and important process, setting the stage for the proper timing and coordination of the swallowing reflex (Wolf & Glass, 1992).

Pharyngeal Phase

The reflex swallow of the pharyngeal phase is thought to take approximately 1 second (Derkay & Shechter, 1998). This is a rapid process when one considers that 26 muscles and six cranial nerves must be correctly coordinated in order for the involuntary pharyngeal swallow to occur safely and efficiently (Wolf & Glass, 1992). After her review of the literature, Logemann (1988) summarized the major neuromuscular characteristics of the pharyngeal phase as: elevation of the velum or soft palate to close off the nasopharynx, laryngeal closure, pharyngeal peristalsis, anterior-superior laryngeal movement to move the larynx out of the bolus's path, and relaxation of the cricopharyngeus muscle to allow the bolus to flow through the sphincter. Kennedy and Kent (1988) summarized three functional components of the pharyngeal phase: (1) closure of the nasal, laryngeal, and oral apertures to avoid fluid leakage and direct the bolus; (2) opening of the upper esophageal sphincter (UES); and (3) creating a pharyngeal pressure gradient strong enough to transport the bolus from the oral cavity to the superior opening of the esophagus. Derkay and Schechter (1998) suggested that the primary component of the pharyngeal phase is the actual reflex swallow and bolus transit through the pharynx. However, airway protection is also of primary importance during this phase. "The two primary functions of pharyngeal swallowing are to transport a swallowed bolus through the pharynx whilst protecting the airway from aspiration" (Dodds et al., 1990, p.960).

Airway Protection for Swallowing

There are many mechanisms that contribute to airway protection during the pharyngeal stage of the swallow that also contribute to bolus transport, reenforcing the highly coordinated interdependent nature of the swallowing process (Dodds et al., 1990). The first stage of the involuntary pharyngeal swallow, after the swallow has been initiated, has been reported to be the closure of the nasopharynx by elevation of the soft palate to meet the posterior wall of the pharynx (Zemlin, 1988; Stevenson & Allaire, 1991). The closure occurs via contraction of the palatopharyngeal sphincter (and upper part of the superior constrictor; Zemlin, 1988). This action results in closure of the nasopharynx, preventing nasal regurgitation of the bolus and creates a closed pharyngeal chamber. The next step is typically thought to be laryngeal closure (Zemlin, 1988).

A study by Shaker, Dodds, Dantas, Hogan, and Andorfer (1990) investigated the coordination of glottic closure during swallowing in healthy young adults via frame-by-frame analysis of a number of procedures including: transnasal videoendoscopy, videofluoroscopy, pharyngeal intraluminal manometry, and submental surface electromyography. They discovered that vocal fold adduction actually began 0.3 seconds *before* the onset of the swallow in the majority of their subjects, and was completed 0.4 seconds before the appearance of the peristaltic wave in the oropharynx, with maximal vocal cord adduction persisting throughout the swallow sequence. They noted that partial vocal fold closure occurred frequently in response to the introduction of liquid into the mouth, suggesting that this action may have resulted from an oroglottal reflex, or may involve higher brainstem centers (Shaker et al. 1990).

Once laryngeal closure begins at the level of the true vocal folds, a sequence is thought to progress superiorly. The sequence comprises: adduction of the false cords, epiglottal closure, and finally the approximation of the aryepiglottic folds (Ardran & Kemp, 1951, 1952, 1956; Fink & Demarest, 1978). Shaker and coworkers (1990) supported this progression, listing four sequential events associated with laryngeal closure: adduction of the true vocal folds associated with the horizontal approximation of arytenoid cartilage, vertical approximation of the arytenoids to the base of the epiglottis, laryngeal elevation, and epiglottal descent.

While the majority of authors agree on the basic progression through to closure of the glottis, there is continuing debate regarding the presence/absence of closure of the false vocal cords. Shaker et al. (1990) found that the false vocal folds generally remain open during swallowing. Previous studies, however, have reported that the folds do indeed close during swallowing (Barclay, 1930; Sasaki & Isaacson, 1988; Sasaki & Masafumi, 1976). Cook (1991) defined the procedure for airway protection as involving a sequence of true vocal cord closure, followed by false cord closure, and finally, closure of the laryngeal vestibule. Derkay and Schechter (1998) stated that as anterosuperior tilting of the true vocal folds occurs, the base of the tongue is moving posteriorly so that closure occurs in the laryngeal vestibule. It has been suggested that it is the aryepiglottic folds (which also contain some thyroarytenoid muscle fibers) that come together at this time to cover the laryngeal vestibule (Cook, 1991). The final actions involved in completing the laryngeal closure sequence are laryngeal ascent (occurring via a shortening of the thyrohyoid and suprahyoid muscles) with concomitant epiglottal inversion (Cook, 1991).

Cook (1991) explained that it is at the level of the larynx, including both elevation and closure, where the most important airway protection occurs. "Laryngeal elevation is a vital component of airway protection since this action not only facilitates closure of the laryngeal vestibule, but also repositions the larynx anterosuperiorly under the tongue base, thereby removing the laryngeal inlet from the direct path of the oncoming bolus" (Cook, 1991, p.249). He also stated that the most important defense in avoiding aspiration is integrity of vocal fold function, whereas neither the presence nor normal function of the epiglottis is essential for airway protection.

Pharyngeal Bolus Transport

Four main forces facilitate bolus transport through the pharynx: (a) momentum of the bolus; (b) translational force on the bolus from the posterior movement of the tongue; (c) peristaltic contractions; and (d) the force of gravity (Miller 1982).

While both momentum and gravity have been recognized as factors contributing to bolus propulsion (Fisher, Hendrix, Hunt, & Murrills, 1978), the majority of researchers have focused on the importance of pharyngeal peristalsis and pressure gradients in assisting this process.

The combined effects of gravity, negative pressure, and sequential contraction of the pharyngeal constrictors are important for inferior stripping of the bolus following entry to the pharynx (Wolf & Glass, 1992; Derkay & Schechter, 1998). Logemann (1988) stated that laryngeal and tongue movements also contribute to pressure generated in the pharynx during the pharyngeal phase of the swallow. Specifically, the rapid pistonlike movements of the posterior tongue are used to drive the bolus through the oropharynx into the hypopharynx (Dodds et al., 1990). Dodds et al. (1990) explained that this rapid pistonlike tongue movement occurs because of the creation of a pharyngeal chamber. The sequential peristaltic wave in the pharyngeal constrictors (superior, middle, inferior) follows the bolus to apply back-pressure to the tail of the bolus as it is moving through the pharynx (Logemann, 1988). Thus, during the pharyngeal phase, bolus transit is facilitated not only via muscle contraction, but also by the force of changing pressure gradients throughout the mouth, pharynx, and esophagus.

The bolus, on reaching the epiglottis, divides in half, with each half moving through the pyriform sinuses at either side of the pharynx (Cumming & Reilly, 1972; Arvedson et al., 1993). These portions then combine again just above the level of the opening to the esophagus (Ardran & Kemp, 1951). There are many labels for the opening to the esophagus, including the cricopharyngeal valve/sphincter, upper esophageal sphincter (UES), and the pharyngoesophageal segment (PE segment). This opening is a musculoskeletal valve made up of the cricoid cartilage and a number of muscles that attach to this cartilage, including the cricopharyngeal muscle, the lower fibers of the inferior constrictor, and the upper fibers of the esophageal constrictor (Logemann, 1988). The bolus tail has a v-shaped configuration in the pharynx, as in the oral cavity (Cook, Dodds, Dantas, Kern et al., 1989). As a result of the head of the bolus traveling faster than the tail, the bolus elongates in the pharynx, becoming a contributing force for UES opening, and subsequently causes rapid entry of the bolus into the proximal esophagus (Cook, Dodds, Dantas, Kern et al., 1989; Dodds et al., 1990).

There is much debate regarding both the sequence of events involved in UES relaxation (or opening) and the innervation and control of the esophageal sphincter. Cook, Dodds, Dantas, Massey et al. (1989) have examined the numerous factors facilitating PE segment opening. It has been suggested that the cricopharyngeal muscle relaxes following reception of a signal originating in the oro- and hypopharynx through vagal sensory fibers (Derkay & Schecter, 1998). Logemann (1988) suggested that laryngeal elevation and anterior movement, and cricopharyngeal region opening are closely related. At rest, closure of the UES is maintained by the positioning of the cricoid lamina touching the posterior pharyngeal wall at the level of the cricopharyngeal region (Logemann, 1988). In regard to UES opening, however, as the larynx moves superanteriorly during the swallow, subsequent stretch is exerted on the cricopharyngeal muscle and its adjacent fibers, stretching the muscular components of the UES, and helping to open the sphincter (Cook, 1991; Kahrilas, Dodds, Dent, Logemann, & Shaker, 1987). Doty (1968), and Derkay and Schechter (1998) also agreed that the relaxation phase was initiated when the larynx moved anterosuperiorly. Another factor contributing to the degree of UES opening is the volume of the swallowed bolus (Cook, Dodds, Dantas, Massey et al., 1989).

The primary sensory and motor functions performed within the pharyngeal phase of swallowing involve three cranial nerves: the glossopharyngeal nerve (velopharyngeal closure), the vagus nerve (velopharyngeal closure, pharyngeal peristalsis, pharyngeal sensation, cricopharyngeal opening, laryngeal closure), and the accessory nerve (laryngeal elevation, laryngeal sensation, pharyngeal sensation; Logemann, 1988).

Esophageal Phase

The esophageal phase begins when the bolus passes through the relaxed cricopharyngeal muscle and enters the cervical esophagus. At the instant of swallowing, relaxation of the cricopharyngeal sphincter allows a bolus of food or liquid to pass from the pharynx into the esophagus. In regard to timing, Cook (1991) reported that relaxation of the UES occurs at the beginning of the pharyngeal phase. He stated that the sphincter opens 150 ms later during laryngeal elevation and remains open for a further 500 ms. The bolus is then carried into the esophagus, initiating the esophageal stage of the swallow by a series of contraction waves that are a continuation of the pharyngeal stripping action (Arvedson et al., 1993).

The primary function of the esophagus is passage of the bolus to the stomach via an automatic peristaltic wave. This wave, along with the tonic contraction of the cricopharyngeus muscle, helps prevent gastroesophageal reflux (GOR), or the reentry of material from the esophagus into the pharynx (Arvedson et al., 1993). An esophageal wave or phase normally occurs in the presence of a definite time delay, following each separate pharyngeal phase of the swallow (Arvedson et al., 1993). These phases or stages follow in rapid succession, and may occur up to 300 times per hour during eating (Zemlin, 1988). Swallow-induced peristalsis usually occurs at about 2 to 4 m/secs and traverses the length of the esophagus in 6 to 10 seconds (Dodds, Hogan, Reid, Stewart, & Andorfer, 1973; Ingelfinger, 1958). Two waves of contraction (known as primary and secondary waves) occur during peristalsis (Logemann, 1983). The primary wave of contraction arises in the pharynx and continues along the length of the esophagus, whereas secondary waves are initiated in the body of the esophagus and travel to the stomach (Derkay & Schecter, 1998). Derkay and Schecter (1998) listed a number of other variables determining movement of the bolus: (a) the bolus moves more quickly in the cervical segment of the esophagus, which contains skeletal muscle, and moves more slowly in the thoracic segment, where it is under the influence of smooth muscle; (b) intrathoracic changes associated with respiration occur whereby inspiration enhances bolus movement, but positive pressure from expiration slows it down; and (c) coughing from primary respiratory problems or aspiration may also slow or reverse the passage of the bolus in the intrathoracic portion of the esophagus.

Neural Control of Swallowing

Dodds (1989) and Dodds et al. (1990) stated that the neural control of swallowing involves four major components: (a) efferent motor fibers contained in cranial nerves and the ansa cervicalis; (b) afferent sensory fibers contained in cranial nerves;

(c) cerebral, midbrain, and cerebellar fibers that synapse within the midbrain swallowing centers; and (d) paired swallowing centers located in the brainstem. "Fibers from the higher CNS centres and oral-pharyngeal sensory fibres send input signals to the brainstem swallowing centers that process the information. Output signals pass via those cranial nerves that operate the muscle machinery of swallowing" (Dodds et al., 1990, p. 954). Cook (1991) reported that voluntary swallowing can occur via cortical pathways, whereas reflexive swallowing is triggered by the appropriate combination of stimuli from oral and pharyngeal sensory receptors. The neural control mechanisms of swallowing may be divided into cortical control, brainstem control, and peripheral sensory factors (Doty, 1968; Jean, 1984; Miller, 1982) and will be discussed under these headings in the sections below.

Cortical Control of Swallowing

The cerebral cortex has a significant role in the initiation of the voluntary oral and pharyngeal phase of swallowing (Plant, 1998). Subcortical regions such as the hypothalamus and midbrain (possibly via dopaminergic pathways) can also elicit swallowing (Bieger, Weerasuriya, & Hockman, 1978). Thus, the cortical and subcortical centers of the amygdolohypothalamic regions which are involved in the integration of eating behavior and visceral responses may modify the volitional initiation of swallowing (Cook, 1991). Difficulties such as altered feeding behavior (e.g., loss of internal regulation of appetite) and problems with swallow initiation are common deficits resulting from damage to these areas (Cook, 1991). Martin and Sessle (1993) provided a thorough discussion of evidence suggesting that the cerebral cortex plays a large role in swallowing. In particular, they included data on the effects of cortical lesions on swallowing, data from neuroanatomical tracing studies, data from neuronal recordings, and a detailed discussion of the effects of cortical stimulation on swallowing. Numerous lesion studies (Alberts, Hornery, Gray & Brazer, 1992; Barer, 1984, 1989; Gordon, Hewer & Wade, 1987; Horner & Massey, 1988; Meadows, 1973; Robbins & Levine, 1988; Willoughby & Anderson, 1984; Veis & Logemann, 1985) and stimulation (Amri, Lamkadem & Car, 1991; Car, 1970, 1973; Huang, Hiraba, & Sessle, 1989; Jean & Car, 1979; Penfield & Rasmussen, 1950; Pritchard, Hamilton, Morse & Norgren, 1986; Scott, Yaxley, Sienkiewcz, & Rolls, 1986) have been perfomed, investigating the cortical control of swallowing. For the purposes of the present chapter only a few key lesion and stimulation studies will be discussed in the following sections.

The voluntary control of swallowing is thought to be primarily the responsibility of the cerebral cortex, whereas muscle contraction during the involuntary phase of swallowing, is thought to be primarily influenced by lower brainstem activity (Plant, 1998). Brainstem regions receive bilateral cortical input, thus it was previously felt that bilateral injury was necessary to impair swallowing (Plant, 1998). However, there has been increasing evidence to show that the cortex may be more heavily involved in orchestrating the swallowing process, and that unilateral brain lesions may indeed cause dysphagia.

Daniels, Foundas, Iglesia, and Sullivan (1996) examined unilateral stroke, investigating eight patients with left hemispheric damage and eight patients with right hemispheric damage. They found that the insular cortex was the most common lesion site, found in 11 of 16 unilateral stroke patients with dysphagia. This new finding led Daniels et al. (1996) to hypothesize that the insula may be crucial to swallowing because of its connectivity to cortical, subcortical, and brainstem sites proven to be important in swallowing (Daniels & Foundas, 1997). In particular, they hypothesized that the insula, and primarily the anterior insula, may contribute to oral and pharyngeal motility. This information was based on previous studies documenting the association between swallowing and nutritional properties, including coordinated interaction of oral musculature, gustation, and autonomic functions through connectivity or inherent properties (Daniels & Foundas, 1997). Daniels and Foundas (1997) further investigated the possible role of the insula in swallowing by studying four cases of unilateral stroke. Three out of four patients with lesions to the anterior insula presented with dysphagia. This finding led the authors to conclude that a lesion in this area may result in dysphagia by disrupting gustatory input processing, which may in turn yield a delay in triggering a swallow response, and subsequently, impair pharyngeal swallowing (Daniels & Foundas, 1997).

Disconnection of sensorimotor information between the nucleus tractus solitarus (NTS) and the anterior insular cortex may result in a delayed pharyngeal swallow (Daniels & Foundas, 1997). Increasing sensory characteristics of a bolus (taste, volume, temperature) have been found to reduce the delay in pharyngeal swallow time in stroke patients (Logemann et al., 1995). Daniels and Foundas (1997) suggested that increasing the magnitude of gustatory signals may facilitate stronger sensory signals from the oropharyneal cavity to the brainstem and subsequently to the anterior insula, assisting the timing of the swallow. However, lesions to the anterior insula may potentially reduce the level of sensory input, resulting in an increased swallowing threshold and delayed elicitation of the reflex swallow (Daniels & Foundas, 1997).

Stimulation studies have also indicated the importance of the cerebral cortex in swallowing. In particular, stimulation studies have identified a consistent relationship between different feeding or swallowing responses and the area stimulated. Martin and Sessle (1993) reviewed a number of stimulation studies to find that stimulation of overlapping areas, such as the anterolateral frontal, lateral pericentral, and insular cortex, may evoke swallowing and a number of related ingestive and alimentary sensorimotor behaviors, such as mastication, sucking, salivation, and gustation (Dubner, Sessle, & Storey, 1978; Miller, 1982,1986).

The cerebral cortex has also been thought to play a role in the modulation of swallowing behavior. Miller and Bowman (1977) studied swallowing responses evoked from cortical stimulation in anesthetized monkeys. They found that stimulation of the lateral and caudal surface of the precentral cortex (including Brodmann's areas 44, 3, 1, and the caudal part of area 6) resulted in swallowing alone or chewinglike movements followed by swallowing. Swallowing alone was more frequently associated with stimulation posterior to the subcentral dimple, and chewing and swallowing movements occurred when the region anterior to this dimple was stimulated (Miller and Bowman, 1977). Due to the close association identified between cortically stimulated chewing and swallowing, Miller and Bowman (1977) concluded that the cortex is involved in monitoring and integrating information for mastication within a complex buccopharyngeal motor pattern.

Brainstem/Central Control of Swallowing

Information projected from oral-pharyngeal sensory fibers and higher central nervous system regions is integrated and analyzed in the swallowing centers located in the brainstem (Stevenson & Allaire, 1991). In order for the swallowing process to be orchestrated, the brainstem swallowing centers then distribute output signals to the corresponding efferent motor fibers located in the cranial nerve nuclei and their axons, which subsequently project signals to the appropriate swallowing musculature (Dodds, et al., 1990; Stevenson & Allaire, 1991). Miller (1982) proposed the existence of two possible theories or hypotheses to explain the central control of swallowing: a) the reflex-chain hypothesis and b) the central pattern generator (CPG) hypothesis. Dodds (1989) suggested that there is support for both theories, and that they are not necessarily mutually exclusive. Dodds et al. (1990) proposed that the reflex-chain hypothesis involves the bolus stimulating sensory receptors as it moves through the mouth and pharynx, which sequentially trigger the next step in the swallowing sequence. These authors maintained that even in the absence of a bolus, the posterior excursion of the tongue is thought to stimulate faucial or pharyngeal mechanoreceptors to initiate the pharyngeal swallow.

The CPG theory, however, proposes that once a swallow is initiated, it is executed in a preprogrammed manner by nerves in the brainstem swallowing centers (Dodds et al., 1990). Swallowing relies on a central patterned program, which is only modulated by, and is not reliant upon, feedback sensory input such as volume and consistency (Dodds, 1989; Dodds et al., 1990). While evidence exists to support elements of both hypotheses, the CPG theory is more commonly used to describe the neuronal control of swallowing.

Findings from both animal and human clinical studies affirm the existence of central pattern generators for swallowing (Dodds, 1989; Kennedy & Kent, 1988). The CPG are believed to consist of groups of interneurons, not organized into discrete focal areas, but into rather poorly defined areas located bilaterally in the medulla, specifically the NTS ventromedial reticular formation and the nucleus ambiguous (NA; Jean, 1972; Cook, 1991; Dodds et al., 1990; Miller, 1982, 1993; Plant, 1998). The NTS is found in the dorsal region of the brainstem, and the NA is found more ventrally in the medulla (Miller, 1993). The cortical inputs to the NA area are thought to be involved in the modulation of activity during swallowing (Plant, 1998). Although the NA receives sensory inputs from the superior laryngeal nerve and more extensive cortical input than the NTS, stimulation of the NA produces the esophageal, but not the pharyngeal phase of swallowing (Plant, 1998).

The NTS and adjacent reticular formation lie dorsally in the medulla oblongata (Plant, 1998). Sensory fibers from the glossopharyngeal nerve (IX), from both branches of the vagus nerve (superior laryngeal and recurrent laryngeal; X), and from higher cerebral centers, synapse in this area (Dodds et al., 1990; Plant, 1998). Taste and sensory information from the tongue and oral-pharyngeal mucosa, along with proprioceptive information from the pertinent musculature are transmitted to the swallowing centers via sensory cranial nerve input. The swallowing centers also receive input from rostral brainstem centers, cerebellum, basal ganglia, and higher cortical centers. Numerous interneurons, found within each swallowing center, receive and process the aforementioned input signals and project a stereotyped response to the cranial nerve motor nuclei and their axons (Dodds et al., 1990). Subsequently, the motor nuclei project signals to the appropriate swallowing musculature in order to initiate the swallowing process (Dodds et al., 1990).

Motor neurons from the swallowing centers synapse in ipsilateral cranial nerve nuclei, with the lower motor neurons for the swallowing musculature being located in cranial nerves V, VII, IX, X, and XII and the ansa cervicalis (c1-c3), which joins to run with the hypoglossal nerve (XII; Arvedson et al., 1993). The swallowing centers maintain coordination and bilateral movement of the musculature involved in swallowing, and help to prevent competing muscle activities, such as speech and respiration, allowing for efficient swallowing (Arvedson, et al., 1993; Kennedy & Kent, 1985). The close proximity of the CPG to the respiratory control centers in the medulla oblongata enables coordination between the initiation of swallowing, glottal approximation, and the cessation of respiration during the pharyngeal phase of swallowing (Ichord, 1994).

Peripheral Sensory Factors

Afferent pathways and their subsequent feedback play a crucial role in stimulating and modifying a swallow (Plant, 1998). The appropriate oropharyngeal sensory input must be projected to both the cortical and medullary swallowing centers in order for the cortical swallow center to initiate a voluntary swallow (Cook, 1991). Cook (1991) explained that the voluntary swallow is dependent on having something, at least saliva, in the mouth. This conclusion has been drawn from the known inability of humans to sustain rapid multiple swallows at the same rate for more than a few swallows. On the basis of this evidence, it has been concluded that peripheral sensory input determines volitional swallow frequency (Cook, 1991).

The oral cavity, pharynx, and larynx are all lined with a variety of different types of sensory cells that play a role in swallowing. Within the oral cavity, the largest concentration and most widespread coverage is provided by the mechanoreceptive cells, which are most numerous at the tip of the tongue and along the midline of the palate (Plant, 1998). Pressure stimulation to the sensory cells of the palate results in peristaltic tongue movements (Plant, 1998). As Plant (1998) described, thermoreceptive and chemoreceptive cells are also found in the oral cavity; however, the role of these receptors in swallowing is not well known. Thermoreceptive cells are found in highest concentration in those areas of the palate and tongue that come in contact with each other during swallowing, while chemoreceptive cells are distributed most densely along the tongue (Plant, 1998).

Throughout the larynx and pharynx, afferent mucosal receptors are found that are sensitive to touch and pressure as well as to taste (Donner et al., 1985). Taste stimulation alone, however, has been reported as a weak stimulus for swallowing (Dodds, 1989; Dodds et al., 1990). Pharyngeal and laryngeal sensation that stimulates and guides swallowing is carried via the glossopharyngeal (IX) and vagus (X) nerves to the nucleus solitarius in the brainstem (Donner et al., 1985). The dorsal surface of the tongue, faucial pillars, pharynx, and posterior larynx are thought to be the origins of the major sensory stimuli needed to elicit swallowing (Miller, 1986), with the tonsillar or faucial pillars being the most sensitive to light touch (Plant, 1998; Shinghai & Shimada, 1976; Storey, 1968; Dodds et al, 1990; Pommerencke, 1928). While the posterior pharynx is sensitive to contact stimulation, this region responds more strongly to heavy pressure (Miller, Biegler, & Conklin, 1997). The larynx, in contrast, has fewer deep pressure mechanoreceptive cells, but more cells with free nerve endings in the epithelium. These receptors respond more to liquid than to pressure stimulation. As previously mentioned, local sensory input, such as bolus volume and consistency, is believed to modulate or alter the swallow (Dodds et al., 1990). Thus, ascending sensory tracts evoke motor programs via the CPG and provide ongoing feedback to monitor the descending motor systems (Ichord, 1994).

The sensory system is connected to motor nuclei in the brainstem by interneurons. The cranial nerve motor nuclei involved in deglutition are: the trigeminal (V), facial (VII), glossopharyngeal (IX), vagus (X), and hypoglossal (XII). Taste fibers for a large proportion of the tongue, and for touch sensation to the lips and face, are provided by the facial nerve. The glossopharyngeal and vagus nerves innervate all intrinsic muscles of the soft palate, pharynx, and larynx, with the exception of the tensor veli palatini, which receives motor fibers from the maxillary branch (V3) of the trigeminal nerve. The somatic motor components of the glossopharyngeal and vagus nerves originate in the nucleus ambiguous, whereas the motor nuclei are close to the NTS in the brainstem. This swallowing center also coordinates swallowing and respiration. Sensory loss in the oropharyngeal isthmus, pharynx, or larynx invariably leads to swallow impairment, and possibly to aspiration. Frequently, the cough reflex in such individuals is also eliminated, resulting in "silent dysphagia" and, even more important, to asymptomatic or "silent" aspiration.

Summary

Swallowing is an extremely complex and highly coordinated process, requiring the integration and modulation of a number of specialized areas. Swallowing occurs with the assistance of cortical and sensory input, brainstem integration, processing and modulation of this input, and finally projection of this information to create the required motor swallowing response. In order to achieve and complete the swallowing sequence, assistance is also required from sensory receptors, cranial nerves, cranial nuclei, cortical pathways, numerous muscles, and other bony and cartilaginous structures.

Kirshner (1989) discussed the potential neurological causes of neurogenic dysphagia as they relate to the model of "upper" and "lower" motor neuron lesion types. Using this model it was evident that both upper motor neuron lesions of the cerebral cortex, cerebral white matter, or upper brainstem white matter, and lower motor deficits, including the motor nerve cells of the brainstem, the vagus nerve, the neuromuscular junction, or the pharyngeal muscles, may lead to dysphagia (Kirschner, 1989). However, as Kirshner (1989) explained, this approach is an oversimplification of the issue since it omits additional factors such as the contribution of sensory deficits from cranial nerve or brainstem damage, coordination impairments from disorders of the cerebellum and its connections, movement disorders such as tremor or hesitancy in initiating swallowing, and irregular movements due to basal ganglia involvement. It is clear that with such expansive neurological control being required for efficient and accurate execution of the swallowing process, the likelihood of dysphagia occurring following TBI is high, and the nature of its presentation diverse. The next chapter of this book outlines the characteristics and methods of assessment of dysphagia occurring subsequent to TBI.

References

Alberts, M.J., Horney, J., Gray, L., & Brazer, S.R. (1992). Aspiration after stroke: Lesion analysis by brain MRI. *Dysphagia, 7,* 170–173.

Amri, M., Lamkadem, M., & Car, A. (1991). Effects of lingual nerve and chewing cortex stimulation upon activity of the swallowing neurons located in the region of the hypoglossal motor nucleus. *Brain Research, 548,* 149–155.

Ardran, G.M. & Kemp, F. (1951). The mechanism of swallowing. *Proceedings of the Royal Society of Medicine, 44,* 1038–1040.

Ardran, G. & Kemp, F. (1952). The protection of the laryngeal airway during swallowing. *British Journal of Radiology, 25,* 406–416.

Ardran, G. & Kemp, F. (1956). Closure and opening of the larynx during swallowing. *British Journal of Radiology, 29,* 205–208.

Arvedson, J., Rogers, B., & Brodsky, L. (1993). Anatomy, Embryology and Physiology. In J. Arvedson and L. Brodsky (Ed.), *Pediatric Swallowing and Feeding: Assessment and Management* (pp. 5–51). San Diego, CA: Singular Publishing Group, Inc.

Barclay, A.E. (1930). The normal mechanism of swallowing. *British Journal of Radiology, 3,* 534–546.

Barer, D.H. (1984). Lower cranial nerve motor function in unilateral vascular lesions of the cerebral hemisphere. *British Medical Journal, 289,* 1622.

Barer, D.H. (1989). The natural history and functional consequences of dysphagia after hemispheric stroke. *Journal of Neurology, Neurosurgery and Psychiatry, 52,* 236–241.

Bieger, D., Weerasuriya, A., & Hockman, C.H. (1978). The emetic action of L-dopa and its effect on the swallowing reflex in the cat. *Journal of Neural Transmission, 42,* 87–98.

Car, A. (1970). La commande corticale du centre deglutiteur bulbaire. *Journal of Physiology Paris, 62,* 361–386.

Car, A. (1973). La commande corticale de la deglutition II. Point d'impact bulbaire de la voie corticifuge deglutitrice. *Journal of Physiology Paris, 66,* 553–576.

Cherney, L.R. & Halper, A.S. (1989). Recovery of oral nutrition after head injury in adults. *Journal of Head Trauma Rehabilitation, 4,* 42–50.

Cook, I.J. (1991). Normal and disordered swallowing: new insights. *Bailliere's Clinical Gastroenterology, 5,* (2), 245-267.

Cook, I.J., Dodds, W.J., Dantas, R.O., Kern, M.K., Massey, B.T., Shaker, R., & Hogan, W.J. (1989). Timing of videofluoroscopic, manometric events and bolus transit during the oral and pharyngeal phases of swallowing. *Dysphagia, 4,* 8–15.

Cook, I.J., Dodds, W.J., Dantas, R.O., Massey, B.T., Kern, M.K., Lang, I.M., Brasseur, J.G., & Hogan, W.J. (1989). Opening mechanisms of the human upper esophageal sphincter. *American Journal of Physiology, 257,* G748–G759.

Cumming, W.A. & Reilly, B.J. (1972). Fatigue aspiration. *Radiology, 105,* 387–390.

Daniels, S.K., Foundas, A.L., Iglesia, G.C., & Sullivan, M.A. (1996). Lesion site in unilateral stroke patients with dysphagia. *Journal of Stroke and Cerebrovascular Disorders, 6,* 30–34.

Daniels, S.K. & Foundas, A.L. (1997). The role of the insular cortex in dysphagia. *Dysphagia, 12,* 146–156.

Derkay, C.S. & Schechter, G.L. (1998). Anatomy and physiology of pediatric swallowing disorders. *Otolaryngologic Clinics of North America, 31*(3), 397–404.

Dodds, W. (1989). The physiology of swallowing. *Dysphagia, 3,* 171–178.

Dodds, W.J., Hogan, W.J., Reid, D.P., Stewart, E.T., & Arndorfer, R.C. (1973). A comparison between primary esophageal peristalsis following wet and dry swallows. *Journal of Applied Physiology, 35,* 851–857.

Dodds, W.J., Stewart, E.T., & Logemann, J.A. (1990). Physiology and radiology of the normal oral and pharyngeal phases of swallowing. *American Journal of Radiology, 154,* 953–963.

Donner, M.W., Bosma, J.F., & Robertson, D.L. (1985). Anatomy and physiology of the pharynx. *Gastrointestinal Radiology, 10(3)*, 196–212.

Doty, R.W. (1968). Neural organization of deglutition. In C.F. Code, (Ed.), *Handbook of Physiology: Alimentary Canal, 4(6)*, 1861–1902).

Dubner, R., Sessle, B.J., & Storey, A.T. (1978). *The Neural Basis of Oral and Facial Function*. New York: Plenum Press.

Fink, B. & Demarest, R. (1978). *Laryngeal Biomechanics*. Cambridge, MA: Harvard University Press.

Fisher, M., Hendrix, T., Hunt, J., & Murrills, A. (1978). Relation between volume swallowed and velocity of the bolus ejected from the pharynx into the esophagus. *Gastroenterology, 74*, 1238–240.

Flowers, C. & Morris, H. (1973). Oropharyngeal movements during swallowing and speech. *Cleft Palate Journal, 10*, 181–191.

Gordon, C., Hewer, R.L., & Wade, D.T. (1987). Dysphagia in acute stroke. *British Medical Journal, 295*, 411–414.

Groher, M. (Ed.). (1997). *Dysphagia: Diagnosis and Management*, third edition. Boston: Butterworth-Heinemann.

Horner, J. & Massey, E.W. (1988). Silent aspiration following stroke. *Neurology, 38*, 317–318.

Huang, C-S., Hiraba, H., & Sessle, B.J. (1989). Topographical distribution and functional properties of cortically induced rhythmical jaw movements in the monkey (Macaca fascicularis). *Journal of Neurophysiology, 61*, 635–650.

Ichord, R.N. (1994). Neurology of Deglutition. In D. Tuchman & R.S. Walter (Eds.), *Disorders of Feeding and Swallowing in Infants and Children: Pathophysiology, Diagnosis, and Treatment*. San Diego: Singular Pub. Group 37(52).

Ingelfinger, F.J. (1958). Esophageal motility. *Physiological Review, 38*, 533–584.

Jean, A. (1972). Localisation et activite des neurones deglutiteurs bulbaires. *Journal of Physiology (Paris), 64*, 227–268.

Jean, A. (1984). Brainstem organization of the swallowing network. *Brain Behaviour, 25*, 109–116.

Jean, A. & Car, A. (1979). Inputs to the swallowing medullary neurons from the peripheral afferent fibers and the swallowing cortical area. *Brain Research, 178*, 567–572.

Kahrilas, P.J., Dodds, W.J., Dent, J., Logemann, J.A., & Shaker, R. (1987). The dynamics of pharyngeal and upper esophageal sphincter function during deglutition. *Gastroenterology, 92*, 1458.

Kennedy, J.G. & Kent, R.D. (1985). Anatomy and physiology of deglutition and related functions. *Seminars in Speech and Language, 6*, 257–273.

Kennedy, J.G. & Kent, R.D. (1988). Physiologic substrates of normal deglutition. *Dysphagia, 3*, 24–27.

Kirshner, H.S. (1989). Causes of neurogenic dysphagia. *Dysphagia, 3*, 184–188.

Larson, C. (1985). Neurophysiology of speech and swallowing. *Seminars in Speech and Language, 6*, 275–290.

Lazarra, G.L., Lazarus, C., & Logemann, J.A. (1986). Impact of thermal stimulation on the triggering of the swallowing reflex. *Dysphagia, 1*, 73–77.

Leopold, N.A. & Kagel, M.A. (1983). Swallowing, ingestion, and dysphagia: A reappraisal. *Archives of Physical Medicine and Rehabilitation, 64*, 371–373.

Leopold, N.A. & Kagel., M.C. (1997). Dysphagia—ingestion or deglutition?: A proposed paradigm. *Dysphagia, 12*, 202-206.

Linden, P., Tippett, D., Johnston, J., Siebens, A., & French, J. (1989). Bolus position at swallow onset in normal adults: Preliminary observations. *Dysphagia, 4*, 146–150.

Logemann, J.A. (1983). Anatomy and physiology of normal deglutition. In J.A. Logemanm (Ed.), *Evaluation and Treatment of Swallowing Disorders* (11–36). San Diego: College-Hill Press.

Logemann, J.A. (1988). Swallowing physiology and pathophysiology. *Otolaryngological Clinics of North America, 21*, 613–623.

Logemann, J.A. (1989). Evaluation and treatment planning for the head-injured patient with oral intake disorders. *Journal of Head Trauma Rehabilitation, 4(4)*, 24–33.

Logemann, J.A., Pauloski, B.R., Colangelo, L., Lazarus, C., Fujiu, M., & Kahrilas, P.J. (1995). Effects of sour bolus on oropharyngeal swallowing measures in patients with neurogenic dysphagia. *Journal of Speech and Hearing Research, 38*, 556–563.

Mackay, L.E., Morgan, A.S., & Bernstein, B.A. (1999). Factors affecting oral feeding with severe TBI. *Journal of Head Trauma Rehabilitation, 14(5)*, 435–447.

Martin, R.E. & Sessle, B.J. (1993). The role of the cerebral cortex in swallowing. *Dysphagia, 8*, 195–202.

Meadows, J.C. (1973). Dysphagia in unilateral cortical lesions. *Journal of Neurology, Neurosurgery and Psychiatry, 38*, 853–860.

Miller, A.J. (1982). Deglutition. *Physiological Reviews, 62*, 129–184.

Miller, A.J. (1986). Neurophysiological basis of swallowing. *Dysphagia, 1*, 91–100.

Miller, A.J. (1993). The search for the central swallowing pathway: The quest for clarity. *Dysphagia, 8*, 185–194.

Miller, A.J., Biegler, D., & Conklin, J.L. (1997). Functional controls of deglutition. In A.L. Perlman & K. Schulze-Delrieu (Eds.), *Deglutition and Its Disorders*. San Diego: Singular Publishing Group Inc.

Miller, A.J. & Bowman, J.P. (1977). Precentral cortical modulation of mastication and swallowing. *Journal of Dental Research, 56*, 1154.

Nelson, J.B. & Castell, D.O. (1988). Esophageal motility disorders. *Disease a Month, 34(6)*, 297–389.

Penfield, W. & Rasmussen, T. (1950). *The Cerebral Cortex of Man*. New York: MacMillan.

Plant, R.L. (1998). Anatomy and physiology of swallowing in adults and geriatrics. *Otolaryngologic Clinics of North America, 31(3)*, 477–489.

Pritchard, T.C., Hamilton, R.B., Morse, J.R., & Norgren, R. (1986). Projections of thalamic gustatory and lingual areas in the monkey, Macaca fascicularis. *Journal of Comparative Neurology, 244*, 213–228.

Pommerenke, W. (1928). A study of the sensory areas eliciting the swallowing reflex. *American Journal of Physiology, 84*, 36–41.

Ramsey, G.H., Watson, J.S., Gramiak, R., & Weinberg, S.A. (1955). Cinefluorographic analysis of the mechanism of swallowing. *Radiology, 64*, 498–518.

Robbins, J.A. & Levine, R.L. (1988). Swallowing after unilateral stroke of the cerebral cortex: Preliminary experience. *Dysphagia, 3*, 11–17.

Sasaki, C.T. & Isaacson, G. (1988). Functional anatomy of the larynx. *Otolaryngology Clinics of North America, 21*, 196–199.

Sasaki, C.T. & Masafumi, S. (1976). Laryngeal reflexes in cat, dog and man. *Archives of Otolaryngology, 102*, 400–401.

Scott, T.R., Yaxley, S., Sienkiewicz, Z.J., & Rolls, E.T. (1986). Gustatory responses in the frontal opercular cortex of the alert cynomolgus monkey. *Journal of Neurophysiology, 56*, 876–890.

Shaker, R., Dodds, W.J., Dantas, R.O., Hogan, W.J., & Andorfer, R.C. (1990). Coordination of deglutitive glottic closure with oropharyngeal swallowing. *Gastroenterology, 98*, 1478–1484.

Shedd, D., Kirchner, J., & Scatliff, J. (1961). Oral and pharyngeal components of deglutition. *Archives of Surgery, 82*, 371–380.

Shinghai, T. & Shimada, K. (1976). Reflex swallowing elicited by water and chemical substances applied in the oral cavity, pharynx, and larynx of the rabbit. *Japanese Journal of Physiology, 26*, 455–469.

Siebens, H., Trupe, E., Siebens, A., Cook, F., Anshen, S., Hanauer, R., & Oster, F. (1986). Correlates and consequences of eating dependency in institutionalized elderly. *Journal of the American Geriatric Society (JAGS), 34*, 192–198.

Stevenson, R.D. & Allaire, J.H. (1991). The development of normal feeding and swallowing. *Pediatric Clinics of North America, 38*, 1439–1453.

Storey, A.T. (1968). A functional analysis of sensory units innervating epiglottis and larynx. *Experimental Neurology, 20*, 366–383.

Veis, S.L. & Logemann, J.A. (1985). Swallowing disorders in persons with cerebrovascular accident. *Archives of Physical Medicine and Rehabilitation, 66*, 372–375.

Willoughby, E.W. & Anderson, N.E. (1984). Lower cranial nerve motor function in unilateral vascular lesions of the cerebral hemisphere. *British Medical Journal, 289,* 791–794.

Wolf, L.S. & Glass, R.P. (1992). *Feeding and Swallowing Disorders in Infancy: Assessment and Management.* Tucson, AZ: Therapy Skill Builders.

Zemlin, W.R. (1988). *Speech and Hearing Science: Anatomy and Physiology,* third edition. Englewood Cliffs, NJ: Prentice-Hall.

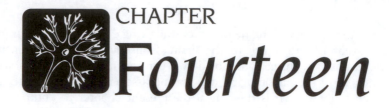

Dysphagia Following Traumatic Brain Injury in Adults and Children: Assessment and Characteristics

Elizabeth C. Ward and Angela T. Morgan

Introduction

Swallowing difficulty, or dysphagia, may result from impaired function of the jaw, lips, tongue, velum, larynx, pharynx, upper esophageal sphincter, and/or esophagus. It may occur during the passage of a solid, semisolid, or liquid bolus at any level from the mouth to the stomach (Freson & Stokmans, 1994). When swallowing impairment results from neurological insult or disease, the term neurogenic dysphagia is commonly used (Horner & Massey, 1991). One form of neurogenic dysphagia, is that resulting from damage to the brain, brainstem, or cranial nerves subsequent to traumatic brain injury (TBI; Field & Weiss, 1989; Groher, 1997; Lazarus & Logemann, 1987; Ylvisaker & Weinstein, 1989). In the patient group with TBI, the nature and severity of the neurogenic swallowing deficit is dependent upon the site and extent of the injury to the brain. Consequently, optimal management of patients with dysphagia following TBI is contingent on a thorough and systematic assessment of the physiological deficits and associated factors affecting swallowing in each individual. It is the aim of the present chapter to outline the process of assessing the disordered swallow of patients following TBI, and to outline the current knowledge regarding the various cognitive, physiological, and other factors influencing swallowing function in both the adult and pediatric TBI populations.

Assessment of Dysphagia in the TBI Population

A thorough feeding and swallowing assessment following head injury typically requires both a clinical bedside assessment and a physiological evaluation, usually a radiographic procedure (Logemann, 1989; Rowe, 1999; Ylvisaker & Weinstein, 1989). The bedside or clinical examination is a subjective method of assessment, commonly involving general observations, an oral motor examination, and a swallowing/feeding trial. This information is typically compared to the clinician's knowledge of the normal swallowing processes and adult oromotor function, with interpretations based on developmental norms for the pediatric patient (Ylvisaker & Weinstein, 1989). The impact of behavioral reactions and language/cognition levels on oral intake are also taken into consideration for both the pediatric and adult client. In addition, of particular clinical value for the pediatric TBI patient is the collection of a comprehensive history of feeding development, patterns, and abilities prior to the injury. This information is referred to as the feeding history.

The instrumental examination of swallowing typically provides objective information on specific areas of the anatomy and physiology of the swallowing process. There are numerous instrumental assessment procedures available, which will be discussed in the following sections, however, to date the videofluoroscopic swallowing study (VFSS) remains the "gold standard" in swallowing evaluation (Bastian, 1998). Videofluoroscopic studies are the most consistently used physiological assessment of swallowing function with the TBI population.

The assessment of the swallowing abilities of the head-injured patient is an ongoing process, necessitating multiple reassessments over the course of the rehabilitative period. Even for patients requiring long-term rehabilitation, best practice management of these cases would involve regular reassessments to evaluate physiological and cognitive status. In the single case study reports of dysphagic management post-TBI in the literature (Drake, O'Donoghue, Bartram, Lindsay, & Greenwood, 1997; Hoppers & Holm, 1999; Rowe, 1999; Tippett, Palmer, & Linden, 1987; Yuen & Hartwick, 1992), the need for multiple reassessments of patient status is highlighted, with the majority of cases undergoing at least two, and sometimes three or four, instrumental studies of swallowing behavior over the rehabilitation period.

The Clinical Approach to Dysphagia Assessment

The clinical assessment of swallowing disorders involves the collection of medical and historical information relating to the swallowing disorder, and the completion of the clinical bedside examination of swallowing. Clinical assessments of swallowing rely on the clinicians' skill in interpreting the information obtained from oromotor assessments and swallowing trials to identify possible underlying deficits and associated factors that may be contributing to the swallowing disorder. Using the information collected during the clinical swallowing assessment, the speech-language pathologist formulates specific diagnostic questions that guide the subsequent instrumental investigations of swallowing (Park & O'Neill, 1994).

The Feeding and Swallowing History

Regardless of any obvious cause for a feeding or swallowing impairment, clinicians agree that a careful review of the patient's general medical, psychosocial, and feeding history should be completed in order to identify any other factors contributing to the oral intake problem. Kramer and Eicher (1993) stated that *any* medical problem may have an effect on feeding, and it is important to understand the dysphagic problems in the context of other medical, psychosocial, and developmental factors. This is particularly important for the pediatric patient with dysphagia following TBI. Kramer and Eicher (1993) proposed that a thorough feeding history should begin at birth and should attempt to record the child's: developmental progress, psychosocial factors, health factors, transition through each phase of oral feeding, transition through the introduction of advancing textures, and premorbid feeding status. Examples of feeding histories to use with the pediatric population have been detailed in Arvedson and Brodsky (1993), Arvedson and Lefton-Greif (1998), Starr (1994) and Wolf and Glass (1992). Following completion of a detailed history, the clinician can begin a direct assessment of the patient's oromotor and swallowing abilities. It is the analysis of the information obtained from the case history that provides the basis for the choice and order of subsequent diagnostic tests (Hendrix, 1993).

Clinical Bedside Examination

On completion of the comprehensive medical and swallowing/feeding history, the clinician may then conduct the clinical bedside examination (CBE) of swallowing. This process involves a series of steps incorporating general observations, an oromotor and oral sensory examination, and finally a swallowing trial. By the end of the CBE the clinician should have an understanding of: the presence of any anatomic abnormalities that may affect the swallow (e.g., scar tissue); the patient's behavioral characteristics; linguistic function; oral reactions to secretions; response to the introduction of oral stimuli including, in some cases, small amounts of food; oral physiology as it may affect swallow function; and the presence of any abnormal oral reflexes (Logemann, 1989).

General Observations.   In both the adult and pediatric populations, a number of observations should be made automatically upon initiation of a CBE. The clinician should note: (a) status of lip closure, (b) oral versus nasal breathing, (c) level of secretions, (d) patient awareness of secretions, (e) patient management of secretions, (f) patient awareness of the clinician's approach, and (g) the nature and content of initial verbalization by the patient (Logemann, 1989). It is particularly important to gain an awareness of the cognitive and behavioral functioning of the patient. Certain evaluation procedures require minimal cognitive prerequisites or presuppose the ability to follow commands (Ylvisaker & Weinstein, 1989). A thorough interdisciplinary, functional, cognitive assessment is typically made. The clinician must be fully aware of the current results of any assessment and may have his/her own informal battery to help determine the patient's current functioning level and assist in tailoring the assessment appropriately to the patient.

Oromotor Examination. Following the general observations, the clinical bed-side examination traditionally begins with a careful oral examination. This evaluation details the structure, relationship, and coordinated function of the component parts of the swallowing mechanism (Bosma, 1980; Bosma & Donner, 1980). Examination of anatomical structure involves observation of any abnormalities in the oral cavity or oropharynx. An oral-motor examination is then conducted to determine the rate, range, accuracy, and speed of voluntary and involuntary movements of the face, lips, tongue, palate, pharynx, and/or respiration (Logemann, 1989). These movements provide information on the level of voluntary control that the patient has over the oropharyngeal area (Logemann, 1989). Voluntary control is important for swallowing; however, it is important that the clinician consider that completion of these movements may not be representative of the control required for the actual swallow (Logemann, 1989).

A thorough examination of oral sensation, including assessment of normal and abnormal oral and pharyngeal reflexes must be included in the CBE (Tuchman, 1989). Oral sensory assessment may be conducted by touching the lips, tongue, buccal mucosa, floor of the mouth, and faucial arches to assess for normal or abnormal movements in response to this contact (Logemann, 1989). The gag reflex is typically examined during this phase of the clinical bedside assessment. This reflex is triggered by the contact of an object (e.g., laryngeal mirror, tongue depressor) with the posterior pharyngeal wall or the back of the tongue behind the faucial arches. This contact causes contraction of the pharyngeal walls, and laryngeal elevation and closure, so as to push the foreign body out of the pharynx (Logemann, 1989). Tuchman (1989) states that the absence of a gag reflex may be a contraindication to feeding. Other authors, however, stress that it is unacceptable to draw conclusions on the function of the swallowing mechanism based on the presence or absence of a gag reflex (Ylvisaker & Logemann, 1985). The gag reflex neither predicts nor protects against an oropharyngeal swallowing disorder; however, the presence of asymmetrical contraction in response to the elicitation of the reflex indicates a unilateral pharyngeal weakness during swallowing, which itself can be a potential contraindication to normal feeding and swallowing (Logemann, 1989). A hyperactive gag reflex, however, may result in severe feeding difficulties (Tuchman, 1989).

Examination of laryngeal functioning is warranted during a clinical bedside assessment. Vocal quality is an important parameter of investigation, as a gurgly quality is an indication of food, liquid, or saliva being present on the vocal folds, placing the patient at risk of aspiration (Linden & Siebens, 1983). A hoarse vocal quality may indicate the need for an otolaryngologic investigation in order to define the presence of any laryngeal pathology or neuromuscular abnormality (Logemann, 1989). Vowel prolongation on a single exhalation at various loudness levels is useful for investigating respiratory and laryngeal control (Logemann, 1989).

The reflexive cough should be triggered when material touches the laryngeal vestibule (Logemann, 1989). A high proportion of head-injured patients, however, are silent aspirators, and do not demonstrate a reflexive cough in the event of food or fluid entering the airway (Horner & Massey, 1991; Lazarus & Logemann, 1987).

Because of this characteristic, the clinical bedside assessment is consequently highly inaccurate for defining or predicting the occurrence of aspiration or identifying its cause (Logemann, 1989). Although active throat clearing or the ability to cough voluntarily does not indicate that the patient will be able to avoid aspiration, observing these behaviors in the CBE provides the clinician with information on respiratory support and the strength of voluntary expectoration (Logemann, 1989).

Evaluations of how the patient handles his/her own secretions in the oral cavity and pharynx should also be made during the clinical bedside evaluation. Evidence of spontaneous swallowing, occurrence of drooling, pooling of secretions in the oral cavity, and the patient's reactions to these secretions should be noted (Logemann, 1989). Evaluation of oral awareness and ability to control secretions may indicate the patient's ability to control food (Logemann, 1989). On completion of the oral-motor and oral sensory examination, the clinician should have developed an oral map that identifies (a) areas of the oral cavity where abnormal, undesirable reflexes or movements are elicited; (b) areas that produce awareness of specific stimuli (i.e., texture, temperature, taste combinations); and (c) areas where specific stimuli elicit desirable oral movements (Logemann, 1989).

For the adult population, no specific, dedicated assessments of oromotor function for swallowing have been developed or marketed. Traditionally, a systematic assessment of oromotor functioning for the adult population follows the cranial nerve assessment as outlined by Darley, Aronson, and Brown (1975) and/or motor and sensory profiles such as those discussed by Sonies et al. (1987). In contrast, a number of specialized oromotor assessments have recently been developed for the pediatric population. The Pediatric Oral Skills Package (Brindley, 1996) is one such newly developed tool for examining oral motor skills in the pediatric population. This assessment includes 12 sections systematically examining posture, reflexes and reactions, breathing, voice, orofacial status, eating, drinking, movement, saliva control, and other elements.

The majority of oral-motor assessments developed and available for use with the pediatric population, however, are limited by poor standardization, have reduced application for mildly impaired populations, and lack of normative data during infancy and early childhood with which to compare oral-motor performance (Reilly, Skuse, Mathisen, & Wolke, 1995). Reilly et al. (1995) recognized the limitations of existing assessments and subsequently developed a new assessment called the Schedule for Oral Motor Assessment (SOMA). The SOMA was designed to be applicable to a wide range of age groups, from children who have just been introduced to mixed feeds (minimum age of 6 months) to those who are totally independent feeders, with a maximum appropriate age in normal children of about 2 years (Skuse, Stevenson, Reilly, and Mathisen, 1995). The upper age limit in those children with developmental disability is to be determined largely by the extent of the subject's handicap, with the assessment being suitable for oral-motor testing of children with general developmental abilities equivalent to a chronological age of 6 months to 2 years (Skuse et al., 1995). It was designed primarily to assess a wide range of oral-motor skills in infancy with a grossly intact neurological system; however, it has been extended to include those children with both minor and major neurological impairment.

The schedule takes approximately 20 minutes to administer and has been designed to be videotaped to allow for the majority of scoring to be performed at a later time (Reilly et al., 1995). The assessment can be administered without special equipment by a trained observer (e.g., a speech-language pathologist), and a simple scoring system makes the assessment an attractive tool for clinical and research use (Skuse et al., 1995). Seven oral motor challenge categories (OMC) have been included, and are designed to evaluate the oral-motor control required for puree, semisolids, solids, cracker, liquid from a bottle, liquid from a trainer cup, and liquid from a cup. Each of the OMC categories can be described on three levels: functional areas (FA), functional units (FU), and discrete oral motor behaviors (DOMs). Functional areas refer to the muscle group or structure being investigated, e.g., lip function. Functional units describe the activity that the muscle group(s) or structure(s) participates in or performs, while discrete oral motor (DOM) behaviors refer to the individual oral-motor movements that prevent food loss. The DOM behaviors are further divided into such areas as: refusals, reactivity, acceptance, initiation, sequencing/rhythmicity, drooling, etc.

Three groups of infants were studied during development of the SOMA, including 58 normal infants, 56 infants with nonorganic failure to thrive (NOFT), and 13 children with cerebral palsy (CP). It was established that the SOMA was a reliable and comprehensive assessment of infant oral-motor function (Skuse et al., 1995). However, although the SOMA has proven to be a valid and reliable tool for use in a number of populations, the clinical application of the SOMA has not yet been established with the pediatric TBI population.

Another recently available tool that may have application in an oromotor assessment for swallowing, is the Verbal Motor Production Assessment for Children (VMPAC; Hayden & Square, 1999). The VMPAC was designed to assess the neuromotor integrity of the speech production mechanism both at rest and during vegetative and volitional nonspeech and speech tasks, and has been constructed to include all parameters of neuromotor integrity typically tested when screening for dysarthria and apraxia of speech disorders. Although the VMPAC was not created or marketed as an assessment tool for oral-motor movement associated with swallowing impairment, the standardized norms provided by the test (standardized on 1434 children between the ages of 3y 0 mths and 12 y 11 mths) provide a reliable and valid method of assessing oral-motor function in children aged between 3 and 12 years.

There are three main areas of assessment in the VMPAC: Global Motor Control, Focal Oromotor Control, and Sequencing. Two supplemental areas are also included: Connected Speech and Language Control, and Speech Characteristics. The Global Motor Control section of the VMPAC investigates neuromotor innervation to peripheral muscles in the torso, neck, head, and orofacial region required for the efficient production of speech (Hayden & Square, 1999) and contains two subsections: (a) General motor control, encompassing assessment of tone, respiration/phonation, reflexes, and vegetative functions, and (b) Oromotor integrity, which assesses muscular symmetry, smoothness of movement, and presence of abnormal movement. The authors of the present chapter advocate the use of items in the Global Motor Control section to help provide norm-referenced data on aspects of oral-motor functioning in children with TBI. These relevant sections of the VMPAC take approximately 5–10 minutes to complete.

The Feeding Trial.   Once the clinician has performed a thorough evaluation of the patient's oral physiology, a feeding trial at the bedside is advocated to observe the oral reactions and visible aspects of swallowing. As mentioned previously, although the clinician can gain an indication of a patient's voluntary oral-motor movements and responses to swallowing saliva from an oral examination, it is imperative that a proper feeding trial be performed during the clinical bedside assessment. Swallowing involves a number of more reflexively mediated processes, which only occur in response to certain food stimuli, hence the necessity of a feeding trial. As Kramer and Eicher (1993) report, observing the consumption of a meal provides information on the level of competency of demonstrated oral skills, coordination, and fatigue associated with swallowing.

A variety of food textures are generally tested during an initial assessment in order to observe how the patient handles particular food and fluid consistencies. It is best to begin the trial for head-injured children with a puree since they tend to cope best with this consistency (Bruce, 1996). For adults, thickened liquids are typically introduced before thin liquid trials, while the consistency of the foods selected for the trial will be dependent on the outcome of the general observation of cognitive and medical status, in addition to oromotor functioning.

When observing the swallow, the clinician should look and feel for strong upward and forward movement of the larynx within one second of initiation of the oral swallow (Logemann, 1989). After the swallow, the clinician should listen to the patient's vocal quality. If residue enters the airway, the patient's voice may become gurgly and wet, indicating that material is pooling at the level of the pharynx, providing the clinician with some insight, albeit limited, concerning the presence of residue in the pharynx. Various techniques, such as head rotation, which places pressure on each pyriform sinus, and chin elevation, which narrows the valleculae, can assist in emptying any residue postswallow.

To complement the observations made during the clinical feeding trial, Takahashi, Groher, and Michi (1994) stated that cervical auscultation may form an important component of the bedside assessment for evaluating the pharyngeal swallow. The authors state that although this is a subjective method of assessment, the acoustic analysis of swallowing sounds may increase the objectiveness of the procedure for detecting swallowing impairment. Despite the current reliance of this procedure on largely perceptual rating, a large number of clinicians have already advocated the use of cervical auscultation as an important adjunct to the clinical bedside evaluation (Hamlet, Nelson, & Patterson, 1990; Selley, Flack, Ellis, and Brooks, 1990; Zenner, Losinski, & Mills, 1995).

Logemann, Veis, and Colangelo (1999) detailed a screening procedure for oropharyngeal dysphagia, which consists of 28 items divided into five sections: (a) four medical history variables, (b) six behavioral variables, (c) two gross motor variables, (d) nine observations from oromotor testing, and (e) seven observations during trial swallows. Screening procedures are used to investigate the symptoms present in a disorder, whereas diagnostic procedures look at anatomy and physiology (Logemann et al., 1999). Logemann et al. (1999) reviewed the limitations of screening assessments in the literature, and subsequently designed a relatively low-risk, inexpensive screening tool with acceptable levels of sensitivity and specificity. Two hundred consecutively referred heterogeneous dysphagia patients, aged from 14 to 97 years (mean = 65 years) were included in the study. Fifty-one patients had dysphagia following a single stroke, 18 patients following multiple strokes, 26 patients following head and neck cancer treatment, 21 patients following spinal cord injuries, and 84 patients following other etiologies that had resulted in their dysphagia (Logemann et al., 1999). Due to the heterogenous nature of the group, the number of patients in each group was too small to allow statistical analysis for each group. As a consequence, the authors were unable to determine whether a ranking of unsafe on one variable was a better predictor than another in certain diagnostic groups (Logemann et al., 1999).

The results of the Logemann et al. (1999) study, revealed that the clinical oropharyngeal screening procedure was able to classify patients correctly, identifying the presence/absence of aspiration 71% of the time, detecting an oral stage disorder 69% of the time, identifying a pharyngeal delay 72% of the time, and revealing pharyngeal stage swallowing problems 70% of the time. Thus while further research is needed into this tool, as a screening procedure for oropharyngeal dysphagia, it appears potentially useful in guiding the clinician's identification of patients at risk for dysphagia. Logemann et al (1999) stated that further research is underway to investigate the use of this tool in separating oral from pharyngeal problems in patients with either one or both of these swallowing phases impaired.

The Instrumental Approach to Dysphagia Assessment

Objective measurement of the oral, pharyngeal, and esophageal phases for swallowing requires utilization of instrumental diagnostic imaging techniques. For clinicians working with the pediatric population, determining "whether, when and how" (Arvedson & Lefton-Greif, 1998, p.3) to involve instrumental assessments with this population is a particularly challenging aspect of patient management. While the clinical bedside assessment is heavily dependent upon subjective external observations, instrumental procedures allow visualization and measurement of the intrinsic physiology.

Instrumental methods are of particular importance to the speech-language pathologist for the evaluation of the pharyngeal phase of swallowing, and for determining the presence of aspiration. Since the risk for aspiration is greatly increased and may have no observable clinical indications (e.g., coughing or choking) in persons with neurologic impairment, the bedside assessment may be inadequate in a high proportion of patients. Therefore, the instrumental or objective assessment is of paramount importance to the clinician in dealing with a patient with head injury. A discussion of assessment techniques that are either used with the TBI population or have potential for use with this population, including videofluoroscopy, scintigraphy, ultrasonography, manometry, electromyography, electroglottography, and endoscopy are outlined below.

Videofluoroscopy

Videofluoroscopic assessments of swallowing function are also commonly referred to as either the modified barium swallow (MBS) procedure or a videofluoroscopic study of swallowing (VFSS). A barium swallow is a study of esophageal motility performed by radiologists. Logemann (1983, 1986) altered this common procedure for investigating swallowing function and developed the MBS procedure, which requires the patient to chew and swallow a number of barium-impregnated mouthfuls of food or fluid, which typically vary in consistency. Dynamic radiographic tracking of the food bolus occurs as it moves through the upper aerodigestive tract, subsequently monitoring the structure and function of the oral, pharyngeal, and potentially the esophageal phases of swallowing. Currently, the MBS is the most widely used and effective technique in evaluating swallowing dysfunction available and is considered the "gold standard" in dysphagia diagnosis (Bastian, 1998; Christensen, 1989; Kramer & Eicher, 1993; Langmore & Logemann, 1991; Logemann, 1983; Loughlin & Lefton-Greif., 1994; Palmer, Kuhlemeier, Tippett, & Lynch, 1993; Sonies, 1991; Sorin, Somers, Austin, and Bester, 1988; Tuchman, 1989). In the research studies of dysphagia in both the adult and the pediatric TBI populations conducted to date, the MBS has been the most frequently used instrumental assessment.

Many authors have tried to detect abnormalities of swallowing (particularly aspiration) using alternate, nonradiographic observation techniques; however, these methods have been shown to have poor sensitivity and specificity (Linden & Siebens, 1983; Loughlin & Lefton-Greif, 1994). The MBS not only determines *whether* the patient is aspirating, but also the *reason* for the aspiration, so that appropriate treatment can be initiated (Groher, 1984; Kramer, 1989; Logemann, 1986). As previously mentioned, the MBS provides dynamic recording of the structures and functions involved in the swallowing process, thus allowing for the identification of a variety of factors affecting the oral, pharyngeal, and esophageal phases of the swallow. The primary focus is typically on the pharyngeal phase since this is the most difficult stage to assess using a clinical bedside examination alone (Sorin et al., 1988).

Linden and Siebens (1983) stated that the clinical examination provides information from which implications must be drawn, for example: wet hoarseness may imply that there is pyriform sinus pooling, or impaired pharyngeal gag reflex may imply poor pharyngeal contractility or pharyngeal sensation. Neurologically impaired persons, however, usually present with multiple clinical findings requiring multiple implications to be drawn from the clinical examination. The MBS allows monitoring of features unable to be observed during a clinical examination, including: velopharyngeal function, laryngeal elevation and closure, pharyngeal motility, pharyngeal transit time, pooling in the pharyngeal sinuses, the number of swallows to clear material, and the presence and timing of aspiration in relation to the swallow (Jones & Donner, 1988; Sorin et al., 1988). Because of the accurate, specific, and detailed information that can be obtained from the MBS procedure, the patient's subsequent management can be based on direct observations of physiological deficit rather than on "clinical inference" alone.

A number of studies confirming that the MBS is a more consistent predictor of aspiration than a clinical bedside examination have been performed. Approximately 40% of aspiration is not detected in adults at the bedside clinical assessment (Logemann, 1983). Splaingard, Hutchins, Sulton, and Chaudhuri (1988) conducted a blinded study to compare the diagnosis of aspiration by speech-language pathologists using videofluroscopy versus bedside clinical evaluations. Of 107 patients, only 10 were children below the age of 15. The authors found that the VFSS revealed that 43 (40%) of the 107 patients aspirated at least one food consistency. Only 18 (42%) of the 43 patients who were found to be aspirating on VFSS were identified as aspirating on the clinical bedside evaluation. In addition, 21 patients of the 107 (20%) were found to be silent aspirators, not coughing or showing any clinical change at the time aspiration was noted during VFSS. Similar results have been found for children. Arvedson, Rogers, Buck, Smart, and Msall (1992) reviewed 186 children from the Children's Hospital of Buffalo with a range of diagnoses, who had been assessed with VFSS from 1989 through 1991. The children had been referred to VFSS due to the presence of possible aspiration and/or respiratory distress during feeding. The review found that 48 (26%) aspirated at least one texture, and of those who aspirated, almost all (94%) had silent aspiration.

In their videofluoroscopic study of swallowing function in head-injured adults, Lazarus and Logemann (1987) identified aspiration in 38% of their patient group. They noted that many of the patients who aspirated did not produce a reflexive cough either during or after they had aspirated, and required prompting to cough and clear the aspirated materials. The lack of reflexive coughing noted among these patients highlighted how, at a clinical bedside examination, such aspiration would go unnoticed. Videofluoroscopy is, therefore, an invaluable tool for assisting the clinician to determine both the nature of the swallowing disorder, and the presence and etiology of aspiration (Lazarus & Logemann, 1987). Rosenbek, Robbins, Roecker, Coyle, and Wood (1996) created a rating scale that can be used to quantify the degree and extent of aspiration noted on the MBS procedure.

A number of differences exist between the application of the MBS procedure for the adult versus the pediatric population. Arvedson and Lefton-Greif (1998) pointed out that the most significant changes to the process for the pediatric population exist in the procedural modifications that must be applied to the videofluoroscopic assessment. Although the procedures used in the videofluoroscopic studies with the adult population are fairly standardized, this protocol may not be appropriate for infants or children (Palmer, Tanaka & Siebens, 1993).

The majority of changes introduced during the pediatric assessment simulate typical feeding routines. These include changes such as: scheduling the procedure to coincide with mealtimes, adjusting positioning to test both the optimal and "typical" postures, the use of familiar foods, altering the order of presentation of food types, and adjusting the method of bolus delivery, e.g., presenting food using familiar utensils or nipples to assist intake (Arvedson & Lefton-Greif, 1998). Studies with children also face the need to motivate the child to participate, often requiring the assistance of the primary caregiver (Arvedson & Lefton-Greif, 1998).

Determining when to conduct a videofluoroscopic procedure with a pediatric patient is also dependent on a number of factors. It has been stated that ideally, the patient must remain sufficiently alert to participate in the procedure, be able to ingest sufficient food/fluid in time to allow for maximal information with minimal exposure to radiation, and be able to remain medically stable (adequate respiratory rates and cardiopulmonary functioning) throughout the assessment (Arvedson & Lefton-Greif, 1998). Determining the readiness of a patient for the procedure is dependent on developmental age rather than chronological age. Ideally, infants should be 37 weeks gestation or older to participate, since prior to this stage the development of coordinated sucking, swallowing, and breathing has not been achieved. By 6 months of age (developmental age) both liquid and puree consistencies can be examined. By 36 months the child should have cognitive and communicative skills to follow some instructions (Arvedson & Lefton-Greif, 1998).

Further detailed discussion of the issues related to conducting videofluroscopy with infants and children can be found in Arvedson and Lefton-Greif's (1998) manual on videofluroscopy for the pediatric patient.

Disadvantages of the MBS procedure for both the adult and pediatric populations include the exposure to radiation, the expense of the system, the indirect assessment of sensation, and the inability to repeat the procedure frequently (Bastian, 1998). Radiation exposure can be easily controlled by limiting the number of repeat procedures over time and reducing the amount of "on" time during the assessment, in order to meet national health standards. For the pediatric population, however, radiation exposure is a significant consideration, since a complete understanding of all long-term effects of radiation exposure on the developing system has not yet been achieved (Arvedson & Lefton-Greif, 1998). As noted by Arvedson and Lefton-Greif (1998), the videofluroscopy procedure with children frequently results in structures such as the ocular lens and the thyroid gland, which are particularly sensitive to the effects of radiation, being exposed in the imaging field. The goal of "maximum information with minimum exposure" (Arvedson & Lefton-Greif, 1998, p. 10), therefore, becomes all the more critical for the pediatric population. Where long-term management requires repeat reassessment, Arvedson and Lefton-Greif (1998) suggested a minimum of 6 months between clinical studies for the pediatric population.

The limitations and disadvantages of the MBS procedure, however, are readily outweighed by the wealth of clinical information gained. Other instrumental techniques are available to assess oropharyngeal swallowing; however, each provides only limited information about the swallow (Logemann, 1989). An evaluation strategy that determines only whether or not aspiration occurs and does not define its cause, is inadequate for the head-injured patient. The MBS study of swallowing is the single best assessment tool for this population, enabling the clinician to develop a swallow rehabilitation plan (Logemann, 1989) to target the oropharyngeal deficits and aspiration frequently noted in these patients.

Cinefluorography

Cineradiography or cinefluorography is a radiographic imaging technique used for assessing the oral and pharyngeal phases of a swallow. As with videofluroscopy, the technique uses barium contrast and dynamic recording to view the swallowing process. In contrast with videofluroscopy, however, cineradiography is recorded on motion picture film, as opposed to videotape, resulting in a clearer image that can be analyzed frame by frame at 60 frames per second. Disadvantages of cineradiography include greater radiation exposure than with videofluroscopy, the inability to record voice on the film, greater time taken, and the high cost of film development.

Scintigraphy

Scintigraphy primarily assesses bolus transit and the presence of aspiration (Bastian, 1998). Scintigraphy involves the ingestion of a single bolus mixed with a short-lived radiopharmaceutical (typically Technetium-99m), and subsequent radionuclide scanning during and after ingestion (Bastian, 1998; Benson & Tuchman, 1994; Holt et al., 1990; Loughlin & Lefton-Greif, 1994; Sonies, 1991). Using a gamma camera, the radiation field is imaged, and the number of the radiation particles in the bolus are counted as it passes through the digestive tract (Bastian, 1998). The main advantage of this procedure is the ability to accurately quantify both the amount of radioactive material present in tissues or structures (such as the pharynx or lungs) and the transit time for the bolus for each area (Holt et al., 1990; Kramer & Eicher, 1993; McVeagh, Howman-Giles, and Kemp, 1987; Sonies, 1991). Sonies (1991) and Bastian (1998) suggested that it remains the only truly quantitative technique in regard to determining the exact amount of bolus aspirated. Although this procedure has the advantage of being truly quantitative and involving less radiation exposure than fluoroscopic procedures (Bastian, 1998; Sonies, 1991), there are a number of limitations to scintigraphy. Disadvantages include: poor resolution of the image with no patient anatomy being visible, only one swallow of one consistency observed, little knowledge of the effects of exposure on the pediatric population, and the need for a physician trained in nuclear medicine (Bastian, 1998; Newman, Cleveland, Blickman, Hillman, & Jaramillo, 1991; Sonies, 1991). While it has been suggested that the VFSS procedure exposes a child to greater radiation exposure, it is able to provide far more clinical information to the therapist than the scintigraphic study. The ability to visualise the dynamic swallowing mechanism in response to different bolus consistencies over a more representative number of swallows, as observed during the VFSS procedure, is invaluable to the speech-language pathologist.

Ultrasonography

Ultrasound, ultrasonography, or sonography is a noninvasive procedure that allows visualization of the movement of the structures in the oral cavity and hypopharynx during feeding (Newman et al., 1991; Sonies, 1991; Tuchman, 1989). In ultrasound imaging, a transducer is used both to generate the sound waves and to receive the ultrasound echoes. These echoes are then electronically converted into an image. Body tissues (such as fat, muscle, fascia, and bone) and fluids (blood, cerebral spinal fluid, and water) have different densities such that sound waves either pass through them or reflect back to the transducer at different intensities. The sound waves cannot pass through bone.

The sound transducer can be placed either under the chin (submental approach) or on the cheek (transbuccal approach; Benson & Tuchman, 1994). The submental approach is most commonly used, since the transbuccal approach is only appropriate for infants with unerrupted teeth (Benson and Tuchman, 1994). From their review of the literature, Arvedson and Christensen (1993) found that this tool has been used for imaging tongue movement and the floor of the mouth during the oral phase of swallowing in infants (Bosma, Hepburn, Josell, & Baker, 1990; Weber, Woolridge, & Baum, 1986) as well as in older children and adults (Shawker, Sonies, Stone, & Baum, 1983; Stone & Shawker, 1986).

Although sonography is an appealing technique due to the absence of radiation exposure, enabling one to assess fatigue effects safely and to repeat procedures if desired, it has limited clinical applicability (Kramer & Eicher, 1993; Newman et al., 1991). Simultaneous imaging of the oral cavity and pharynx is not technically possible. The pharynx is not seen easily, thus penetration and aspiration cannot be definitively detected due to shadows cast by laryngeal structures (Kramer & Eicher, 1993; Tuchman, 1989). Bastian (1998) stated that ultrasonography is segmental and subsequently cannot compete with the comprehensiveness of VFSS in regard to providing panoramic anatomic detail.

Manometry

Benson and Tuchman (1994) describe manometry as being a test of function, rather than an imaging study; it allows measurement of motor activity of muscle by measuring the strength, speed, direction, and duration of muscle contraction. Manometry is used to assess the pressure dynamics of motor function in the pharynx and upper esophagus (Bastian, 1998; Loughin & Lefton-Greif, 1994; Sonies, 1991; Tuchman, 1989). Measurements include: pharyngeal peristalsis, esophageal peristalsis, intraluminal pressures in the oropharynx, upper esophageal sphincter (UES) response to swallowing, and cricopharyngeal sphincter tone and relaxation. Clinically, manometry has mainly been used in children for investigation of esophageal function (Tuchman, 1989). The technique involves the transnasal insertion of a catheter (which holds a series of intraluminal solid-state transducers), which records pressure changes resulting from swallowing at various intervals along its length (Bastian, 1998). A gastroenterologist performs the procedure and requires specialized training to insert the catheter, apply anesthetic to the nasopharynx, and analyze the results (Sonies, 1991). Because of the inability to view anatomic landmarks with this procedure, manometry is often paired with videofluoroscopy so that the etiology of pressure changes can actually be identified (Bastian, 1998; Loughlin & Lefton-Greif, 1994; Sonies, 1991). This combined procedure is often referred to as manofluorography. Not only does this procedure require numerous personnel and equipment coordination, it is expensive, invasive, and generally not recommended in children (Bastian, 1998; Logemann, 1994; Newman et al., 1991; Sonies, 1991; Tuchman, 1989).

Electromyography

Electromyography (EMG) provides information on the onset of muscle activity, the frequency of motor neuron firing, and muscle contraction (Benson & Tuchman, 1994; Logemann, 1994; Palmer, 1989; Sonies, 1991), allowing measurement of the myoelectric activity of a single muscle or group of muscles. Palmer (1989) noted that EMG has the potential to contribute greatly to an understanding of the processes of swallowing. The technique has a number of applications for swallowing diagnosis, though it is currently used more as a research tool, and is not yet used routinely in the conduct of clinical evaluations of swallowing function (Benson & Tuchman, 1994; Cooper & Perlman, 1997). There is, however, potential for EMG to assist in the assessment of the severity of muscular impairment resulting from damage to the swallowing mechanism, and therefore provide useful information to the clinician for prognostic decisions and diagnosis of severity of impairment.

A seminal article by Palmer (1989) explained the "basic concepts" of electromyography needed for investigating oropharyngeal swallowing. In simple terms, electromyography records the electrical activity of muscle (Palmer, 1989). The two main applications of EMG relevant to swallowing are: EMG kinesiology and analysis of individual myoelectric potentials (Palmer, 1989). Electromyographic kinesiology involves observing specific muscles or groups of muscles during particular actions, e.g., looking at the pharyngeal constrictor during deglutition (Palmer, 1989). In this way, the researcher is able to interpret the strength and timing of myoelectrical events. Electromyographic kinesiology is therefore useful for examining muscle coordination in both normal and disordered populations (Basmajiaan, 1978). There have been numerous reports on the myoelectric activity of various muscles involved in the deglutitive process in both humans and animals (Palmer, 1989). From his review of the literature, Palmer (1989) found that the suprahyoid muscles (especially geniohyoid, genioglossus, and digastric muscles), palatal muscles, tongue muscles, laryngeal muscles, pharyngeal constrictor muscles, and cricopharyngeus muscle have all been investigated (Basmajian, 1978; Doty, 1968; Miller, 1982; Palmer, et al., 1989; Tanaka, Palmer, & Siebens, 1986).

Tanaka, et al. (1986) developed bipolar suction electrodes to examine surface EMG (SEMG) of the pharynx and esophagus. The authors stated that this technique had advantages over traditional hooked wire and needle electrodes for a number of reasons, including: simple verification of placement, easier recording of pharyngeal constrictors than with needle electrodes due to the thinness of these muscles, minimal pain, and ease of swallowing with little traction on the tubing or movement artifact. However, despite these advantages measurement of these muscle groups remains an invasive procedure, requiring anesthetization of the nares and pharynx and insertion of the electrodes through the nose, and has the potential to cause punctate trauma in the area of suction (Tanaka, et al., 1986). Such an invasive and potentially traumatic procedure is not appropriate for children or adults with severe impairment, such as a head injury.

Gupta, Reddy, and Canilang (1996) investigated whether SEMG with basic surface electrodes could be used to measure swallowing via the surface tissues at the throat. They hypothesized that there would be a difference in measurement between dry and wet swallowing. In their study, 35 adult subjects were assessed with three measurements each for dry (saliva only) and wet swallows (5 ml water—spoon presentation). They found that while the duration of SEMG was the same during dry and wet swallows, there was a mean power spectrum of significantly larger magnitude for wet ($3.489 \times 10{-}9$) than for dry ($2.6377 \times 10{-}9$) swallowing. They concluded that their study represented successful measurement of SEMG at the throat during swallowing and advocated further research in the area.

Simultaneous measurements of SEMG with needle EMG would be useful in order to determine the contribution of individual muscles to the SEMG (Gupta et al., 1996). In this way, SEMG could potentially be used to determine which muscle or muscles are not activated and whether the dysphagia is due to a neurologic or muscular disorder (Gupta et al., 1996). Gupta et al. (1996) also suggested that a combination of SEMG with other noninvasive measures, such as ultrasound and acceleration testing, may provide a more reliable method of noninvasive clinical bedside evaluation.

Reimers-Neil, Logemann, and Larson (1994) investigated SEMG in the normal swallow, looking at the effects of viscosity on total swallow duration, maximum and average EMG activity of the submental and infrahyoid muscle groups, and the frequency with which each muscle group initiated and terminated the swallow. They supported the use of noninvasive SEMG over other instrumental procedures, including radiography, manometry and endoscopy. In their study, five normal subjects, aged between 25 and 42, were tested with two foods in three consistencies: liquid, thin paste, and thick paste. Five electrodes were used for each subject; one ground, one pair placed under the chin, and the other pair placed above the right superior border of the thyroid cartilage. Electrodes under the chin recorded SEMG activity for the submental group: anterior belly of the digastric, mylohyoid, and geniohyoid. Those placed above the thyroid recorded activity from the infrahyoid (predominantly thyrohyoid) muscles. Submental muscle activity initiated the swallows 84.52% of the time, and the infrahyoid muscle activity most frequently terminated the swallows (71.51%) (Reimers-Neil, et al., 1994). The study revealed that subjective judgements regarding differences in food consistencies are not a valid method for selecting food for inclusion in a dysphagia evaluation or treatment protocol. They found that liquids versus thin pastes were not significantly different on any of the EMG measures. However, the study identified a number of significant differences between the thickest and the two thinner food categories. These results highlighted the need for consideration of the rheological characteristics of boluses in future studies.

Surface EMG has been used with a number of populations in swallowing rehabilitation (Crary, 1995; Huckabee & Cannito, 1999; see Chapter 15), and patients with TBI are one population group for whom this technique may prove useful. Although, at present, limited information is available on the use of SEMG in the assessment and diagnosis of oropharyngeal swallowing disorders, with further research, this tool may prove to be an important adjunct to the clinical bedside evaluation. It has been acknowledged that the increasing emphasis on medical care cost containment and noninvasive diagnosis has created the need for assessment tools that provide quick, reliable, and accurate evaluations of swallowing function that can be conducted at the bedside (Gupta et al., 1996).

Electroglottography

Electroglottography (EGG) is a technique best known for measuring vocal fold vibration during speech phonation (Sonies, 1991), specifically the impedance change as the focal folds adduct and abduct during phonation (Perlman & Grayhack, 1991). This procedure involves electrode placement on each side of the neck, and over the thyroid cartilage (Sonies, 1991), with one electrode transmitting a signal, and the other receiving the signal after it has been modulated by impedance of the neck. In this way, information is obtained on vocal fold movement. With slight modification, however, EGG can also be used for the investigation of laryngeal elevation during swallowing. Logemann (1994) stated that monitoring laryngeal elevation can be useful in determining the beginning and end of a pharyngeal swallow, as well as for use as a biofeedback therapy technique when working on the extent and duration of laryngeal elevation. At this stage, EGG has been used predominantly for research purposes (Perlman & Grayhack, 1991). Sonies (1991) proposed that while this method remains under study at the present time, it may provide investigators with a method for studying laryngeal elevation in a more specific manner.

Fiberoptic Endoscopic Evaluation of Swallowing

Fiberoptic endoscopy is commonly used for observation of the vocal folds; however, this procedure has been modified to examine aspiration and laryngeal function during swallowing (Sonies, 1991). The fiberoptic endoscopic evaluation of swallowing (FEES) procedure involves the use of a flexible fiberoptic endoscope with an endoscopic video camera and a light source (Sonies, 1991). Using this equipment, the scope is passed via a patent nasal passage, through the nasopharynx and hypopharynx, until it is positioned above the false vocal folds, superior to the epiglottis (Sonies, 1991). All food consistencies are typically dyed in order to monitor their movement during the swallow, and to facilitate easy visualization of any residue in the laryngeal area and pharyngeal sinuses. The presence of pharyngeal dysphagia, and such clinical symptoms as excess residue, aspiration, and laryngeal penetration can be examined using this technique (Langmore, Schatz, & Olson, 1991). Although the image of the larynx is entirely obscured when the vocal folds adduct and the epiglottis descends, laryngeal anatomy is visible before the swallow, providing information on the presence or absence of supraglottic laryngeal penetration (i.e., premature spillage into the hypopharynx and laryngeal vestibule; Sonies, 1991). This technique is useful for those patients unsuited to videofluorographic studies (Langmore et al., 1991).

Hoppers and Holm (1999) have reported on the use of FEES with the adult brain-injured population. These authors noted that in their rehabilitation setting twice as many FEES studies are conducted than are MBS procedures. Using the FEES technique, Hoppers and Holm (1999) were able to identify a variety of oropharyngeal deficits in their brain-injured populations, including premature spillage, delayed or absent swallow reflex, residue, and aspiration. These characteristics were similar to those deficits identified on videofluroscopic studies of this population (Lazarus & Logemann, 1987). Hoppers and Holm (1999) concluded that FEES is "an effective tool to evaluate all of the common physiologic dysphagia symptoms in the population with brain injury" (p. 481).

Leder (1999) reported the use of FEES with a group of 47 TBI patients in an acute care setting. The author concluded that FEES was a valuable technique for assessing dysphagia and aspiration status in acute TBI patients, providing objective information on which feeding recommendations could be based. Leder (1999) argued that because FEES is a flexible bedside assessment tool that uses real foods, can be videotaped for review, and is repeatable, it makes it an ideal diagnostic and therapeutic tool for acute TBI patients who are at risk of aspiration and are often still fluctuating in medical status. While Leder (1999) states that the FEES procedure is the "cogold standard" (p. 449) with MBS, and that it "is uniquely suited for assessing patients with acute TBI" (Leder, 1999, p. 449), the authors of the present chapter caution that the FEES procedure does not allow visualization of tongue control or oral phase deficits, which have been identified as physiological deficits contributing to impaired swallowing in the TBI population (Field & Weiss, 1989; Lazarus, 1989; Lazarus & Logemann, 1987). The MBS remains the most widely used procedure with the TBI population due to its ability to provide the most complete information about the physiology of both the oral and pharyngeal phases of the swallow (Langmore & Logemann, 1991; Lazarus & Logemann, 1987; Mackay, Morgan, & Bernstein, 1999a).

Kidder, Langmore, and Martin (1994) stated that there are a number of patients for whom FEES is contraindicated, and that several potential risks associated with FEES exist for the general population. Hypotension, bradycardia, or cardiac dysryhthmia may all occur as a result of stimulation of the nose, pharynx, or larynx (Kidder, et al., 1994). Resuscitation equipment and individuals trained in cardiopulmonary resuscitation must be available during the FEES procedure in case of such complications (Kidder, et al., 1994). It is also imperative that patients with cardio-vascular disease receive continual monitoring of blood pressure and cardiac rhythm during the FEES procedure. Tactile stimulation of the endolaryngeal mucosa via the tip of the endoscope, or from saliva, liquid, or food entering the endolarynx, may trigger a laryngospasm (Kidder, et al., 1994). Laryngospasm may occur quite easily in patients with a low threshold to this reflex (Kidder, et al., 1994). Although laryngospasm is often self-limiting, some patients may require positive pressure ventilation with a mask, or even endotracheal intubation (Kidder, et al., 1994). Nasal hemorrhage may also occur as a result of abrasion of a mucosal arteriole when passing the flexible endoscope through the nose. Although Kidder et al. (1994) indicated that nasal hemorrhage is uncommon if certain measures are taken, including the use of a topical decongestant, they also recognised that topical decongestants may on rare occasions cause an allergic, toxic, or idiosyncratic reaction. Furthermore, this procedure is not recommended for patients who are agitated, are hostile, or have movement disorders (all conditions that may be present following head injury), because some degree of cooperation is required from the patient (Kidder, et al., 1994). For further specific details regarding the use of endoscopy in the investigation of dysphagia, we refer the reader to the chapter by Langmore and McCulloch (1997).

Characteristics of Dysphagia in the Adult and Pediatric TBI Populations

The signs of dysphagia vary from person to person (Rosenbek, et al., 1996) and in terms of their clinical significance. This issue is particularly relevant for the TBI population, where diffuse and differential patterns of neurological damage among patients may result in dysphagia with variable characteristics and severity. From the literature reported to date, the incidence of swallowing disorders in both the adult and pediatric TBI population is high, with the presenting dysphagia typically characterized by a combination of oral and pharyngeal stage deficits (discussed in detail in the following sections). Particularly in the TBI population, it is recognized that coexisting cognitive and behavioral deficits further compromise swallowing safety.

Incidence Data

Early studies that have reported on or investigated the frequency of dysphagia in the adult population with head injury were inconsistent in their findings. Winstein, in 1983, reported that 25% (55) of their 201 patients with brain injury in a rehabilitation setting had dysphagia. Cherney and Halper (1989) reported a similar rate of 26% of dysphagia in their sample of 189 patients, while Field and Weiss (1989) noted that 30% (9/30) of patients in a rehabilitation program had swallowing difficulties. Lazarus and Logemann (1987), however, estimated that approximately 50% of head trauma patients exhibited dysphagia, while Yorkston, Honsinger, Mitsuda, and Hammen in 1989, reported even higher figures, noting that 82% of patients with brain injury in acute care medical settings, 78% of those in acute care rehabilitation hospitals, and 14% of those in outpatient rehabilitation settings were dysphagic.

During the past five years, however, more consistent incidence figures for dysphagia in the adult TBI population have been reported. Cherney and Halper (1996) found an incidence rate of 41.6%, while Schurr et al. (1999) found that 51% of the 47 patients with TBI had dysphagia. Mackay, et al. (1999a) reported an incidence figure of 61% for their TBI group, and Halper, Cherney, Cichowski, and Zhang (1999) noted that 65% of people with TBI in their study had dysphagia. It has been suggested that the higher incidence figures reported in the more recent literature may reflect the trend for earlier admission of TBI patients to acute rehabilitation (Halper, et al., 1999).

In most areas of dysphagia research, there is limited information available on pediatric aspects of the disorder when compared to the adult literature. This finding holds true in regard to incidence data on pediatric dysphagia associated with closed head injury. Presently in the literature, there is no evidence of the incidence of dysphagia following closed head injury in children. While authors suggest that dysphagia is "common" or "typical" in children with an acquired brain injury (Ylvisaker & Logemann, 1985), no specific figures are provided. Because of the limited investigation of dysphagia in children with head injuries, it is impossible to determine whether findings for the adult population can be applied to children. Consequently, there is a clear need for further research to determine the incidence of dysphagia in children with TBI.

Factors Affecting Swallowing Function Following TBI

"Historically the association between dysphagia and head injury has been poorly delineated, most likely because the diagnosis of head injury actually represents many diverse diagnoses with different degrees of severity" (Field & Weiss, 1989, p.19). However, research is continuing to define those factors that may potentially determine the presence and severity of dysphagia following TBI (Cherney & Halper, 1996; Halper, et al., 1999; Mackay, Morgan, & Bernstein, 1999 a,b; Morgan & Mackay, 1999). The main areas of focus have tended to include the extent of injury, presence of tracheostomy and/or duration of ventilation, and cognitive impairment. Other factors are also recognized as having a significant role in influencing swallowing function in this population, including: disorders of positioning and control for self-feeding; physical damage to the oral, laryngeal, and pharyngeal structures; oral and/or pharyngeal sensory disorders; and the presence of any oral and/or pharyngeal movement disorders. While no quantitative studies have been performed in order to assess these factors in children, a review of the literature to date, reported for the adult TBI population, is presented in the sections below.

Extent of Injury

One may assume that the greater the extent of brain injury, the greater the impairment to the swallowing mechanism. Duration of coma is one determinant of the extent of head injury, and indeed, a relationship has been documented relating greater duration of coma to a greater degree of swallowing impairment (Lazarus & Logemann, 1987). While no direct statistical evaluation of the relationship between coma duration and swallowing severity was conducted, Lazarus and

Logemann (1987) documented swallowing impairment and coma duration data on 53 adult TBI patients, and found that the severity of swallowing impairment increased along with increases in coma duration. It was noted that patients who had been in a coma for longer than 24 hours exhibited more severe swallowing problems than patients whose coma lasted less than 24 hours. The authors were cautious to point out, however, that this relationship was not direct, and some patients with no coma history or only short durations of coma were also found to present with severe swallowing problems. There was also a cohort of patients who were not comatose yet presented with dysphagia and those who were comatose for an extended duration who only demonstrated mild swallowing difficulties.

Similarly to coma duration, a lower Glasgow Coma Score (GCS) score on admission (GCS 3, 4, or 5) is also indicative of greater neurological impairment, and subsequently places a patient at greater risk for swallowing impairment and aspiration (Mackay et al., 1999a). Research into the factors affecting swallowing ability following TBI has revealed that patients with GCS scores of between 3 and 5 on admission have significantly longer durations until the initiation of oral feeding, longer durations until achieving total oral intake, and almost three times the duration between initial oral trials and achieving total oral feeding (Mackay et al., 1999b). They also have almost twice as many swallowing abnormalities identified on VFSS than patients with GCS scores of 6 to 8 (Mackay, et al., 1999b). Direct comparisons between the mean admitting GCS of TBI patients with abnormal and normal swallowing following TBI revealed a significantly higher mean score in the normal swallowing group (Mackay, et al., 1999b). Similarly, comparisons between patients demonstrating aspiration on assessment compared to nonaspirating patients, revealed significantly higher GCS scores in the nonaspirating TBI group (Mackay, et al., 1999b).

The CT scan can provide information as to the extent of head injury. Mackay, et al. (1999b) found that patients with more severe CT scans (those denoted as midline shift, brainstem injury, or intracranial bleeds requiring emergent operative intervention) had more than twice as many swallowing abnormalities on VFSS than patients with other, less severe CT scan results. Patients with more severe CT scan results also presented with significantly longer durations before achieving oral feeding and had significantly longer intervals from initiation to total oral feeding (Mackay et al., 1999b).

Intubation, Tracheostomy and Ventilation

Increased duration of ventilation and endotracheal intubation (ETT) and the presence of a tracheostomy may also have a negative impact on swallowing function. Duration of ventilation has been documented to significantly affect the number of abnormal swallowing characteristics observed on videofluoroscopic studies and the incidence rate of aspiration in the TBI population. Specifically, it has been reported that ventilation durations of 15 days or more resulted in statistically higher percentages (90%) of abnormal swallowing, compared to 75% in the 8 to 14 day ventilated group and only 42.9% in the 7 day ventilated group. It also was found to be associated with statistically higher incidence rates of aspiration (60%), compared to 56% in the 8 to 14 day ventilated group and only 25% in the 7 day ventilated group (Mackay et al., 1999b).

Physiologically, endotracheal (ETT) intubation and increased duration of ETT intubation may lead to additional laryngeal trauma, such as reduced mobility of the vocal cords, which may range from mild dismobility to unilateral or bilateral paresis (Logemann, Pepe, & Mackay, 1994). Formation of vocal nodules, granulomas, or polyps as a result of laryngeal irritation from the intubation are additional complications. Furthermore, prolonged intubation may create a tracheoesophageal fistula from tissue breakdown resulting from irritation and rubbing of the end of the tube on the tracheoesophageal party wall (Logemann et al., 1994).

The presence of a tracheostomy may also complicate swallowing due to possible anchoring of laryngeal movement and or additional difficulty arising from the presence of an inflated tracheostomy cuff. Morgan and Mackay (1999) in a recent review of the literature, revealed that airway complications following translaryngeal intubation may affect glottic anatomy and precipitate swallowing dysfunction. Hauck (1999) outlined the potential effects of tracheostomy/ventilation on the swallowing mechanism, indicating that the presence of a tracheostomy tube/and or ventilator support may have an impact on the laryngeal processes of the lifting and tilting of the larynx, vocal fold closure, and the cough reflex, which are all critical processes for prevention of aspiration and protection of the airway. Long-term tracheostomy may result in additional complications, including: further movement limitations, large trache tubes or overinflation of a cuff negatively affecting laryngeal and esophageal movements, and the presence of an open subglottic airway, which may affect subglottic pressure and adequate airway protection provided by sustained vocal fold closure (Hauck, 1999). Even when the tracheostomy is removed, the initial surgical incision that was performed for placement of the tubing may have damaged nerves and muscles that function in laryngeal elevation and vocal cord function, further compromising the swallowing system and increasing the risk of laryngeal penetration or aspiration (Hauck, 1999).

Morgan and Mackay (1999) supported the concept that injuries due to the translaryngeal intubation or tracheostomy may contribute to swallowing dysfunction in the TBI patient. However, as Tolep, Gretch, and Criner (1996) commented, much of the negative effects of the tracheostomy on swallowing function can be modified to some degree by ensuring the use of appropriately sized tracheostomy tubes and avoiding overinflation of the cuff. Indeed, Lazarus and Logemann (1987) reported that none of the 14 subjects in their study who had a tracheostomy tube at the time of the swallow evaluation demonstrated swallowing problems directly related to the presence of the tracheostomy tube.

Mackay et al. (1999a) found that TBI patients with a tracheostomy presented with a higher incidence (17 out of 19) of disordered swallowing than nontracheostomy patients (16 out of 35). They also found a significant difference in the duration of ventilation between the TBI patients with and without swallowing disorders. The average duration of ventilation was found to be higher in the swallowing disordered group, with the normal swallowing group found to be ventilated for a mean of 5.5 days, while those with swallowing disorders found to have been ventilated for a mean duration of 13.9 days. Mackay et al. (1999a), concluded that while the presence of a tracheostomy and increased duration of ventilation were not the main causative factors, they may increase the risk of swallowing impairment.

Cognitive Impairment and Behavioural Dysregulation

Cherney and Halper (1989) noted that severe cognitive and communication disorders tend to cooccur with severe oral intake problems in the TBI population. Cognitive and behavioral impairments, such as poor memory, limited insight, reduced alertness and attention, poor organization and sequencing skills, impulsivity, poor judgment and reasoning, and communication deficits, compound the physical causes of dysphagia (Cherney & Halper, 1989; Logemann, 1990). Specific details of the impact these cognitive deficits can have upon oral intake has been outlined elsewhere in an excellent review by Cherney and Halper (1989).

Indeed recently, more emphasis has been placed on the importance of cognition in the return to oral intake. Winstein (1983) was the first to investigate the impact of cognition on swallowing impairment using a more defined measurement tool: the Ranchos Los Amigos Hospital (RLA) cognitive scale (Hagen, 1981). She found that impaired cognition was the problem most frequently identified as interfering with swallowing following TBI in the adult population. Findings from this study suggested that while oral feeding may be indicated earlier, progression to a functional eating level is usually not seen until the patient reaches at least level V (confused and inappropriate). Mackay et al. (1999a) also investigated the relationship between cognition (measured using the RLA scale) and return to oral intake in their two-phase study, which focused on the factors affecting oral feeding in 54 patients with severe traumatic brain injury. Mackay et al. (1999a) found an association between level of cognitive function and oral intake. Regardless of the presence of a swallowing disorder, they noted that patients had to be functioning at least at RLA level IV (confused and agitated) in order to commence oral feeding, and RLA level VI (confused but displaying more appropriate behavior) to manage full oral intake.

In the second phase of their study, Mackay et al (1999b) found that of the 54 patients, patients with RLA levels of II at the time of admission had a statistically higher percentage of abnormal swallowing than patients with admission RLA levels of between III to IV. It was also noted that the RLA II group took significantly longer to initiate oral feeding, to maintain a full oral diet and to progress from initiating the diet to tolerating a full diet. Percentage of aspiration was the only factor not found to differ statistically between the two TBI groups (Mackay et al., 1999b).

Lazarus and Logemann (1987) highlighted the potential detrimental impact of coexisting cognitive issues on swallowing disorders. They conducted a study of swallowing disorders in 53 closed head trauma patients and found that a number of patients who had shown clinical difficulties such as coughing during mealtimes, did not aspirate during the VFSS. They suggested that this may have been due to the small amount of material used during VFSS and the controlled nature of the procedure in comparison to real-time meals with less stringent controls on bolus size and delivery. Lazarus and Logemann (1987) expressed concern in regard to the potential additional risk of impulsivity for some dysphagic TBI patients, leading to the rapid intake of large amounts of food without the existing physiological control to handle food at that rate of ingestion. Cherney and Halper (1989) stressed the importance of considering the impact of cognition on swallowing, stating that cognitive deficits can interfere with the eating process to the extent that they may cause aspiration, even in the *absence* of a physiological cause for dysphagia. Halper et al. (1999) outline a number of cognitive-communicative deficits and behavioral deficits that may occur following TBI, and their potential impacts on oral intake.

Physical Damage to Swallowing Structures

Additional complications in swallowing function may result from physical damage to the oral, pharyngeal, laryngeal, and esophageal structures. In their review of the nature of the swallowing impairments following TBI, Logemann et al. (1994) summarized a number of potential complications. Common examples of structural trauma that may cooccur with TBI include: fractures of the jaw, affecting jaw opening and movement; laryngeal trauma, which may lead to reduced laryngeal elevation or closure; scar tissue formation on the tissues of the pharynx, leading to possible pooling or reduced pharyngeal wall movement; and wounds to the chest, which may cause esophageal perforation or fistula formation (Logemann et al., 1994). Particularly in the initial stages of acute hospital management, the coexistence of such physical damage can significantly affect swallowing function and impede, or even delay, the initial stages of swallowing rehabilitation.

Positioning and Control for Self-Feeding

Dysphagia may occur through inadequate airway protection, oral and pharyngeal dysfunction, or difficulties with self-feeding, all of which may occur with improper positioning and body alignment (Groher, 1997). In brain injury, abnormal muscle tone, reflexes, and sensory deficits may result in postural problems that may affect the ability to assume and maintain a seated upright position. Close liaison with physiotherapy and occupational therapy services can help maximize posture and control for feeding. Where optimal positioning cannot be achieved, a thorough assessment of swallowing function in alternate postures is critical.

Drake et al.(1997) reported a single case study of a 26-year-old male head-injury patient who was observed to aspirate when eating in an upright position; however, when in a side-lying posture, he was able to safely manage an oral diet without aspiration. From 4 months postinjury, the patient gradually increased oral intake in the side-lying position. By 9 months, all intake was achieved in this side-lying position and supplemental feeding was ceased. Safe self-feeding in the upright position without aspiration was not achieved until 12 months postinjury. During the course of rehabilitation, the patient underwent repeat videofluroscopy studies to ensure aspiration was not occurring in the side-lying posture and to assess the degree of aspiration occurring in the upright positions. This case study demonstrated how alternate posturing may be appropriate for some patients. The authors of the paper noted that feeding in a side-lying position is actively discouraged in most situations; however, with videofluoroscopic support, its use in the management of this patient facilitated an early return to an oral diet. Drake et al. (1997) proposed that patients who may benefit from such compensatory postures are patients with poor base of tongue motion, affecting delivery of a cohesive bolus to the pharynx, and those who have impaired pharyngeal clearance of the bolus. It is critical, however, that if alternate positioning or postures are to be used with a patient videofluoroscopic evidence be obtained to ensure that aspiration is not occurring.

Oral and Pharyngeal Sensory Disorders

Patients, following TBI, may display disorders of oral or pharyngeal sensation, displaying either hyper- or hyposensitive responses to touch. Winstein (1983) identified disordered sensory function in 73% of the 30 nonoral feeders identi-fied in her retrospective chart review of adult patients with dysphagia following head injury. In this group of patients, primitive orofacial reflexes and reactions such as biting, pursing, and rooting were observed. Bruce (1996) summarized the potential characteristics of hypersensitivity subsequent to trauma in pediatric TBI patients to be: lip pursing or retraction, jaw clenching or hyperextension, tongue protrusion or retraction, head hyperextension or deviation, distress, and aversion. Both pediatric and adult patients with head injury presenting with hyposensitivity tend to display characteristics such as loss of food from the mouth, pooling of food in the buccal cavities, loss of food particles in the mouth, and premature entry of the bolus into the pharynx.

Absent or limited sensation is thought to be responsible for a poor motor response to bolus presentation or leftover bolus in the mouth, although inattention of motor deficits may also be implicated (Lazarus & Logemann, 1987; Veis & Logemann, 1985). The resulting neglect of food in the mouth can create potential for aspiration (Groher, 1984). Foods possess a wide array of sensory qualities with respect to tem-perature, texture, and taste. These sensory qualities in combination probably stimu-late oral movements and trigger the swallowing reflex. Changing the volume and viscosity of boluses, which can be done through the use of different foods, has been shown to change oral movement responses (Dantas, Kern, et al., 1990; Dantas, Dodds, Massey, & Kern, 1989; Dodds et al. 1988). In the presence of reduced oral sensitivity, the swallow reflex may often be absent or delayed. Alternately, hyper-sensitivity may be associated with abnormal reflexive responses to oral stimulation, including tonic or clonic bite reflex, hyperactive gag reflex, rooting reflex, and tongue thrusting.

Reduced pharyngeal sensation can also cause severely impaired swallowing (Morgan & Mackay, 1999; Pommerencke, 1928). Pharyngeal peristalsis may be weak or uncoordinated resulting in residue in the pharynx and possible aspiration after the swallow. The patient may also have reduced airway protection due to an absent or delayed cough reflex. Lazarus and Logemann (1987) noted decreased pharyngeal sensation, whereby patients did not produce a reflexive cough during or after aspiration of material into the airway. These patients needed to be instructed to cough in order to facilitate airway protection.

Oral and Pharyngeal Movement Disorders

A wide array of oral and pharyngeal movement disorders, often occurring in combination, are seen after brain injury (Morgan & Mackay,1999). In closed head trauma these include: limited tongue control, reduced oral and pharyngeal propulsion of the bolus, and a reduced or absent swallowing reflex (Lazarus & Logemann, 1987). Apraxia or motor planning deficits may also be manifested as a movement deficit during eating, at either the oral or pharyngeal level. Abnormality of movement may also result in dysarthria, resulting from hypo- or hypertonicity of muscle tone in the lips, cheeks, jaw, tongue, velum, and larynx, depending upon the site of the damage (upper or lower motor neuron) and the cranial nerve damaged. Specific features of the oral and pharyngeal movements disorders associated with swallowing impairment in the TBI population will be discussed in more detail in the following sections.

Characteristics of Dysphagia Following TBI in Children

While no incidence data for swallowing or feeding disorders for the pediatric TBI population has been reported, authors have noted that transient swallowing impairments in the early stage of the recovery process are pervasive, and persistent deficits necessitating long-term intervention are also common (Ylvisaker & Logemann, 1985). A number of authors assume that the characteristics of pediatric dysphagia are identical to those of adults following trauma to the brain (Ylvisaker & Weinstein, 1989). However, few researchers have investigated the pediatric population or contrasted their findings with the adult population in order to confirm or negate this assumption. Ylvisaker and Weinstein (1989) in their paper documenting clinical experience with the pediatric population, state that differences do exist between children and adults in regard to the recovery of oral intake following head injury. They proposed that significant cognitive-behavioral issues are more likely to interfere with the reestablishment of oral feeding in children than in adults. Little mention is made, however, of the exact physiological deficits or of the resolution of swallowing disorders in children.

Although they agree that some behavioral and cognitive differences exist, Ylvisaker and Weinstein (1989) proposed that the physiological deficits are similar between children and adults. They reiterated that while the research literature does not include specific reports of pediatric swallowing outcome, their experience with children supports Lazarus and Logemann's (1987) investigation of swallowing disorders in adult closed head trauma patients, which revealed that oral feeding and pharyngeal swallowing problems typically occurred in combination, and that the most common problems included reduced lingual control and bolus manipulation, delayed triggering of the pharyngeal swallow (swallowing reflex), and inefficient transport of food through the mouth and pharynx. A combination of the aforementioned difficulties may cause characteristic movement disorders following pediatric head injury. These may include: difficulty opening the mouth to receive food, difficulty closing the lips around a cup or utensil, loss of food from the mouth, loss of food in the pharynx prior to initiation of the swallow, a suckle-swallow pattern that excludes tongue lateralization and limits bolus formation, and reduced speed and control of anterior-posterior tongue movement (Bruce, 1996). Ylvisaker and Logemann (1985) noted that following head injury, the presence of suckle-swallow and munch patterns are not uncommon and may lead to bolus dispersion, and inefficient and slowed anterior-to-posterior movement of the tongue.

Although it has been noted that children with head injuries are "particularly susceptible to feeding and swallowing impairments as a consequence of cognitive and neurologic difficulties" (Arvedson & Lefton-Greif, 1998, p. 51), to date only one article has documented the exact nature of the swallowing impairment following pediatric TBI. Rowe (1999) presented single case study data on the characteristics of dysphagia in five male children with closed-head injury. Each of the five case studies varied dramatically in age at presentation (2 months, 19 months, 5 years 10 months, 13 years 8 months, and 16 years 10 months), severity of injury (severe[3], moderate [1], no GCS data available [1]), and cause of injury (motor vehicle accident [2], fall [1], hit by baseball bat [1], and nonaccidental trauma [1]), with differential patterns of dysphagia severity and recovery.

Rowe (1999) used a combination of clinical bedside examination and videofluroscopy to examine swallowing function in all cases except for one patient where clinical bedside data only was reported because further radiological investigation was not indicated. Analysis of the videofluroscopic data presented by Rowe for 4 of the 5 cases, revealed a number of deficits including: disorganized oral preparatory phase (1/4), disorganized oral phase/oral phase delay (2/4), decreased tongue to palate seal (1/4), variable bolus control (1/4), nasopharyngeal reflux (1/4), premature spillage of consistencies into the pharyngeal area/valleculae/pyriform sinus (4/4), delayed initiation of swallow (4/4), moderate amounts of pharyngeal residue (2/4), and laryngeal penetration or aspiration (4/4). While this pattern of physiological deficits appears comparable to those reported in the adult TBI dysphagic population (Lazarus & Logemann, 1987), large group studies are still required to determine whether or not it can be assumed that the physiological deficits of adult and pediatric TBI patients are indeed similar as suggested by Ylvisaker and Weinstein (1989). In addition, the cases described in the article by Rowe (1999) have been retrospectively analyzed, and the author stressed the importance of prospective studies to investigate the relationship between different features of neuropathology and swallowing deficit.

The authors of the present chapter have been prospectively studying the swallowing characteristics of the pediatric TBI population, during both the acute and rehabilitation phases of recovery. Subjects comprise those children admitted to either of two major children's hospitals with severe head injury. Children included in the study are aged between 4 and 12 years, have no previous neurological or feeding impairment, and have been referred to speech pathology for a swallowing evaluation. A clinical feeding assessment is completed upon initial referral, comprising of a standard test battery of oromotor and feeding trial assessment procedures, and is conducted biweekly until the swallowing disorder is resolved. Following a clinical trial in which the child meets criteria denoting that they can safely undergo videofluoroscopy, a modified barium swallow is conducted within 24 hours of that clinical trial. Children are then reassessed 6 months postinjury using both clinical bedside and MBS procedures.

Pediatric Case Studies

The following three cases, taken from larger group data compiled to date, are presented in the following sections to document the differential patterns of dysphagia rehabilitation across pediatric TBI patients, and also to highlight patterns of residual deficit persisting at 6 months postinjury. These three cases were selected from the group data because each presented with severe TBI on admission to the hospital following an accident involving a motor vehicle, and each child was of a comparable age at the time of the accident (10, 9, and 7 years of age).

Case 1

Juanita was a 10-year-old female who sustained a severe closed head injury (GCS of 7) following a motor vehicle accident. On admission, CT confirmed a 4 cm diameter, 2 cm thick disk-shaped right extradural hematoma, which was relieved via craniotomy, as confirmed by the follow-up CT conducted at 18 hours postinjury. The child was intubated at admission, and extubated on her second day. Her chest remained clear at all times during her admission. A severe generalized left hemiparesis was noted initially, which resolved quickly over the first week postinjury. Juanita was fed via total parentral nutrition (TPN) for the first 3 days before commencing nasogastric feeds and was referred to speech pathology for a swallowing assessment on the third day of admission. This assessment, consisting of a clinical bedside evaluation and an MBS procedure, revealed a number of deficits in the oral preparatory and oral stages of the swallow including: hesitation in eating; reduced mouth opening in anticipation of the spoon; reduced lip seal; reduced range, rate, and strength of tongue movement; repetitive tongue pumping, piecemeal deglutition; reduced posterior tongue movement; impaired bolus formation, increased oral transit time; oral residue; and delayed triggering of the swallow. Examination of the pharyngeal phase of the swallow revealed delayed swallow trigger, pooling in the valleculae, throat clearing, multiple swallows to clear the bolus through the pharynx, and increasing fatigue with multiple swallows, resulting in weaker and further delayed swallows. Following this initial assessment, Juanita was placed on supervized pureed diet trials, using small amounts of puree only, with continual monitoring and prompting of swallowing strategies (i.e., keep your lips closed, swallow again, cough and swallow, etc), and dysphagia therapy was commenced. Specific intervention to assist in focusing attention during mealtimes was only required for the first few days following the initial feeding assessment. Swallowing function was continually reassessed throughout her management, with biweekly standardized clinical bedside assessments. Diet upgrades were systematically introduced once safely tolerated. At 6 weeks postinjury, Juanita was tolerating a full oral diet of normal consistencies. At 6 months post injury, a repeat MBS was conducted for research purposes. Despite the fact that Juanita had been tolerating a full normal diet for approximately 4 and a half months, the MBS assessment identified continuing physiological deficits in her swallowing behavior. The 6-month reassessments revealed a slight delay in oral transit time for both soft and hard chewable foods, piecemeal deglutition for both soft and hard chewable foods, and delayed swallow trigger for soft and hard chewable foods. The pharyngeal phase of the swallow revealed pooling of food in the valleculae, multiple swallows to facilitate pharyngeal clearance, and reduced overall coordination of the oral and pharyngeal phases of swallowing. Although no aspiration was noted during Juanita's swallowing rehabilitation, her dysphagia characteristics, both acutely and at 6 months postinjury, continued to place her at risk of aspiration.

Case 2

Sarah was a 9-year-old female who sustained a severe closed head injury (GCS of 4 at the scene; 3 on admission) after being struck by a car. On admission, an initial CT scan revealed just 2 small foci in the left cerebellum, which were absent in the follow-up CT conducted at 18 hours postinjury. Sarah's chest remained clear at all times during her hospital stay. She was fed via TPN for the first 3 days and commenced nasogastric feeds on the fourth day. Seven days postinjury, she was referred to speech pathology and received a clinical bedside assessment, with the initial MBS conducted on the following day. The swallowing assessments revealed preparatory and oral phase difficulties including: hesitancy toward eating, anterior spillage, poor lip seal, failure to chew/swallow/manipulate bolus, impaired chewing, impaired bolus formation, piecemeal deglutition, decreased range and strength of tongue movement, repetitive tongue pumping, impaired oral transit, impaired posterior tongue movement, oral residue requiring numerous swallows to clear, and a delayed onset of the swallow reflex leading into the pharyngeal phase. The pharyngeal phase was characterized by pooling of food in the valleculae and pyriform sinuses, vallecular and pyriform residue postswallow, impaired pharyngeal peristalsis, and the need for multiple swallows to clear residue from the pharynx. Following assessment, she was placed on supervized pureed diet trials using small amounts of puree only following this assessment. As is standard practice, she also commenced dysphagia therapy and daily swallowing trials. Continual prompting was required in order to keep Sarah focused on the meal and the task of eating, and a reduction of external distracters during mealtimes was required for a number of weeks. Even upon discharge, distraction and a lack of focus on the mealtime was one of the largest concerns. However, although Sarah had initial issues with self-monitoring, she had always accepted that it was not safe for her to try certain foods and adhered to modified diets as requested. Sarah achieved a normal oral diet just over 2 months postinjury.

The follow-up clinical beside examination and MBS were conducted at 6 months postinjury, and revealed that Sarah was still demonstrating a number of physiological deficits, despite tolerating a normal diet for around 4 months. Similarly to Case 1, the primary deficits involved the preparation and clearance of soft and hard chewable foods including: impaired bolus preparation/chewing, piecemeal deglutition, increased oral transit time, delayed swallow trigger, pooling of food in the valleculae, multiple swallows to facilitate pharyngeal clearance, and reduced overall coordination of the oral and pharyngeal phases for these consistencies. Sarah had demonstrated more care with eating at this time, however, and was capable of monitoring her own eating. She tended to take smaller amounts of the more difficult consistencies and was aware that multiple swallows were needed in order to clear the food from her "throat". Thus, although Sarah was still displaying characteristics placing her at risk of aspiration, her improved cognitive status and understanding of her eating difficulties improved the functional status of her eating, and decreased the likelihood of her experiencing further complications as a result of her residual physiological deficits.

Case 3

Jason was a 7-year-old male who sustained a severe head injury (GCS 4 at scene, 6 at admission) after being struck by a car. On admission, the CT scan revealed one small foci in the left cerebellum. However, the follow-up CT conducted 18 hours postinjury revealed an area of attenuation in the right temporal lobe. Jason was intubated at admission and extubated on his third day. He had a chest infection upon admission that had resolved by day 5. Some small areas of lung collapse were noted at this time. As with the other cases, Jason was initially fed via TPN for the first few days, and commenced nasogastric feeding on the third day. He was referred to Speech Pathology and received a swallowing assessment on his seventh day. Clinical bedside evaluation and subsequent initial modified barium swallow assessments revealed the following oral phase difficulties: anterior spillage from lips due with poor lip seal, decreased range rate and strength of tongue movement, repetitive tongue pumping with poor base of tongue movement, impaired bolus formation/chewing, piecemeal deglutition, impaired oral transit, premature spillage into the valleculae and pyriform sinuses, oral residue, multiple swallows to clear the oral cavity, and delayed swallow trigger leading into the pharyngeal phase. In regard to the pharyngeal swallowing deficits seen, Jason demonstrated vallecular and pyriform residue, impaired peristalsis, multiple swallows to help clear the pharynx, and throat clearing. One of the most pervasive features of Jason's swallowing difficulties, however, was his lack of attention to feeding. Jason's lack of self-monitoring for feeding extended into continually requesting inappropriate food items from *his mother, the nursing staff, and the speech pathologists involved in his intervention. Jason's focus on attempts to obtain other food items served as another distraction to his feeding for the first few weeks of intervention in particular. In regard to general attention and self-monitoring, however, Jason required continual redirection to the task of eating or drinking in some form for the entire duration of his hospital stay (over 2 months) and beyond. He demonstrated a continual pattern of attempting to rush the feeding process beyond his level of physiological functioning, placing him at an increased risk of aspirating. He required continual prompts such as "chew carefully", "move your tongue to both sides of your cheeks", "swallow", "take a small sip", "just one sip at a time," etc. As with the previous two cases, Jason was initially placed on a pureed diet, with supervision and individually appropriate swallowing prompts. He required supervision during feeding for over 2 months because his impulsive nature placed him at greater risk of complications. He did not achieve normal diet status until 2 and a half months postinjury and at this stage it was still suggested that Jason be monitored regularly and prompted when necessary. The largest area of concern with Jason was his poor oral preparation of solids, and poor control and pacing of thin fluids.*

At 6 months postinjury, the MBS and clinical assessments revealed that JH still had difficulty with oral preparation/chewing of hard and soft chewable foods, leading to increased oral transit time. He also demonstrated reduced triggering of the swallow for both thin fluids and soft and hard chewable foods, and multiple swallows for soft and hard chewable foods. The most striking clinical feature observed at this time was Jason's continued lack of containment and self-monitoring during the mealtime. In contrast to the previous case, Jason continued to demonstrate pervasive difficulties in this area. Although Jason's swallow was quite functional during periods of monitoring and supervision, feeding at school and in other environments where he was not being externally focused on the mealtime, placed him at continued risk of aspiration.

Summary of case studies

Although a number of the physiological deficits observed in the three pediatric TBI cases discussed are similar to those reported by Rowe (1999), unlike Rowe's cases, no subject experienced any aspiration during their acute or follow-up MBS assessments. In light of their complex physiological and cognitive deficits, however, each child remained at potential risk for aspiration. In addition, although none of the cases experienced decreased tongue to palate seal or nasopharyngeal reflux, these characteristics have been observed in other cases presently under review in our larger group study. The present case data also highlights the individual nature of the dysphagic impairment and rehabilitation as discussed by Rowe (1999).

One strikingly variable feature of all three cases is the date of recommencement of a normal oral diet. Each child achieved a full oral diet at quite different stages of their recovery, despite having similar initial presentations. Another aspect of particular interest is the finding that these children continued to display disordered swallowing physiology at 6 months postinjury despite achieving normal oral intake. This finding is a cause for concern, considering that in our experience, some children are discharged from the hospital as early as 6 weeks postinjury on a normal diet with minimal/no strategies, or on a slightly modified diet. Children may appear to handle the normal diet well clinically, and it is often expected that any minor residual deficits will continue to resolve over ensuing months, consolidating the child's return to normal feeding. We believe that a follow-up modified barium swallow may prove invaluable at 6 months postinjury in order to highlight any persisting deficits and areas of weakness, allowing the clinician the opportunity to provide further strategies or for swallowing regulatory controls over oral intake (e.g., rate of intake, size of bolus), in order to prevent further complications.

Both the present case studies and the work reported by Rowe (1999) highlight the unique features of each case of pediatric traumatic brain injury, and the fact that problems may occur in all phases of the swallow and may be compounded further by coexisting cognitive and behavioral deficits. Rowe (1999) states that in her experience, patients with brainstem involvement have both motor and sensory aspects of their swallowing affected, and that a MBS is necessary in this case to rule out silent aspiration. It was noted that fewer swallowing problems are seen in patients with extradural hematomas than in those with subdural hemorrhages because of the depth of the injury, and in general, those patients with diffuse axonal injury often have swallowing issues related to arousal, attention, and cognition (Rowe, 1999). As one might expect, patients with combined multifocal and diffuse injuries present as being very complex, with a multitude of swallowing issues (Rowe, 1999).

Although swallowing skills and abilities are generally similar across individuals in the adult population, children or infant's feeding skills may be influenced by chronological age and developmental factors (Rowe, 1999). Variations of only months in chronological age may produce wide variations in the feeding ability of the pediatric population (Rowe, 1999). Because of these considerations, Rowe (1999) states that the awareness of premorbid feeding skills is *essential* in managing children with dysphagia subsequent to TBI. Ylvisaker and Weinstein (1989) reported difficulties comparing children and adults in regard to the recovery of oral intake following head injury, listing nutrition/hydration factors, sociological differences in rehabilitation management (i.e., parental nurturing issues), cognitive/behavioral issues, and anatomical/physiological differences as influencing factors.

Ylvisaker and Weinstein (1989) proposed that significant cognitive-behavioral issues associated with TBI are more likely to interfere with the reestablishment of oral feeding in children than in adults. Rowe (1999) supported this view, stating that cognitive/behavioral factors may have a marked impact upon the reestablishment of oral feeding in the pediatric population, especially with the overlay of normal developmental and behavioral skills. This issue was also highlighted in the previous three cases where coexisting cognitive deficits further complicated dysphagia management. Bruce (1996) stated that a child's level of consciousness is usually affected following a head injury, though the degree and duration to which it is affected will vary widely. However, as with adults, Bruce (1996) advocated that the child be aware of and be able to follow simple instructions before commencing oral feeds. Unfortunately intervention for the pediatric TBI population is further limited by the developmental state of the child. Memory strategies to encourage safe feeding may not even be possible in children because of their cognitive restrictions. Similarly, many of the compensatory swallowing strategies widely used with adults may not be well adapted to children, since these tasks require a certain level of comprehension and execution (Rowe, 1999).

As evidenced by the present review, large group scientific studies have yet to be performed to investigate the acute swallowing deficits present, and the resolution of swallowing impairment subsequent to traumatic brain injury in the pediatric population.

Further research is required in order to reliably confirm or negate present reports of clinical experience and single case study findings regarding the physiological deficits of pediatric TBI patients. While authors such as Arvedson and Lefton-Greif (1998) suggested that the frequency of silent aspiration in the population with neurogenic dysphagia may actually be higher than the figures reported for the adult population, we have yet to see evidence that this is true. Studies examining the impact of associated factors, such as severity of injury, cognitive status, ventilation, intubation, and others, on swallowing function, are also necessary to aid prognostic decisions for the pediatric TBI population.

Characteristics of Dysphagia Following TBI in the Adult Population

In contrast to the absence of literature regarding the characteristics of dysphagia in the pediatric population, a number of articles have documented the nature of the swallowing deficit identified in adult patients following TBI. To date, one of the largest systematic studies of swallowing function following TBI was conducted by Lazarus and Logemann (1987). With a subject cohort of 53 patients, swallowing function was examined fluoroscopically, and levels of severity were compared with aspects of medical status such as presence and duration of coma. The results of this study revealed the presence of nine swallowing motility problems, which were identified in varying patterns of concurrence across all patients. The most frequently occurring disorder, observed in 81% of the group, was an absence of, or a delay in, triggering of the swallow reflex. Reduced lingual control was observed in 53% of the group, while 32% of cases were identified as having reduced pharyngeal peristalsis. Much smaller percentages of patients (14%) were found to have disorders relating to laryngeal function, such as reduced closure, elevation or spasm, and 6% were observed to display cricopharyngeal disorders. Across the subject group, 29% of patients were observed to present with one motility disorder, 47% with two, 21% with three, and 2% noted to present with four cooccurring disorders. The high incidence of disorders involving the swallowing reflex in this sample of TBI patients may reflect the importance of cortical as well as brainstem input into triggering a swallow reflex. Although the reticular formation in the brainstem controls the swallowing center, voluntary tongue initiation of the swallow also plays a role in triggering the reflexive swallow.

Field and Weiss (1989) reported that the most common swallowing problems they identified in their nine adult TBI patients were prolonged oral transit and a delay in the swallowing reflex, which was observed in 87.5% of their cases. Additional deficits were noted on videofluoroscopy, including pooling in the valleculae and pyriform sinuses in five of the eight cases, late triggering of the swallow at pyriform sinus in four of the eight, and the premature entry of the bolus into the hypopharynx prior to the swallow in three cases. Two patients were observed to have reduced pharyngeal peristalsis (Field & Weiss, 1989). Mackay et al. (1999a) found loss of bolus control and reduced lingual control as the main characteristics of the swallowing disorders identified in 26 of their 33 severely head-injured patients.

Hoppers and Holm (1999) discussed the results of the use of FEES with the brain-injured population. These authors reported that the most common deficits identified in their patient group (approximately 60 cases per year of which 20% require instrumental assessments) were premature spillage of the bolus, delayed swallow, and pharyngeal residue (identified in 75% of cases). Aspiration with reflexive cough was noted in 33% of the group, while silent aspiration occurred 20% of the time. Unfortunately, no specific group numbers to which these percentages can be referenced were provided by these authors. Logemann, et al. (1994) summarized the characteristics of the oropharyngeal deficits as follows: the presence of increased muscle tone and abnormal oral reflexes, affecting mouth opening and movement; reduced lip closure leading to drooling and loss of saliva control; pooling of food in the lateral sulcus due to unilateral buccal weakness; reduced range of tongue movement and coordination, resulting in increased oral transit times and inefficient clearing; delayed or absent trigger for the pharyngeal swallow, causing aspiration; impaired velopharyngeal closure, leading to nasal regurgitation; reduced movement of the base of tongue, resulting in poor clearance of the valleculae; and reduced laryngeal elevation, leading to pooling of foods in the pyriform sinus and laryngeal entrance.

In a conference paper examining lingual control for speech and swallowing, Lazarus and Logemann (1987, cited in Lazarus, 1989) examined the lingual control for swallowing and for speech in a group of 20 TBI patients. They classified patients by their severity of tongue dysfunction during swallowing, and found severe tongue dysfunction (oral transit delays of 11 to 15 seconds) in seven patients, moderate lingual dysfunction in six patients (delays of 6 to 10 seconds), and mild tongue dysfunction (delays of 1 to 5 seconds) in the remaining seven patients. Additional measures were collected, including: the number of repetitive tongue movements required to initiate the pharyngeal swallow, the range of movement (expressed as a percentage) of the base of tongue relative to posterior pharyngeal wall, and the range of vertical movement (expressed as a percentage) of the tongue tip, mid-tongue, and back relative to the hard and soft palate. Using this information the authors found that 25% of the subject group failed to achieve normal posterior tongue to palate contact, concluding that deficits in the elevation of the tongue were a major factor contributing to poor oral transit of the bolus. The range of tongue movement to the posterior pharyngeal wall was also impaired in most subjects. Comparisons between rating of severity of tongue function during speech (classified using a dysarthria rating scale) revealed no clear pattern or relationship between lingual function in speech and in swallowing. The authors noted that the 15 patients with severe dysarthria presented with an almost equal distribution of mild, moderate, and severe lingual dysfunction in swallowing. Patients with normal or mild dysarthria (4), however, were found to have similar mild or normal lingual function during swallowing.

In a later study of 14 patients with TBI, Lazarus (1989) reported preliminary data that examined the effects of tongue movement on the oral and pharyngeal stages of the swallow. They found that the degree of lingual dysfunction observed during the oral stage of the swallow was not a good predictor of the degree of tongue base dysfunction observed during the pharyngeal stage of the swallow. In light of the preliminary nature of this data and the minimal subject numbers, however, the authors called for further research into the area of tongue control and swallowing ability in the TBI population. As yet, studies of this nature have not been conducted.

"Silent" aspiration is a significant issue in the TBI population, with a number of authors identifying evidence of frank aspiration on videofluoroscopic investigations with no coughing or distress observed (Horner & Massey, 1991; Lazarus & Logemann, 1987). Leder (1999) examined the swallowing function of TBI patients in an acute care setting using FEES. Within the group of 47 patients studied, 17 (36%) were found to be aspirating, with nine (53%) of these silently aspirating.

Aspiration rates in the adult TBI population have been consistently noted to be high, with figures of up to 71% reported in some studies (Schurr, et al., 1999). The primary physiological cause of the aspiration, however, has varied between studies. Lazarus and Logemann (1987) found an aspiration rate of 38% in their group of 53 dysphagic patients, with the majority of aspiration events occurring before the swallow in 13 patients due to either an absent or delayed swallowing reflex or a combination of reduced lingual control with a delayed reflex. Two of the 53 patients were found to be aspirating during the swallow as a result of reduced laryngeal closure. Aspiration after the swallow was observed in four cases due to reduced pharyngeal peristalsis and in one case due to cricopharyngeal dysfunction (Lazarus & Logemann, 1987). A slightly higher aspiration rate of 41% (22 of 54) was documented by Mackay et al. (1999a). In contrast to Lazarus and Logemann's (1987) findings, Mackay et al. (1999a) noted that the majority of the aspiration occurred during the swallow (77%), before the swallow (41%), and in a few cases after the swallow (18%). Field and Weiss (1985) similarly reported aspiration rates of 37.5% in their group of eight subjects, however, no details were provided as to whether this aspiration occurred before, during, or after the swallow.

Summary

As noted by a number of researchers, the long-term prognosis of severe head injury, in both the pediatric and adult TBI population, has both practical and theoretical implications (Costeff, Groswasser, Landon, & Brenner, 1985). Long-term rehabilitation of TBI patients has financial as well as sociological implications for families, the community, and governments. Hence, it is important that robust research analyzes both the nature of the swallowing disorders and the rehabilitative process of the presenting dysphagia, as well as any sequelae that may have an impact on recovery. While the body of knowledge regarding dysphagia in the adult TBI population is growing, particularly as a result of excellent large group studies conducted in the last few years, the present chapter highlights the current lack of large group studies in the area of dysphagia in the pediatric TBI population. As yet, no studies have systematically examined the patterns of physiological deficit, the factors influencing oral intake, or the long-term outcomes for this group. In the absence of information specific to the pediatric population, the clinician is forced to draw from literature related to the adult population, a situation that is less than satisfactory.

Logemann (1989, p.32) noted "that many head injured individuals, for whom long term non-oral feeding is advised and therapy terminated because of lack of progress, have recovered normal swallowing after one or two years." As yet, no studies have followed the long-term swallowing outcomes of patients following TBI with respect to either spontaneous recovery or response to rehabilitation. In the absence of definitive data on the duration of the postinjury recovery period, there is a need for clinicians to continue to monitor the long-term patterns of recovery and any change in physiological or cognitive function, in order to continue to maximize functional swallowing for these patients. The pediatric case study data presented in this chapter revealed that physiological deficits remain, and may continue to compromise swallowing function long after the patient returns to a full oral diet. Clinicians and researchers must conduct further clinical research in these areas if we are to provide an optimal and coordinated therapeutic service for patients following TBI.

References

Arvedson, J. & Brodsky, L. (1993). *Pediatric Swallowing and Feeding: Assessment and Management.* San Diego, CA: Singular Publishing Group.

Arvedson, J.A. & Christensen, S. (1993). Instrumental Evaluation. In J.A. Arvedson and L. Brodsky (1993). *Pediatric Swallowing and Feeding.* San Diego, CA: Singular Publishing Group, Inc. 293–326.

Arvedson, J. & Lefton-Greif, M. (1998). *Pediatric Videofluoroscopic Swallow Studies: A Professional Manual with Caregiver Guidelines.* San Antonio, TX: Communication Skill Builders/Psychological Corporation.

Arvedson, J., Rogers, B., Buck, G., Smart, P., & Msall, M. (1992). Aspiration by children with dysphagia. *Developmental Medicine and Child Neurology. 34(9), (Suppl. 66),* 37.

Basmajian, J.V. (1978). *Muscles alive: their functions revealed by electromyography,* fourth edition. Baltimore, MD: Williams & Wilkins.

Bastian, R.W. (1998). Contemporary diagnosis of the dysphagia patient. *Otolaryngologic Clinics of North America, 31(3),* 489–506.

Benson, J.E. & Tuchman, D.N. (1994). Other diagnostic tests used for evaluation of swallowing disorders. (pp. 201–207). In D.N. Tuchman and R.S. Walter (1994). (Eds.), *Disorders of Feeding and Swallowing in Infants and Children: Pathophysiology, Diagnosis, and Treatment.* San Diego, CA: Singular Publishing Group.

Bosma, J.F. (1980). Physiology of the mouth, pharynx, and esophagus: physiology of the mouth. In M.A. Paparella and D.A. Shumrick (Eds.), *Otolaryngology,* second edition. pp. 319–331, Philadelphia: W.B. Saunders.

Bosma, J.F. & Donner, M.W. (1980). Physiology of the mouth, pharynx, and esophagus: physiology of the pharynx. In M.A. Paparella and D.A. Shumrick (Eds.), *Otolaryngology,* second edition. pp. 332–345, Philadelphia: W.B. Saunders.

Bosma, J.F., Hepburn, L.G., Josell, S.D. & Baker, K. (1990). Ultrasound demonstration of tongue motions during suckle feeding. *Developmental Medicine and Child Neurology, 32(3),* 223–229.

Brindley, C. (1996). *Paediatric Oral Skills Package.* San Diego: Singular Publishing Group.

Bruce, T. (1996). Head injury, gastro-oesophageal reflux, congenital heart disease. In T. Anderson, S. Starr, J. Hemmings, T. Bruce, L. Fordham, R. Hunt, P. Dempsey, and A. Slater, *The Graduate Pediatric Feeding Education Program.* Sydney, NSW Australia: St. George Hospital, Kogarah.

Cherney, L.R. & Halper, A.S. (1989). Recovery of oral nutrition after head injury in adults. *Journal of Head Trauma Rehabilitation, 4,* 42–50.

Cherney, L.R. & Halper, A.S. (1996). Swallowing problems in adults with traumatic brain injury. *Seminars in Neurology, 16(4),* 349–353.

Christensen, J.R. (1989). Developmental approach to pediatric neurogenic dysphagia. *Dysphagia, 3,* 131–134.

Cooper, D.S. & Perlman, A.L. (1997). Electromyography in the functional and diagnostic testing of deglutition. In A.L. Perlman and K. Schulze-Delrieu (Eds.), *Deglutition and Its Disorders, Anatomy, Physiology, Clinical Diagnosis and Management.* pp. 255–284, San Diego: Singular Publishing.

Costeff, H., Groswasser, Z., Landon, Y., & Brenner, T. (1985). Survivors of severe traumatic brain injury in childhood. II. Late residual disability. *Scandinavian Journal of Rehabilitation Medicine: Supplement, 12,* 10–15.

Crary, M. (1995). A direct intervention program for chronic neurogenic dysphagia secondary to brainstem stroke. *Dysphagia, 10,* 6–18.

Dantas, R.O., Dodds, W.J., Massey, B.T., & Kern, M.K. (1989). The effect of high- vs low-density barium preparations on the quantitative features of swallowing. *American Journal of Roentgenology, 153(6),* 1191–1195.

Dantas, R.O., Kern, M.K., Massey, B.T., Dodds, W.J., Kahrilas, P.J., Brasseur, J.G., Cook, I.J., & Lang, I.M. (1990). Effect of swallowed bolus variables on oral and pharyngeal phases of swallowing. *American Journal of Physiology, 258,* G675–G681.

Darley, F.L, Aronson, A.E., & Brown, J.R. (1975). *Motor Speech Disorders.* Philadelphia: W.B. Saunders.

Dodds, W.J., Man, K.M., Cook, I.J., Kahrilas, P.J., Stewart, E.T., & Kern, M.K. (1988). Influence of bolus volume on swallow-induced hyoid movement in normal subjects. *American Journal of Roentgenology, 150(6),* 1307–1309.

Doty, R.W. (1968). Neural organisation of deglutition. In C.F. Code, (Ed.), *Handbook of Physiology: Alimentary Canal 4(6).* 1861–1902

Drake, W., O'Donoghue, S., Bartram, C., Lindsay, J., & Greenwood, R. (1997). Eating in side-lying facilities rehabilitation in neurogenic dysphagia. *Brain Injury, 11(2),* 137–142.

Field, L.H. & Weiss, C.J. (1989). Dysphagia with head injury. *Brain Injury, 3(1),* 19–26.

Freson, M. & Stokmans, R. (1994). The Radiologic Investigation of Dysphagia. *Acta-Oto-Rhino-Laryngologica Belgica, 48,* 127–137.

Groher, M.E. (1984). *Dysphagia: Diagnosis and Management.* Stoneham: Butterworth.

Groher, M. (Ed.). (1997). *Dysphagia: Diagnosis and Management,* third edition. Boston: Butterworth-Heinemann.

Gupta, V., Reddy, N.P., & Canilang, E.P. (1996). Surface EMG measurements at the throat during dry and wet swallowing. *Dysphagia, 11(3),* 173–179.

Hagen, C. (1981). Language disorders secondary to closed head injury: Diagnosis and management. *Topics in Language Disorders, 1,* 73–87.

Halper, A.S., Cherney, L.R., Cichowski, K., & Zhang, M. (1999). Dysphagia after head trauma: The effect of cognitive-communicative impairments on functional outcomes. *Journal of Head Trauma Rehabilitation, 14(5),* 486–496.

Hamlet, S.L., Nelson, R.J., & Patterson, R.L. (1990). Interpreting the sounds of swallowing: Fluid flow through the cricopharyngeus. *Annals of Otology, Rhinology and Laryngology, 99,* 749–752.

Hauck, K.A. (1999). Communication and swallowing issues in tracheostomized/ventilator-dependent geriatric patients. *Topics in Geriatric Rehabilitation, 15(2),* 56–70.

Hayden, P. & Square, D. (1999). *Verbal Motor Production Assessment for Children (VMPAC).* United States of America: The Psychological Corporation, Harcourt Assessment Company.

Hendrix, T.R. (1993). Art and science of history taking in the patient with difficulty swallowing. *Dysphagia, 8(2),* 69–73.

Holt, S., Miron, S.D., Diaz, M.C., Shields, R., Ingraham, D., & Bellon, E.M. (1990). Scintigraphic measurement of oropharyngeal transit in man. *Digestive Diseases and Sciences, 35,* 1198–1204.

Hoppers, P. & Holm, S.E. (1999). The role of fiberoptic endoscopy in dysphagia rehabilitation. *Journal of Head Trauma Rehabilitation, 14(5),* 475–485.

Horner, J. & Massey, E.W. (1991). Managing dysphagia: Special problems in patients with neurologic disease. *Postgraduate Medicine, 89(5),* 203–213.

Huckabee, M.L. & Cannito, M.P. (1999). Outcomes of swallowing rehabilitation in chronic brainstem dysphagia: A retrospective evaluation. *Dysphagia, 14(2),* 93–109.

Jones, B. & Donner, M.W. (1988). Examination of the patient with dysphagia. *Radiology, 167,* 319–326.

Kidder, T.M., Langmore, S.E., & Martin, B.J.W. (1994). Indications and techniques of endoscopy in evaluation of cervical dysphagia: Comparison with radiographic techniques. *Dysphagia, 9(4)*, 256–261.

Kramer, S.S. (1989). Radiologic examination of the swallowing impaired child. *Dysphagia, 3*, 117–125.

Kramer, S.S. & Eicher, P.M. (1993). The evaluation of pediatric feeding abnormalities. *Dysphagia, 8*, 215–224.

Langmore, S.E. & McCulloch, T.M. (1997). Examination of the pharynx and larynx and endoscopic examination of pharyngeal swallowing. In A.L. Perlman, and K. Schulze-Delrieu, (Eds.), *Deglutition and Its Disorders, Anatomy, Physiology, Clinical Diagnosis and Management.* pp. 201–226, San Diego: Singular Publishing.

Langmore, S.E., Schatz, K., & Olson, N. (1991). Endoscopic and videofluoroscopic evaluations of swallowing and aspiration. *Annals of Otolaryngology, Rhinolology and Laryngology, 100*, 678–681.

Langmore, S.E. & Logemann, J.A. (1991). After the clinical bedside swallowing examination: What next? *American Journal of Speech-Language Pathology*, September, 13–19.

Lazarus, C. & Logemann, J.A. (1987). Swallowing disorders in closed head trauma patients. *Archives of Physical Medicine and Rehabilitation, 68(2)*, 79–84.

Lazarus, C.L. (1989). Swallowing disorders after traumatic brain injury. *Journal Head Trauma Rehabilitation, 4(4)*, 34–41.

Leder, S.B. (1999). Fiberoptic endoscopic evaluation of swallowing in patients with acute traumatic brain injury. *Journal of Head Trauma Rehabilitation, 14(5)*, 448–453.

Linden, P. & Siebens, A. (1983). Dysphagia: Predicting laryngeal penetration. *Archives of Physical Medicine and Rehabilitation, 64(6)*, 281–284.

Logemann, J.A. (1983). Anatomy and physiology of normal deglutition. In J.A. Logemann (Ed.), *Evaluation and Treatment of Swallowing Disorders* (pp. 11–36). San Diego: College-Hill Press.

Logemann, J.A. (1986). *Manual for the Videofluorographic Study of Swallowing.* Boston: College-Hill.

Logemann, J.A. (1989). Evaluation and treatment planning for the head-injured patient with oral intake disorders. *Journal Head Trauma Rehabilitation, 4(4)*, 24–33.

Logemann, J.A. (1990). Factors affecting ability to resume oral nutrition in the oropharyngeal dysphagic individual. *Dysphagia, 4(4)*, 202–208.

Logemann, J.A. (1994). Non-imaging techniques for the study of swallowing. *Acta Oto-Rhino-Laryngologica Belgica., 48(2)*, 139–142.

Logemann, J.A., Pepe, J., & Mackay, L.E. (1994). Disorders of nutrition and swallowing: Intervention strategies in the trauma center. *Journal of Head Trauma Rehabilitation, 9(1)*, 43–56.

Logemann, J.A., Veis, S., & Colangelo, L. (1999). A screening procedure for oropharyngeal dysphagia. *Dysphagia, 14(1)*, 44–51.

Loughlin, G.M. & Lefton-Greif, M.A. (1994). Dysfunctional swallowing and respiratory disease in children. *Advances in Pediatrics, 41*, 135–162.

Mackay, L.E., Morgan, A.S., & Bernstein, B.A. (1999a). Swallowing disorders in severe brain injury: Risk factors affecting return to oral intake. *Archives of Physical Medicine and Rehabilitation, 80*, 365–371.

Mackay, L.E., Morgan, A.S., & Bernstein, B.A. (1999b). Factors affecting oral feeding with severe TBI. *Journal of Head Trauma Rehabilitation, 14(5)*, 435–447.

McVeagh, P., Howman-Giles, R., & Kemp, A. (1987). Pulmonary aspiration studied by radionuclide milk scanning and barium swallow roentgenography. *American Journal of Diseases of Children, 141(8)*, 917–921.

Miller, A.J. (1982). Deglutition. *Physiological Reviews, 62(1)*, 129–184.

Morgan, A.S. & Mackay, L.E. (1999). Causes and complications associated with swallowing disorders in traumatic brain injury. *Journal of Head Trauma Rehabilitation, 14(5)*, 454–461.

Newman, L.A., Cleveland, R.H., Blickman, J.G., Hillman, R.E., & Jaramillo, D. (1991). Videofluoroscopic analysis of the infant swallow. *Investigative Radiology, 26(10)*, 870–872.

Palmer, J.B. (1989). Electromyography of the Muscles of Oropharyngeal Swallowing: Basic Concepts. *Dysphagia, 3(4)*, 192–198.

Palmer, J.B., Kuhlemeier, K.V., Tippett, D.C., & Lynch, C. (1993). A protocol for the videofluoro-scopic swallowing study. *Dysphagia, 8(3),* 209–214.

Palmer, J.B., Tanaka, E., & Siebens, A.A. (1989). Electromyography of the pharyngeal muscula-ture: technical considerations. *Archives of Physical Medicine and Rehabilitation, 70(4),* 283–287.

Park, C. & O'Neill, P.A. (1994). Management of neurological dysphagia. *Clinical Rehabilitation, 8,* 166–174.

Perlman, A.L. & Grayhack, J.P. (1991). Use of electroglottograph for measurement of temporal aspects of the swallow: Preliminary observations. *Dysphagia, 6(2),* 1–6.

Pommerencke, W. (1928). A study of the sensory areas eliciting the swallowing reflex. *American Journal of Physiology, 84,* 36–41.

Reilly, S., Skuse, D., Mathisen, B., & Wolke, D. (1995). The objective rating or oral-motor func-tions during feeding. *Dysphagia, 10(3),* 177–191.

Reimers-Neils, L., Logemann, J., & Larson, C. (1994). Viscosity effects on EMG activity in normal swallow. *Dysphagia, 9(2),* 101–106.

Rosenbek, J.C., Robbins, J.A., Roecker, E.B., Coyle, J.L., & Wood, J.L. (1996). A penetration-aspiration scale. *Dysphagia, 11(2),* 93–98.

Rowe, L.A. (1999). Case studies in dysphagia after pediatric brain injury. *Journal of Head Trauma Rehabilitation, 14(5),* 497–504.

Selley, W.G., Flack, F.C., Ellis, R.E., & Brooks, W.A. (1990). The Exeter dysphagia assessment technique. *Dysphagia, 4(4),* 227–235.

Schurr, M.J., Ebner, K.A., Maser, A.L., Sperling, K.B., Helgeson, R.B., & Harms, B. (1999). Formal swallowing evaluation and therapy after traumatic brain injury improves dysphagia outcomes. *The Journal of Trauma: Injury, Infection and Critical Care, 46(5),* 817–821.

Shawker, T.H., Sonies, B.C., Stone, M., & Baum, B.J. (1983). Real-time ultrasound visualization of tongue movement during swallowing. *Journal of Clinical Ultrasound, 11(9),* 485–490.

Skuse, D., Stevenson, J., Reilly, S., & Mathisen, B. (1995). Schedule for Oral Motor Assessment (SOMA): Methods of validation. *Dysphagia, 10(3),* 192–202.

Sonies, B.C. (1991). Instrumental procedures for dysphagia diagnosis. *Seminars in Speech and Language, 12(3),* 185–197.

Sonies, B.C., Weiffenbach, J., Atkinson, J.C., Brahim, J., Macynski, A., & Fox, P.C. (1987). Clinical examination of motor and sensory functions of the adult oral cavity. *Dysphagia, 1,* 178–186.

Sorin, R., Somers, S., Austin, W., & Bester., S. (1988). The influence of videofluoroscopy on the management of the dysphagic patient. *Dysphagia, 2(3),* 127–135.

Splaingard, M.L., Hutchins, B., Sulton, L.D., & Chaudhuri, G. (1988). Aspiration in rehabilita-tion patients: Videofluoroscopy vs bedside clinical assessment. *Archives of Physical Medicine and Rehabilitation, 69(8),* 637–640.

Starr, S. (1994). Case History. In *Feeding Assessment Resources Management (F.A.R.M) Supplement.* Sydney Australia: Westmead Adults Hospital.

Stone, M. & Shawker, T.H. (1986). An ultrasound examination of tongue movement during swal-lowing. *Dysphagia, 1(2),* 78–83.

Takahashi, K., Groher, M., & Michi, K. (1994). Methodology for detecting swallowing sounds. *Dysphagia, 9,* 54–62.

Tanaka, E., Palmer, J., & Siebens, A. (1986). Bipolar suction electrodes for pharyngeal elec-tromyography. *Dysphagia, 1,* 39–40.

Tippett, D.C., Palmer, J., & Linden, P. (1987). Management of dysphagia in a patient with closed head injury. *Dysphagia, 1,* 221–226.

Tolep, K., Getch, C.L., & Criner, G.J. (1996). Swallowing dysfunction in patients receiving pro-longed mechanical ventilation. *Chest, 109(1),* 167–172.

Tuchman, D.N. (1989). Cough, choke, sputter: The evaluation of the child with dysfunctional swallowing. *Dysphagia, 3(3),* 111–116.

Veis, S.L. & Logemann, J.A. (1985). Swallowing disorders in persons with cerebrovascular acci-dent. *Archives of Physical Medicine and Rehabilitation, 66, 6,* 372–375.

Weber, F., Woolridge, M.W., & Baum, J.D. (1986). An ultrasonic study of the organization of sucking and swallowing by newborn infants. *Developmental Medicine and Child Neurology, 28(1)*, 19–24.

Winstein, C.J. (1983). Neurogenic dysphagia: Frequency, progression, and outcome in adults following head injury. *Physical Therapy, 63(12)*, 1992–1997.

Wolf, S. & Glass, R.P. (1992). *Feeding and Swallowing Disorders in Infancy: Assessment and Management.* Tucson, AZ: Therapy Skill Builders.

Yorkston, K.M., Honsinger, M.J., Mitsuda, P.M., & Hammen, V. (1989). The relationship between speech and swallowing disorders in head-injured patients, *Journal of Head Trauma Rehabilitation, 4(4)*, 1–16.

Ylvisaker, M. & Logemann, J.A. (1985). Therapy for feeding and swallowing disorders following head injury. In M. Ylvisaker, (Ed.), *Head Injury Rehabilitation: Children and Adolescents,* pp. 195–215, Boston: College Hill Press.

Ylvisaker, M. & Weinstein, M. (1989). Recovery of oral feeding after pediatric head injury. *Journal of Head Trauma Rehabilitation, 4(4)*, 51–63.

Yuen, H.K. & Hartwick, J.A. (1992). Diet manipulation to resume regular food consumption for an adult with traumatic brain injury. *The American Journal of Occupational Therapy, 46(10)*, 943–945.

Zenner, P.M., Losinski, D.S., & Mills, R.H. (1995). Using cervical auscultation in the clinical dysphagia examination in long-term care. *Dysphagia, 10(1)*, 27–31.

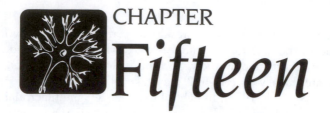

CHAPTER
Fifteen

Rehabilitation of Dysphagia Following Traumatic Brain Injury

Elizabeth C. Ward & Angela T. Morgan

Introduction

It is recognized that a formal swallowing management service should be included as an active component of rehabilitation for the patient with TBI, in order to prevent or minimize the incidence and risk of aspiration, and to restore safe oral intake or establish optimal nonoral feeding routines (Schurr et al., 1999). The rehabilitation of the dysphagic TBI patient is challenging and requires individualized intervention programs that reflect the extent of both the physiological and the cognitive deficits of the patient. Depending on the nature and severity of deficits in each TBI patient, the clinician must make informed and sensitive decisions regarding the needs for additional supplementary feeding and/or ways to maximize safe oral intake. Because of the complex nature of the coexisting deficits, an interdisciplinary team approach, combining medical, speech pathology, physiotherapy, occupational therapy, dietetics, nursing, psychology, social work services, and the family, is essential for achieving optimal swallowing and feeding outcomes for the dysphagic patient (Logemann, 1994).

Traumatic brain injury frequently results in permanent disability for those who survive. Indeed, the spectrum of injury is wide, with frequent need for prolonged hospitalization (Scott-Jupp, Marlow, Seddon & Rosenbloom, 1992). The patterns of recovery are equally diverse and may take place over a long period of time (Klonoff, Low, & Clark, 1977). In light of the complex, multifactorial nature of the swallowing deficit following TBI, researchers and clinicians are continually striving to develop an increased understanding of the interplay of factors that influence the extent and rate of recovery of swallowing for this population. It is acknowledged that the importance of the early assessment of, and intervention for, the presenting swallowing disorders cannot be overestimated in the neurological recovery of patients with severe TBI (Mackay, Morgan & Bernstein, 1999a; Logemann, Pepe, & Mackay, 1994). Detailed information regarding the nature and type of deficit contributing to the swallowing dysfunction is essential in providing accurate diagnosis of swallowing impairment and maximizing the efficacy of intervention strategies. This in turn will lead to improved recovery and enhanced quality of life (Groher, 1992).

The present chapter has been compiled to outline the current knowledge of the prognostic indicators and factors influencing swallowing rehabilitation and the dysphagia outcomes of patients following TBI. In addition, the range and types of supplemental feeding options, frequently required in the early stages of the rehabilitative process, are discussed. Finally, an outline of the various treatment approaches, and specific therapy techniques reported in the literature to date, with application to the rehabilitation and management of the dysphagic patient following TBI will be detailed.

Prognostic Indicators and Dysphagia Outcomes Following Traumatic Brain Injury

Oral nutritional intake requires normal, or at least functional swallowing anatomy and physiology along with enough behavioral control to accept food or liquid into the mouth (Logemann, 1989). Although some strong relationships between medical condition, cognitive state, ventilatory status, and other factors have been reported in relation to swallowing outcomes, researchers and clinicians are still attempting to determine those factors most important for indicating the presence of a persistent, severe swallowing impairment (Greenspan & Mackenzie, 1994). Such research is of paramount importance for the speech-language pathologist in a time of needs-based practice. Clinicians must be able to provide evidence for prioritization of patients, and feel confident in the role of helping to determine the optimal form of oral or supplemental feeding. By defining those factors following TBI that will lead to severe swallowing impairment and the need for long-term swallowing rehabilitation, we will be closer to more quantifiable, objective practice.

Mackay et al. (1999a) undertook a systematic study of the factors affecting oral feeding for patients following TBI. They found that increased severity of injury, as indicated by lower GCS scores (GCS 3 to 5) and CT scan results indicating midline shift, brainstem pathology, and operative procedures, in addition to lower Ranchos

Los Amigos (RLA; Hagen, 1981) cognitive levels (RLA II versus RLA III to IV), were associated with aspiration. These factors were also associated with twice as many swallowing disorders in TBI patients. Patients with severe injury were found to have an increased delay in the initiation of swallowing trials and a delay in oral feeding that was almost twice as long as other patients with less severe injury. Longer durations of ventilatory support, specifically 15 or more days, were also associated with abnormal swallowing and delays in the initiation and achievement of oral feeding. From studying the various factors available on each patient at admission (e.g., CT data, GCS, and RLA), the RLA was found to be the most important independent predictor of the number of days before the patient achieved total oral intake. Mackay et al. (1999a) noted that as more information becomes available from acute care management, the ability to predict oral intake improves. Ventilation duration, the CT scan results, and whether or not aspiration was noted on a videofluoroscopic study, were all factors independently associated with the number of days to achieving oral feeding and the duration of the delay between initial swallowing trials and total oral intake.

As mentioned in the previous chapter, there are a number of coexisting factors that can influence swallowing function and swallowing outcomes in the TBI patient. Aspiration (the penetration of food or fluid into the lungs) is one of the most significant complications of dysphagia. Aspiration may lead to the medical complications of chronic pulmonary disease, aspiration pneumonia, and even death (Martin, et al., 1994). Incidence rates of 37.5% (Field & Weiss, 1989) and more recently 41% (Mackay, et al, 1999a) have been reported for adults with dysphagia following traumatic brain injury, with the risk of aspiration noted to be increased in those trauma patients who undergo orotracheal intubation and prolonged mechanical ventilation (Leder, Cohn, & Moller, 1998). While figures have not been reported for the pediatric population, it is assumed that the rate of aspiration in this population is also high (Arvedson & Lefton-Greif, 1998).

Aspiration pneumonia has been found to: increase length of ICU stay for the TBI patient (Hsieh et al., 1992), increase the overall length of hospital stay, and increase patient mortality (Logemann, et al., 1994). Consequently, the presence of aspiration remains a negative prognostic factor for the TBI patient. Risk factors identified as being associated with early onset pneumonia in the severely brain-injured patient have been identified to include: GCS scores of less than 5, evidence of a swallowing disorder, documented aspiration, and field intubation (Woratyla, Morgan, Mackay, Bernstein & Barba, 1995).

The rehabilitation of dysphagia, however, can be maximized with accurate evaluation tools (Logemann, 1996; Logemann, 2000; Martin et al., 1994). Martin et al. (1994) stated that the use of accurate diagnostic tools contributes to a reduction or elimination of aspiration, and provides guidance for achieving adequate and appropriate nutrition, hydration, and medical management. Field and Weiss (1989) found that videofluoroscopy was instrumental in determining when their head-injured clients could safely receive oral feeding and in achieving earlier discharge. Identification of swallowing potential and progress allows the therapist to interact with the physician in regulating decisions regarding transition to alternative or supplemental feeding sources.

It has been documented that the nature of intervention provided for the patient with TBI can alter the duration of hospitalization and patient outcomes (Cope & Hall, 1982; Mackay et al., 1992). Cope and Hall (1982) followed the outcomes of 16 severe head-injured patients who were admitted to rehabilitation less than 35 days postinjury, and compared their outcomes to a group of 20 patients admitted at greater than 35 days postinjury. They found that, although both groups had comparable outcomes at 2 years postinjury, the patients admitted late to rehabilitation stayed an average of 144 days, in comparison to the early admission group, who had a significantly shorter length of stay of only 64 days (Cope & Hall, 1982).

A number of authors have reported an increased hospital stay (at least twice as long) for those patients with dysphagia subsequent to TBI, as compared to that for TBI patients without a swallowing impairment (Field & Weiss, 1989; Cherney & Halper, 1996; Halper, Cherney, Cichowski, & Zhang, 1999). Field and Weiss (1989) reported that the average length of stay for patients without dysphagia was 52.3 days, and it was 126.7 days for those with swallowing abnormalities. Cherney and Halper (1996) and Halper, et al. (1999) have investigated length of stay in two studies, reporting that patients with severe dysphagia have a mean length of stay approximately 20 days greater than those without swallowing difficulty. In a sample of 195 patients with TBI, the average length of stay for the dysphagic patients was found to be 40.6 days, while the nondysphagic patients were discharged after an average of 27.5 days (Cherney & Halper, 1996). In their study of 148 TBI patients, Halper et al. (1999) found that patients with more severe dysphagia had an average length of stay of 39.83 days, while patients with less severe dysphagic stayed only 19.3 days on average. The authors cited this finding as an indicator that the presence and severity of dysphagia at admission may be an important factor in predicting length of stay. In contrast to these findings, Schurr et al. (1999) found no difference in the duration of stay between patients with and without swallowing dysfunction.

Formalized early intervention programs that include early and aggressive trauma rehabilitation, family education and involvement in patient care, and coordination between medical and rehabilitation professionals have also been shown to have beneficial long-term physical and cognitive outcomes for the patient with TBI (Mackay, et al., 1992). Research has revealed that patients managed in facilities with formalized TBI programs have significantly improved outcomes, compared to patients managed in nonformalized programs. Specifically, reduced coma duration (formalized programs = 18.9 days, nonformalized programs = 53.8 days), shorter rehabilitation stays (formalized = 106.5, nonformalized = 239.5 days), and higher cognitive levels on discharge (Mackay et al., 1992) have been reported. It has also been found that an increased proportion of patients managed under a formalized TBI service are discharged to home rather than to extended care facilities (Mackay et al., 1992).

Acute Care Outcomes for Dysphagia Following TBI in Adults

With respect to overall swallowing outcomes, Winstein (1983) noted that functional swallowing recovery is good following head injury. From her data, she identified an average time from nonoral intake at admission to successful oral intake to be approximately 3 months, with a range of between 5 and 21 weeks. Of the total group of 55 dysphagic patients studied, Winstein (1983) found that 94% of those patients with dysphagia on admission achieved functional oral intake, the majority within 5 months postinjury.

The first author of the current chapter and colleagues have recently conducted a 3-year study of the swallowing outcomes of adult TBI patients in the acute care setting. All patients were admitted to a formal acute care service for patients following TBI, were classified with a primary diagnosis of head injury, and were referred to speech pathology for swallowing assessment and management. Data collection for each patient involved compiling details of swallowing disability measures at admission and discharge from speech pathology management and overall outcome classification ("reached goal" or "still progressing") using the Royal Brisbane Outcome Measure for Swallowing (RBHOMS; Ward & Conroy, 1999). Information regarding ventilation, GCS, CT findings, supplementary feeding requirements, and speech pathology service has been determined from a retrospective chart review following the patients' discharge.

Preliminary analysis of the first 52 consecutive patients (covering approximately a 1-year period of admissions) has revealed an overall average length of stay in the acute care facility of 43.5 days ($SD = 32$, *range* 9–162). With respect to swallowing disability levels, statistical comparisons between RBHOMS scores on admission ($M = 3.4$, $SD = 1.7$) and discharge ($M = 7.2$, $SD = 1.9$) revealed that the group demonstrated a significant improvement in swallowing disability by the time of discharge from the acute management facility. At the initial speech pathology assessment, all patients presented with some degree of swallowing compromise. Specifically, 54% (28/52) were judged clinically to be unsafe for oral trials (RBHOMS levels 1–3), 31% (16/52) were able to safely swallow small amounts of oral intake while still requiring supplementation (RBHOMS levels 4 & 5), and 15% (8/52) were able to be placed on a modified oral diet (RBHOMS level 6). At the point of discharge 38% (20/52) of patients had returned to their premorbid swallowing function, while 62% (32/52) were still progressing with dysphagia rehabilitation. Of the 62% still progressing, 6% (2/32) were discharged still requiring full supplemental feeding, 19% (6/32) were on supplemental feeding plus small amounts of oral intake, and 75% (24/32) were capable of managing a full oral intake of modified consistencies.

A series of T-tests and proportions tests were used to compare those patients who achieved normal swallowing during their acute admission and those who were still progressing with dysphagia rehabilitation on discharge. These statistical comparisons revealed that the subjects with normal swallowing on discharge had significantly higher GCS results (Normal: $M = 8.3$, $SD = 4.2$; Dysphagic: $M = 5.8$, $SD = 3.4$) and a significantly lower proportion of CT scan results indicating midline shift, brainstem pathology, or operative procedures (Normal: 1%, Dysphagic: 63%). The group with normal swallowing on discharge also had significantly fewer days of intubation (Normal: $M = 11.1$, $SD = 10.1$; Dysphagic: $M = 22.4$, $SD = 20.9$), higher RBHOMS scores on admission (Normal: $M = 4.2$, $SD = 1.5$; Dysphagic: $M = 2.9$, $SD = 1.7$), and significantly shorter durations until the first safe oral intake (Normal: $M = 10.1$, $SD = 7.3$; Dysphagic: $M = 24.5$, $SD = 21.2$) than those patients discharged with a swallowing disorder. No significant differences were observed between the two groups with respect to age, length of stay in the acute center, number of days of total speech pathology management, proportion of patients with tracheostomies, or length of mechanical ventilation.

The average length of stay in our facility compares favorably to previously reported figures for dysphagic TBI patients (40.6 days, Cherney & Halper, 1996; 39.8 days, Halper et al., 1999), and with figures reported for dysphagic patients managed within formalized acute care programs (M = 51.5, SD = 6.8 days, Mackay et al., 1992). Overall, the swallowing outcome measures for the TBI group indicated that the large majority of patients were discharged from acute management safely tolerating some oral intake, with just over one-third of patients having returned to their premorbid diets. Only two patients were discharged on full supplementary feeding. As documented previously by Mackay et al. (1999a) increased severity of injury (determined from GCS and CT results) has been associated with more severe swallowing problems, and this finding was also observed in our group data to be associated with continuing swallowing disorders on discharge. An increased duration of intubation was also found to be associated with those patients with persisting swallowing disorders on discharge. Although many authors have discussed the potential effects of endotracheal and tracheostomy tubes on laryngeal sensitivity and swallowing function (see Chapter 14), to date this parameter has not previously been reported as a factor associated with reduced swallowing outcome.

Nutrition and Hydration: Transition to Oral Feeding

Aside from the maintenance of good general medical status (especially respiratory function), the maintenance of adequate nutrition is an essential foundation for maximizing recovery from TBI. It is the aim of the rehabilitation team to identify those patients at risk of aspiration, to lessen the impact of the dysphagia, and to assist in the provision of adequate nutrition and hydration (Groher, 1992). It is well accepted that the duration of nutritional supplementation is lengthy in the TBI population. Mackay, Morgan, and Bernstein (1999b) found that patients with normal swallowing post-TBI required between 2 to 3 weeks of nonoral supplementation, while patients with abnormal swallowing required approximately 8 weeks of supplementation. Similarly, in the current study being conducted by the first author of the present chapter and colleagues (Ward et al, in preparation) the average duration of supplementary feeding for the TBI patients was approximately 2–4 weeks. Specifically, those patients who attained normal swallowing on discharge required on average 14.3 days (SD = 12 days) of supplementary feeding, while the group who were discharged with a continuing swallowing disorder (excluding those eight patients discharged still on supplementary feeding on discharge) required feeding for 25 days (SD = 22 days).

Patients who have acquired traumatic brain injury require vigilant monitoring of their nutritional support because of increased metabolic needs (Pepe, Morgan, & Mackay, 1997), gastric difficulties complicating nutritional intake, and swallowing impairments effecting oral intake. Brooke and Barbour (1986) studied the nutritional status of 56 head injury patients consecutively admitted to a rehabilitation facility. Their study found that from the time of injury to admission to a rehabilitation facility, the TBI patients were found to have lost an average of 29 lbs. The TBI patient group was also, on average, found to be only 82% of their ideal body weight, with 31% of the group identified with protein malnutrition. Within this group 56% of the patients were identified as having dysphagia. Brooke and Barbour (1986) noted that without appropriate monitoring of nutritional status, TBI patients are at risk for malnutrition, further impeding their recovery process.

The difficulty of obtaining early nutritional stability post-TBI is, however, acknowledged, considering the number of potential coexisting problems that may limit the attainment of this goal, including: hypermetabolism, aspiration, gastric dysfunction, cognitive/behavioral problems, and swallowing disorders (Logemann et al., 1994). When determining the optimal method of nutritional support, early evaluation of swallowing ability and aspiration risk is of paramount importance, along with a multidisciplinary approach involving the physician, dietitian, respiratory therapist, and speech-language pathologist (Logemann, 1994; Logemann, et al., 1994). The degree of swallowing impairment in particular will help to guide the medical team in their determination of how nutritional support can safely be provided, and whether or not nonoral nutritional support or supplementary feeds are required in the short or long term. Ylvisaker and Logemann (1985) detailed four main options for nutritional support introduced to the dysphagic client, depending on ability. These include: nasogastric or gastrostomy feeds with swallowing therapy not involving food; nasogastric or gastrostomy feeding with swallowing intervention involving oral food trials; a combination of oral and tube feeding, systematically reducing nonoral supplementation as oral intake improves; and full oral intake, with some modifications (Ylvisaker & Logemann, 1985).

Although oral feeding is the optimal method of enteral nutrition, both nonoral enteral (via the gastrointestinal system) and parenteral (via the blood stream) feeding can provide adequate nutrition for critically injured patients. Total parenteral nutrition (TPN), is administered via specific veins, such as the superior vena cava, selected because of high blood flow rate. This form of nutritional support is typically used for patents with intestinal failure that prohibits ingesting nutrition via the gastrointestinal tract. In contrast, enteral feeding is used for patients who have a functional gastrointestinal tract, but are unable to maintain intake via the mouth. Enteral feeding is commonly accepted to be superior to parenteral feeding, because the use of the gastrointestinal tract is a more natural physiological way of providing nutrition, maximizing intestinal absorption and immune function, and providing nutrition not present in TPN (Akkersdijk, Roukema, & vd Werken, 1998; Ergun & Kahrilas, 1997). Enteral feeding is also significantly less expensive in comparison to parenteral feeds (Ergun & Kahrilas, 1997). As Borzotta et al. (1994) stated, TPN is typically recommended early postinjury due to gastric feeding intolerance (Ott, McClain & Young, 1989). However, recently it has been proposed that enteral nutrition, most commonly administered via nasogastric (NG) feeding or percutaneous endoscopic gastrostomy (PEG), may be successfully used in the early stages after head injury (Kirby et al., 1991). Enteral access distal to the stomach is often used for early nutritional intervention (Logemann, et al., 1994). For further discussion of enteral and parenteral feeding the reader is referred to Ergun and Kahrilas (1997).

Nasogastric tube feeding is frequently used for nutritional support for patients on admission to the intensive care unit (Kiel, 1994), and its use is often prolonged throughout the rehabilitation period as many patients tolerate it well (Annoni, Hubert, Frischknecht, & Uebelhart, 1998). It had been suggested, however, that the presence of a NG tube may delay therapy and aggravate swallowing dysfunction (Ciocon, Silverstone, Graver, & Foley, 1988). Annoni et al. (1998) described the NG tube as having negative effects on vocal fold, laryngeal, and pharyngeal function. Specifically, vocal cord paralysis and other deleterious effects, including damage to the whole pharyngeal and laryngeal complex and laryngeal inflammations, granulations, and muscle lesions have been found to occur from NG tube use (Ibuki, Ando, & Tanaka, 1994; Har-El & Balwally, 1995).

Aspiration pneumonia has been listed as an additional side effect from tube feedings (Norton et al., 1988), although incompetence of the lower esophageal sphincter in patients with brain injury also appears to contribute to this risk (Norton et al., 1988). From their review of the literature, Akkersdijk, et al. (1998) found that the risk of aspiration, frequently associated with NG feeding, has not been eliminated by choosing PEG placement (Burtch & Shatney, 1985; Ciocon et al., 1988; Fay, Poplausky, Gruber, & Lance, 1991). However, Parathyras and Kassak (1983) stated that using PEG, rather than NG feeds, may reduce the risk of overnight aspiration.

Along with the impact that tube feeding may have on the laryngeal and pharyngeal structures and the return to a normal diet, gastroesophageal reflux (GOR) is another common problem frequently associated with tube feeding. Gastroesophageal reflux often occurs in children with neurological disorders, including TBI, and may be more noticeable following placement of a gastrostomy tube in these patients (Ylvisaker & Weinstein, 1989). Ylivsaker and Weinstein (1989) stated that a developmental regression in feeding behavior may occur in young children following stress and prolonged duration of tube feedings.

Prognosis regarding the potential duration of nonoral feeding is a significant factor in the decision-making process to select the optimal nonoral feeding route (Arvedson & Lefton-Greif, 1998). In the literature to date, there has been a recent trend advocating the use of PEG over NG feeding for both the adult and the pediatric patient with brain injury with temporary to long-term nonoral nutritional needs. Akkersdijk, et al. (1998) acknowledged this change, reporting that nasogastric tubes are being replaced by PEG with increasing frequency to provide semi-long-term enteral nutrition because of the various advantages of PEG in daily use.

Winstein (1983) conducted a retrospective chart review of 55 dysphagic patients following head injury and found that 84% of the patients were managing oral intake at the time of discharge from the facility, and that subsequently 94% of patients had become functional oral feeders within 5 months postinjury. On the basis of this finding, she suggested that the prognosis for functional recovery within the first 5 months was good, and therefore may preclude the introduction of a more permanent feeding tube until after this initial period postinjury. In direct contrast to this statement, however, Winstein (1983) noted that clinical experience with the TBI population suggests that gastrostomy feeding and *not* nasogastric, actually facilitates more rapid progression to oral feeding. Winstein (1983) hypothesized that alleviation of the irritation of the NG tube, allowance for normal nasopharyngeal movement previously not permitted by the tube, and resolution of the pharyngeal dysethesia caused by the accommodation of the tube could account for such improvement.

If oral feeding is not possible or effective for longer periods of time, the PEG or Percutaneous Endoscopic Jejunostomy (PEJ) feeding tube is often used to avoid the deleterious effects of NG tube use. Annoni et al. (1998) examined the outcomes of replacing NG tube feeding with PEG in six patients with severe neurological impairment who required hospitalization for rehabilitation or supportive care for at least 1 year. The patients in the study had been receiving enteral feeding via NG for between 15 months and 4 years postimpairment. Annoni et al. (1998) stated that the PEG was performed in these patients for two reasons: to achieve full energy intake in the absence or ineffectiveness of oral feeding, and to allow better rehabilitation of oropharyngeal functions. The study revealed that three of the patients demonstrated improved swallowing/voicing following PEG placement (Annoni et al., 1998).

Aside from the fact that PEG feeding does not interfere with the swallowing mechanism, further advantages of the PEG procedure include allowing bolus feeds (allowing greater freedom for therapeutic rehabilitation), and the cosmetic advantage of the PEG, which can be worn invisibly underneath clothes (Akkersdijk, et al., 1998). Akkersdijk, et al. (1998) advocated a liberal use of PEG for patients with severe cerebral injury who do not recover within 14 days. However, these authors also acknowledged that PEG was associated with a number of risks including: 1 to 3% mortality rate, 3 to 9% major complication rate, and 5 to 45% minor complication rate (Akkersdijk et al, 1995; Bussone, Lalo, Piette, Hirsch, & Senecal, 1992; Larson, Burton, Schroeder, & DiMagno, 1987; Miller, Castlemain, Lacqua, & Kotler, 1989; Steffes, Weaver, & Bouwman, 1989; Stiegmann et al., 1990). For further information regarding NG and PEG feeding, we refer the reader to Wicks et al. (1992), Park et al. (1992), and Allison, Morris, Park, and Mills (1992).

As evidenced by the existing the literature, no particular type of alternative nutritional support method is optimal or without complications. Depending upon the individual presentation of the patient, both enteral and parenteral methods of support are necessary at certain times, in order to be compatible with the gastric functions and heightened energy needs of the TBI patient. However, the early evaluation of swallowing function and aspiration risk enables the earliest possible recommencement of oral diet (Logemann, et al., 1994; Mackay et al., 1992; Morgan, 1994; Mackay, 1994; Schwartz-Cowley, Swanson, Chapman, Kitik, & Mackay, 1994).

Rehabilitation Techniques and Treatment Programs for Dysphagia Following TBI

In the rehabilitation of the patient with TBI, the clinician must implement a range of therapeutic techniques in order to eliminate the risk of aspiration and remediate the physiological and cognitive issues compromising swallowing function and safety.

Intervention strategies, consisting of adjustments in diet or positioning, or elimination of foods can reduce the risk of aspiration and the potential for the development of aspiration pneumonia. In addition, an increasing array of treatment techniques designed to target the physiological impairments underlying the swallowing disorder have also been reported for the management of oropharyngeal dysphagia. These specific techniques and their application in the course of managing the patient with dysphagia following TBI will be outlined in the following sections.

Intervention Techniques for the Rehabilitation of Dysphagia

Logemann (1999) divided the range of available therapeutic strategies applied in dysphagia management into two distinct categories: (a) *compensatory* treatment techniques and (b) *therapy* techniques. Compensatory treatment procedures include those techniques that do not involve direct treatment of the swallowing disorder, and may not change the physiology of the swallow. Instead they eliminate the dysphagic symptoms and risk of aspiration by altering the way the food "flows" (Logemann, 1991; Logemann, 1999). Logemann (1999) noted that the various types of compensatory strategies include: (a) postural adjustments of the head, neck, and body to alter the dimensions of the pharynx and the direction of the flow of the bolus; (b) sensory stimulation techniques designed to increase sensory input either prior to or during the swallow; (c) altering consistency and viscosity of foods; (d) varying the volume and rate of presentation of the food/fluid; and (e) intraoral prosthetics (see Table 15-1).

In contrast to the compensatory techniques, the second group of strategies, the *therapy* techniques, are those techniques that are designed to change the swallow physiology (Logemann, 1999). These techniques include range-of-motion and bolus control tasks that are designed to improve neuromuscular control without actually swallowing. The therapy techniques also include swallowing maneuvers, which target specific aspects of the pharyngeal stage of the swallow. In an earlier paper, Logemann (1991) included medical and surgical management techniques under direct therapy techniques. These more extreme forms of intervention are typically only introduced once trials with more traditional behavioral treatment techniques have proven unsuccessful.

A compilation of the various therapy strategies that have been employed for patient groups presenting with oropharyngeal deficits, has been presented in Table 15-2. Unfortunately, the efficacy of a large majority of these techniques has not been demonstrated for the head-injured population. The present techniques, however, have been included here based on their prior application with other adult populations with neurogenic oropharyngeal dysphagia. Further research into the efficacy of these techniques with the TBI population is necessary, as "treatment without established efficacy may at best not be helpful and at worst may actually impede recovery" (Arvedson, 1983, p.368). Clinicians are therefore advised to be cautious and ensure the careful evaluation of each technique with individual patients. Specific procedures/instructions for the majority of the therapeutic strategies have been reported in detail in a number of existing publications (Groher, 1992; Linden, 1989; Logemann, 1983, 1991, 1993, 1997, 1999).

Table 15-1. Compensatory therapy strategies for managing the TBI patient with oropharyngeal dysphagia.

Therapy Strategy	Rationale	Deficit Targeted	References
(a) Postural Changes			
Tilting head forward, chin down	• Tongue base and epiglottis move back toward posterior pharyngeal wall • Widens vallecular space and narrows laryngeal entrance to prevent bolus entering airway, thereby reducing risk aspiration • Increases epiglottic angle to anterior tracheal wall	• Reduced tongue base to posterior wall contact • Delayed pharyngeal swallow • Reduced airway protection	Logemann (1993, 1997); Rasley et al. (1993); Shanahan, Logemann, Rademaker, Pauloski and Kahrilas (1993); Welch, Logemann, Rademaker, and Kahrilas (1993)
Head rotation	• Rotation moves cricoid cartilage away from posterior pharyngeal wall facilitating opening of the cricopharyngeal sphincter • Causes bolus to lateralize away from the direction of rotation and directs bolus down pharyngeal wall opposite to rotation	• Cricopharyngeal dysfunction • Unilateral oropharyngeal dysphagia	Logemann (1997); Logemann, Kahrilas, Korbara, and Vakil (1989); Rasley et al (1993)
Head rotation to damaged side with chin down	• Closes pyriform sinus on the that side • Leads to improved vocal fold approximation • Directs bolus away from impaired side to the stronger side, maximizing bolus transit down stronger side	• Unilateral vocal fold weakness • Unilateral pharyngeal paresis	Logemann (1993, 1997), Logemann et al. (1989)
Head tilt head to stronger side	• Directs bolus, by gravity, to the stronger side of the oral cavity and pharynx	• Unilateral oral and pharyngeal weakness on the same side	Logemann (1993, 1997); Rasley et al. (1993)

(continues)

Table 15-1. *(continued)*

Therapy Strategy	Rationale	Deficit Targeted	References
(a) Postural Changes			
Lying down on one side or on back	• Alters the effects of gravity on pharyngeal residue, forcing it to remain on the pharyngeal walls to prevent aspiration post swallow	• Patients who aspirate after the swallow—reduced pharyngeal contraction or laryngeal elevation leading to residue thoughout pharynx that is not cleared by successive swallows placing patient at risk of residue entering airway on inhalation postswallow	Logemann (1993, 1997); Rasley et al. (1993)
Tilting head backward/chin up	• Directs bolus, by gravity, into the pharynx, clearing the oral cavity • Improves speed of oral transit time	• Poor tongue control • Delayed oral transit, usually the result of inefficient posterior propulsion of the bolus by the tongue	Logemann (1993, 1997); Rasley et al. (1993)
(b) Sensory Stimulation Techniques			
Cold stimulation to base of anterior faucial arch	• Improves speed of triggering of the pharyngeal swallow, which continues for several successive swallows	• Delayed pharyngeal swallow	Lazzara, Lazarus, and Logemann (1986); Logemann (1991, 1993)
Pressure stimulation on delivery of bolus	• Additional pressure on the tongue with the back of the spoon on delivery of the bolus to heighten sensory awareness	• Reduced oral sensory awareness	Logemann (1991, 1993) Arvedson and Lefton-Greif (1998)

(continues)

Table 15-1. *(continued)*

Therapy Strategy	Rationale	Deficit Targeted	References
(b) Sensory Stimulation Techniques			
Altering bolus temperature (cold)	• Heightened sensory awareness of bolus	• Reduced sensory awareness of bolus	Bisch, Logemann, Rademaker, Kahrilas, and Lazarus (1994)
Altering taste of the bolus (sour)	• Heightened sensory awareness of bolus • Facilitates increased oral transit times • Reduces pharyngeal delay	• Reduced sensory awareness of bolus • Delayed oral transit • Pharyngeal delay	Dodds et al (1988); Lazzara et al. (1986); Lazarus et al. (1993); Logemann et al. (1995), O'Gara (1990)
Altering texture of bolus (smooth or textured)	• Either enhances or minimizes sensory feedback	• Reduced texture for hypersensitivity • Increased texture for hyposensitivity	Arvedson and Lefton-Greif (1998), O'Gara (1990)
(c) Altering Consistency and Viscosity			
Thickened liquids	• Bolus remains cohesive, transition through oral cavity is slowed	• Reduced lingual control and range of motion of the tongue • Delayed triggering of pharyngeal swallow • Reduced airway protection • Unilateral tongue and pharyngeal weakness on same side • Reduced oral awareness	Logemann (1993, 1997), O'Gara (1990)

(continues)

Table 15-1. (continued)

Therapy Strategy	Rationale	Deficit Targeted	References
(c) Altering Consistency and Viscosity			
Thin liquids	• Transit easily through oral cavity to pharynx	• Reduced tongue strength • Reduced tongue to posterior wall contact (in the presence of adequate protection of airway) • Severe pharyngeal dysfunction—reduced pharyngeal wall contraction • Reduced posterior propulsion of the bolus by the tongue • Cricopharyngeal dysfunction	Logemann (1997), O'Gara (1990)
Vitamized/puree consistencies	• Require minimal to no mastication • Remain as a cohesive bolus • Have reduced oral transit times compared to liquids	• Reduced laryngeal closure • Reduced laryngeal elevation • Reduced lingual control, strength, and posterior propulsion • Impaired chewing • Pharyngeal dysfunction • Cricopharyngeal dysfunction	Dantas, Dodds, Massey, and Kern (1989), Dantas et al. (1990), Logemann (1993), O'Gara (1990)
Soft foods (with gravy/sauce)	• Require reduced mastication • Remain as a cohesive bolus • Moisture content facilitates movement through oral cavity	• Impaired chewing ability • Reduced lingual control, range of motion, and coordination • Delayed pharyngeal swallow • Reduced airway protection	O'Gara (1990)

(continues)

Table 15-1. (continued)

Therapy Strategy	Rationale	Deficit Targeted	References
(d) Varying Volume and Rate			
Altering bolus volume (increase)	• Heightens sensory awareness of bolus • Prolongs pharyngeal reconfiguration from a respiratory to a deglutitive pathway • Facilitates pharyngeal transit times • Increases laryngeal closure and cricopharyngeal opening durations • Decreases duration of tongue base to posterior wall contact	• Reduced sensory awareness • Incoordinated swallow • Delayed pharyngeal swallow	Bisch et al. (1994); Kahrilas, Lin, Chen, and Logemann (1996); Kahrilas and Logemann (1993); Lazarus et al. (1993)
Multiple swallows per bolus	• Facilitates clearance of residue • Slows rate of intake	• Residue in the valleculae, pyriform fossa, and/or pharynx	Logemann (1991)
Washing food through pharynx	• Facilitates clearance of residual material from pharynx • Slows rate of intake • Also improves intraoral hydration	• Excessive residue in pharynx postswallow	Logemann (1993)
Altering rate of presentation including—additional techniques: (a) reducing bolus size per mouthful, (b) pausing for vocalization between each mouthful, (c) checking the mouth after each swallow, (d) pacing the meal by placing portions out of reach or sight, (e) double swallow and cough after each swallow	• Assists clearance of any oral or pharyngeal residue • Reduces risk of overloading to unsafe oral or pharyngeal volumes	• Oral and pharyngeal residue • Inability to maintain safe swallowing with larger bolus sizes	Arvedson (1993), Rowe (1999), Tippett, Palmer and Linden (1987, Ylvisaker and Logemann (1985)

(continues)

Table 15-1. (continued)

Therapy Strategy	Rationale	Deficit Targeted	References
(e) Intraoral Prosthetics			
Palatal drop prosthesis	• Intraoral prosthetic devices can be used to improve tongue to palate contact and enhance the effect of tongue movement to facilitate oropharyngeal forces on the bolus during the swallow	• Significantly reduced tongue to palate contact • Bilateral hypoglossal paralysis	Logemann (1991, 1993, 1999)
Palatal lift prosthesis	• Interoral prosthetic device used to improve velopharyngeal closure, facilitate oropharyngeal forces on the bolus during the swallow, and minimize nasal regurgitation	• Moderate to severely compromised velopharyngeal closure during the swallow • Palatal paralysis	Logemann (1991, 1993, 1999)

Table 15-2. Therapy procedures with application for the TBI population with oropharyngeal dysphagia.

Therapy Strategy	Rationale	Deficit Targeted	References
(a) Resistance, range-of-motion, and bolus control exercises			
Range of motion, resistance and coordination exercises for lips, tongue and jaw	• Targeting improved oromotor function relative to swallowing	• Impaired function of the lips, tongue or jaw • Reduced coordination of oromotor components during chewing/swallowing	Huckabee and Cannito (1999), Logemann (1991), Ylvisaker and Logemann (1985)
Chewing exercises	• Improved jaw strength and movement for chewing	• Jaw weakness • Rapid fatigue on chewed boluses	Logemann (1991), Ylvisaker and Logemann (1985)
Manipulation of objects in the mouth	• Facilitates improved bolus control	• Poor oral control/tongue control of bolus • Reduced ability to formulate a cohesive bolus	Logemann (1991), Ylvisaker and Logemann (1985)
Vocal fold adduction exercises	• Improve vocal fold adduction and airway protection	• Impaired laryngeal adduction	Huckabee and Cannito (1999), Logemann (1991), Ylvisaker and Logemann (1985)
(b) Swallowing Maneuvers			
Supraglottic swallow	• Facilitates closure of the true vocal folds both before and during the swallow to prevent penetration	• Delayed pharyngeal reflex • Laryngeal compromise or damage leading to late or incomplete vocal fold closure	Logemann (1983, 1991, 1993); Martin, Logemann, Shaker, and Dodds (1993); Ohmae, Logemann, Kaiser, Hanson, Kahrilas (1996)

(continues)

Table 15-2. (*continued*)

Therapy Strategy	Rationale	Deficit Targeted	References
(b) Swallowing Maneuvers			
Extended supraglottic swallow, "dump and swallow"	• Facilitates oral transit of the bolus while still protecting airway	• Severe reductions in tongue mobility	Logemann (1993)
Super-supraglottic swallow	• Tilts arytenoid cartilage anteriorly to base of epiglottis to close airway before and during the swallow to prevent penetration • Produces earlier cricopharyngeal opening • Alters extent of vertical laryngeal position before swallow	• Delayed pharyngeal reflex • Laryngeal compromise or damage leading to reduced closure of airway • Delayed cricopharyngeal opening • Reduced laryngeal elevation	Martin et al. (1993); Logemann (1991, 1993); Ohmae et al. (1996)
Mendelsohn maneuver	• Extends and prolongs laryngeal elevation during the swallow • Indirectly results in prolonged cricopharyhgeal opening • Technique also assists in normalizing timing of pharyngeal events during the swallow	• Reduced hyolaryngeal movement • Reduced cricopharyngeal sphincter opening • Pooling of food/fluids in pyriform sinus • Impaired bolus transport into cervical esophagus • Weakened or discoordinated pharyngeal contraction	Cook et al. (1989); Huckabee and Cannito (1999); Jacob, Kahrilas, Logemann, Shah, and Ha (1989); Kahrilas, Logemann, Krugler, and Flanagan (1991); Lazarus, Logemann and Gibbons (1993); Logemann (1991, 1993); Logemann and Kahrilas (1990)
Effortful swallow (modified valsalva)	• Improves tongue base movement posteriorly. This action generates increased pressure to improve clearance of the bolus from the oral and pharyngeal regions	• Reduced posterior movement of tongue base • Weakened or discoordinated pharyngeal contraction • Reduced laryngeal excursion resulting in pharyngeal residue	Huckabee and Cannito (1999); Kahrilas, Lin, Logemann, Ergun, and Facchini (1993); Kahrilas, Logemann, Lin and Ergun (1992); Logemann (1991, 1993)

(*continues*)

Table 15-2. *(continued)*

Therapy Strategy	Rationale	Deficit Targeted	References
(b) Swallowing Maneuvers			
Head-lifting maneuver	• Facilitates improved upper esophageal sphincter opening	• Impaired upper esophageal sphincter opening resulting in post swallow residue in pyriform sinus	Huckabee and Cannito (1999); Shaker, Kern, Bardan, Arndorfer, et al. (1997); Shaker, Kern, Bardan, Taylor, et al. (1997).
Masako (tongue-holding) maneuver	• Increases anterior bulging of posterior pharyngeal wall • Develops improved posterior pharyngeal wall adduction to tongue base	• Reduced tongue base to posterior pharyngeal wall contact	Fujiu and Logemann (1996)
(c) Medical & Surgical Management			
Reduction of saliva production	• Various medications designed for alternate purposes such as managing depression (e.g., the tricyclic group of drugs), anxiety, as well as antihistamines and bronchodilators, are associated with decreased saliva production and may be tried under strict medical supervision to reduce excessive secretions (Caution—introduction of some medications may be contraindicated in some patients)	• Patients with excessive secretions, leading to poor saliva and secretion management	Dikeman and Kazandjian (1995)

(continues)

Table 15-2. (continued)

Therapy Strategy	Rationale	Deficit Targeted	References
(c) Medical & Surgical Management			
Facilitation of improved saliva production	• Elimination or alteration of various medications associated with reduced saliva production as side effects e.g., antihistamines, decongestants, sedatives and antidepressants	• Insufficient saliva • thick saliva • difficulty managing and clearing oral intake due to poor oral lubrication	Dikeman and Kazandjian (1995)
Vocal Fold Injection (teflon, absorbable gelatin sponge)	• Moves the paralyzed cord to the median position to facilitate improved laryngeal adduction	• Unilateral vocal fold weakness	Workman, Pillsbury, and Hulka (1997)
Cricopharyngeal myotomy	• Division of cricopharyngeal muscle fibers to improve opening of the cricopharyngeal sphincter	• Premature contraction or spasm of the cricopharyngeus	Workman et al. (1997)
Permanent tracheostomy	• Cuffed tracheostomy tube minimizes risk of aspiration	• Recurrent aspiration • Aspiration of oral secretions	Workman et al. (1997)
Laryngeal closure	• Surgical closure of larynx prevents aspiration. Can be reversed following significant neurological change	• Recurrent aspiration • Aspiration of oral secretions	Sasaki et al. (1980); Workman et al. (1997)

In the management of the pediatric TBI patient, a number of the direct therapy techniques outlined in Tables 15-1 and 15-2 may have limited application, because of the cognitive requirements necessary to understand the instructions and apply the techniques (Arvedson, 1993). In addition, some specific techniques such as the chin tuck maneuver, which can be used with adults and older children, is actually contraindicated in young infants, as this position may lead to pharyngeal collapse, increasing the probability of an apnoeic event (Arvedson & Lefton-Greif, 1998). Application of compensatory techniques, however, such as positioning, method of food presentation, and altering food textures, has been suggested for use with the pediatric population (Arvedson, 1993; Arvedson & Lefton-Greif, 1998). However, as in the adult TBI population, no research data have yet been presented to substantiate these recommendations.

Arvedson and Lefton-Greif (1998) advised that pediatric dysphagic patients are likely to respond in a similar manner to the adult population to increases of bolus volume. Changes in bolus texture and viscosity can also be manipulated to facilitate improved oromotor control and safe swallowing (Arvedson & Lefton-Greif, 1998; Ylvisaker & Logemann, 1985). Similarly alteration of taste and temperature of the bolus may also be applicable with children, with chilled temperatures having been reported to improve pharyngeal phase timing in infants (Wolf & Glass, 1992). For some pediatric patients, however, the use of cold temperatures and strong flavors may be aversive (Arvedson & Lefton-Greif, 1998). Similarly thermal stimulation techniques should also be introduced with caution to the pediatric patient since they may frighten the young child (Arvedson, 1993). Employing adaptive equipment and utensils to deliver the bolus may also be useful for pediatric patients with oral phase deficits (Arvedson & Lefton-Greif, 1998).

Indirect treatment techniques that target the physiological functioning of the oromotor system can also be applied with the pediatric population where patient compliance is possible (Alexander, 1987; Arvedson & Lefton-Greif, 1998; Morris & Klein, 1987; Ylvisaker & Logemann, 1985). In addition, therapeutic techniques that improve awareness and alertness, normalize muscle tone, improve head and neck control, and increase appropriate responses to sensory stimulation are also recommended (Arvedson, 1993; Ylvisaker & Logemann, 1985). Arvedson (1993) advised a cautious approach with children in the early stages of recovery from head injury. The authors noted that the goal of therapy should be to achieve a pleasurable experience for the child, ideally without the use of forced or invasive intervention strategies (Arvedson & Lefton-Greif, 1998; Arvedson, 1993; Ylvisaker & Logemann, 1985). Where oral feeding needs to be forced in order to meet the nutritional needs of the child, supplementary nutrition, such as tube feeding, should be considered as an option to prevent the establishment of negative routines during mealtimes, which may lead to further food refusal. Altered feeding routines can be used to maximize the child's appetite and interest in oral intake (Arvedson & Lefton-Greif, 1998).

In both the adult and pediatric populations, the initial stage of dysphagia intervention in the acute care setting, may be further complicated by the presence of a tracheostomy tube (complications resulting from the presence of a tracheostomy tube have been discussed in detail in the previous chapter). Techniques such as digital occlusion of the tracheostomy, however, may improve swallowing ability and eliminate aspiration in some patients (Logemann, Pauloski & Colangelo, 1998). Research has shown that with the tracheostomy tube occluded, duration of base of tongue contact to posterior pharyngeal wall is reduced, maximal laryngeal elevation is increased, laryngeal and hyoid elevation is increased at the time of initial cricopharyngeal opening, and the onset of anterior movement of the posterior pharyngeal wall relative to the onset of cricopharyngeal opening is delayed (Logemann et al., 1998). The patients in a study by Logemann et al. (1998) had undergone head and neck surgery, and presented with differential responses to the application of digital occlusion. It is possible, however, that light digital occlusion may facilitate improved swallowing and airway protection in other patient groups. However, considering that the patients in the Logermann et al. (1998) study demonstrated differential responses to digital occlusion, the benefits of this technique for any patient should be examined during videofluoroscopy.

Rehabilitation Programs for Dysphagic TBI patients

Determining which of the various therapeutic strategies to introduce with each patient is dependent on the nature of the presenting swallowing impairment and the patient's ability to participate in active therapeutic programs. Logemann (1999) distinguishes between different types of treatment programs for dysphagia, classifying them as either a direct or an indirect rehabilitation program. Indirect therapy, is the use of therapy techniques (mentioned in the previous section) completed without the ingestion of any food or liquid. This type of therapy is necessary for patients who aspirate on all food and fluid consistencies and cannot safely undergo oral trials. Direct therapy, in contrast, involves completing the maneuvers or techniques with varying amounts of food or fluid. This stage is only introduced once the patient is able to swallow small amounts of oral intake without aspiration (Logemann, 1999).

Winstein (1983) commented on the use of three different types of rehabilitation programs with dysphagic patients following head injury, depending on the status of swallowing function on admission to therapy. The first of these programs was referred to as a nonfeeding program, designed as a stimulation program for very low-level patients, in preparation for later feeding. This program was described as encompassing desensitization techniques, such as stroking, and applying pressure or stretching, to facilitate normal swallowing, sucking and interoral responses. The second was a facilitation and feeding program, used to facilitate normal feeding patterns using a small amount of puree consistency food. The third program reported was classified as a progressive feeding program, in which specialized techniques (not detailed by the author) were used to help the patient build swallowing endurance by systematically increasing the amount of oral intake. This progressive feeding program was continued until the patient could manage a whole meal within half an hour without any difficulties (Winstein, 1983).

The article by Winstein (1983) highlighted the issue that dysphagia intervention programs for the TBI patient can be undertaken at all stages of the rehabilitation process regardless of the functional swallowing status of the patient. While it is recognized that there is no benefit in introducing oral feedings when this may place the patient at risk, many authors (Arvedson and Lefton-Greif, 1998; Winstein, 1983; Ylvisaker & Logemann, 1985) strongly support the aggressive early introduction of indirect treatment strategies designed to improve neuromotor function for swallowing. Arvedson and Lefton-Greif (1998) noted the importance of non-nutritive oral-motor programs for those children who receive nutritional intake though nonoral feeding. They suggested the use of techniques such as stroking, stretching, brushing, icing, taping, and vibrating areas of the face and mouth to provide pleasurable oral experiences for these patients and to allow normalization of oral-motor function to whatever degree is possible with these patients (Arvedson & Lefton-Greif, 1998).

To date, there is little reported evidence of the efficacy of dysphagia therapy programs for patients following TBI. Schurr et al. (1999) detailed the various therapeutic modifications introduced with a subgroup of 13 patients with TBI identified as aspirating on videofluroscopic study. In their article they tabulate the various compensatory strategies (diet modification, postural adjustments, and head flexion) introduced to prevent aspiration in each of the 13 cases. Each of the cases also underwent dysphagia therapy; however, the exact details of the therapeutic interventions were not stated. They found that dysphagia therapy, involving dietary, postural, and behavioral modifications, facilitated the return to oral intake in 20 of 24 patients (83%) from their total subject group.

Crary (1995) reported efficacy data on an intervention program conducted with six patients with chronic, severe dysphagia following brainstem stroke. While this population differs from the TBI population in its etiology, aspects of the oropharyngeal swallowing disorder of this patient group are not unlike the physiological deficits identified following TBI, and therefore the results of the study will be discussed in detail. The aim of the program reported by Crary (1995) was to increase the duration and strength of the pharyngeal aspects of swallowing and to improve swallow coordination. All patients were between 5 and 54 months postonset, received all nutrition via gastrostomy tubes, and no patient was able to manage their own saliva at onset of intervention. Videofluroscopic examinations of swallowing in all patients revealed a characteristic pattern of: delayed initiation of the pharyngeal response, reduced duration and extent of hyolaryngeal elevation, reduced and asymmetric pharyngeal contraction, limited opening of the cricopharyngeal sphincter, temporal incoordination of the oral and pharyngeal components, residue in the valleculae and piriform recesses, and aspiration. The swallowing program designed for this group consisted of the use of techniques, including protective head postures where required, with surface electromyography (SEMG) to provide biofeedback of the strength of the pharyngeal response.

The majority of patients reported by Crary (1995) were seen on a daily basis for 3 weeks with three additional daily home practice sessions each day, although some patients received variable treatment schedules (daily, varied, biweekly, monthly) and treatment durations (two patients received 2 months and 7 months of therapy, respectively). Following intervention, changes in swallowing physiology were observed with improved swallowing coordination, longer duration, and increased effort noted. Functionally, at the end of 3 weeks, three patients returned to full oral intake (defined as foods ranging from thin liquids to solids requiring mastication). By the end of each individual treatment program, five of the six patients were able to resume full oral intake and had their gastrostomies removed. The sixth patient resumed limited oral intake, however, continued to require supplemental feeding. These results were maintained up to 2 years posttherapy.

Huckabee and Cannito (1999) reported similar success with an intensive, structured swallowing treatment program, referred to as the Outpatient Accelerated Swallowing Treatment program (Huckabee & Cannito, 1999). They presented data on a group of 10 patients with chronic (at least 8 months postonset, range 8 to 84 months) dysphagia following brainstem infarct, who underwent an intensive block of 10 hours of therapy in a week. This therapy targeted physiological impairments, and again incorporated techniques such as SEMG and cervical auscultation as tools to provide the patient with biofeedback of swallowing maneuvers.

In the intensive therapy program, patients underwent 2 hours of therapy, one in the morning, one in the afternoon, each day for a period of 5 days. Following the intensive treatment, patients were referred for follow-up treatment, however only 3 of the 10 patients continued formal therapy. All reported continuing their rehabilitation exercises at home. Although the rehabilitative exercises used in the intensive therapy program differed slightly for each client, they included: effortful or valsalva swallow, the Mendelsohn maneuver, the Masako maneuver, and head-lifting maneuvers. All were conducted with simultaneous SEMG or auditory feedback as well as oromotor exercises and vocal adduction exercises. Frequent repetition and multiple trials of each technique were conducted. Oral intake trials were introduced for each client to heighten neurosensory stimulation and increase relevance for the patient. Each therapy session included a combination of direct rehabilitative techniques and compensatory management of oral feeding trials delivered in alternating, intensive, 15-minute blocks.

Prior to the treatment program, all patients were on nonoral diets. Following the intensive treatment program, statistically significant improvements in swallowing physiology, functional diet status, and pulmonary status were observed and were maintained up to 12 months posttreatment. 8 of the 10 patients returned to full oral feeding, with termination of gastrostomy feeding on an average of 5.3 months following treatment (range 1 to 12 months; Huckabee & Cannito, 1999).

The results of these two studies (Crary, 1995; Huckabee & Cannito, 1999) raise a number of important issues for the management of patients with dysphagia following TBI. First, this work validates the introduction of intensive therapy programs for patients with dysphagia, even those who are long term postinjury, presenting with chronic dysphagic symptoms, and unable to manage oral intake. Huckabee and Cannito (1999) noted that the severity of the swallowing disorder does not necessarily predict the outcome of intervention. However, in traditional clinical management of chronic dysphagic patients, there has been a tendency to discharge these patients from therapy services with limited long-term follow-up or intervention. In light of the significant changes reported in both Crary and Huckabee and Cannito's patient groups, there is now preliminary evidence to support trials of short-term (1 to 3 weeks) periods of intensive therapy, even with patients with chronic, severe long-term swallowing disorders.

The second major issue raised by these efficacy studies is the importance of designing dysphagia therapy programs that target the underlying physiological swallowing deficit. Both programs focused on altering the physiology of the swallow, not simply on providing compensatory techniques to minimize the risk of aspiration. The outcome of this intervention was that the majority of patients in both studies were able to resume oral intake. It is important to note that, although the use of compensatory strategies may result in immediate changes in swallowing safety and reduce the risk of aspiration, they are only compensatory adjustments and as such provide only a transient approach to the underlying physiological deficit (Huckabee & Cannito, 1999; Logemann, 1993). In order to achieve long-term changes in swallowing physiology, rehabilitative exercises must be targeted in combination with such compensatory techniques. Regular reassessment of swallow physiology should provide the clinician with information on when compensatory strategies are no longer required (Logemann, 1993).

A third issue, is the incorporation of biofeedback techniques to maximize intervention. Biofeedback has been defined as "a process of transducing some physiologic variable, transforming the signal to extract useful information, and displaying that information to the subject in a format that will facilitate learning to regulate the physiological variable" (Rubow, 1984, p. 207). The use of SEMG in these studies has served as the instrumental technique through which immediate feedback regarding the patient's physiological performance on various swallowing maneuvers has been provided. Huckabee and Cannito (1999) discussed at length the possible models of motor learning that may be introduced to facilitate the rehabilitative process. Biofeedback therapy techniques rely on continuous closed-loop learning processes, requiring continuous and immediate reinforcement (Rubow, 1984), which enables the patient to learn to exert control over a physiological process (Prosek, Montgomery, Walden, & Schwartz, 1978). It is possible then, that the incorporation of biofeedback techniques into the treatment programs of these patients may be enhancing the patients ability to gain control over physiological aspects of their swallow, and in doing so be maximizing the rehabilitative process for the patient.

A final key element raised by Crary (1995) and Huckabee and Cannito's (1999) treatment programs, is the use of short-term, intensive programs maximizing repeated daily practice, and intensive repetitions of swallowing maneuvers within the session. The issue of high-intensity therapy was highlighted earlier by Ylvisaker and Logemann (1985), who stated that it was preferable that the clinician administer several short 10 to 15 minute swallowing therapy sessions per day than one or two extended sessions. In addition, with patients who can complete therapeutic exercises independently, Ylvisaker and Logemann (1985) recommend completing the exercises at least five times each day. Unfortunately in busy clinical settings this aspect of therapeutic management often becomes compromised. In other areas of speech pathology management, treatment programs that target high-intensity, repeated, daily practice have supported the fact that this treatment model can result in significant change in the physiological functioning of the motor components targeted (Ramig, Countryman, Thompson, & Horii, 1995; Ward, Theodoros, Murdoch, & Silburn, in press). It is, therefore, possible that the intensive nature of the therapeutic intervention is an additional factor contributing to the positive outcomes reported by Crary (1995) and Huckabee and Cannito (1999).

At present, however, there is insufficient evidence to confirm whether or not the change observed in the dysphagic patients reported in the two studies (Crary, 1995; Huckabee & Cannito, 1999) is the result of the incorporation of biofeedback techniques, the use of intensive therapy models, or a combination of both elements. Another factor that has been suggested as potentially contributing to the positive outcomes observed, is the timing of the therapy service. Crary (1995) suggested that perhaps therapy programs that demand high degrees of patient interaction may work best once a certain amount of poststroke recovery has been achieved. Huckabee and Cannito (1999) stressed the need for further prospective randomized treatment studies to determine which elements (i.e., biofeedback, intensive treatment, stage of intervention, or combinations of these factors) are required in designing "optimal" treatment programs for dysphagic patients.

Finally, with the introduction of any form of swallowing intervention program, the importance of involving family members, along with the patient in the process of goal setting and daily therapy, cannot be overemphasized. Where cognitive and behavioral issues compound the difficulties of ensuring safe oral intake, educating family members about the nature of the patients swallowing difficulties and teaching them strategies to counteract these difficulties during mealtimes can facilitate the rehabilitative process. Where possible, education of the family/caregiver can be enhanced with clear explanations using videofluroscopic recordings (Ylvisaker & Logemann, 1985). Particularly for the families of the pediatric TBI patient, where strong emotional and nurturing feelings may be attached to the process of feeding their child, sensitive and comprehensive education is required at each stage of the rehabilitation process to gain the families' acceptance and continued support of the modified nutritional program (Ylvisaker & Logemann, 1985).

Managing the Cognitive and Behavioral Deficits of Dysphagic TBI Patients

In addition to implementing treatment strategies targeting the physiological basis of the swallowing impairment, the presence of cognitive deficits, affecting safe swallowing need to be addressed in the TBI population. It is recognized that coexisting cognitive and communicative deficits may, in some cases, influence the type of management program and its functional outcomes more than the extent of physiological impairment in the swallowing mechanism (Cherney & Halper, 1989; Mackay et al., 1999b; Halper et al., 1999). The existence of cognitive deficits may limit the application of various techniques in the process of rehabilitation. Training a patient to employ compensatory strategies and incorporate them into their mealtime routines requires a level of cognitive function in areas such as attention, concentration, and memory, which frequently are compromised after head injury (Tippett, Palmer & Linden, 1987). In addition, ability for new learning may also be depressed following head injury, further complicating the introduction and learning of various rehabilitative techniques (Ylvisaker & Logemann, 1985). Ylvisaker and Logemann (1985) outlined the need to consider the environment, the patient's behavior and judgment, as well as his/her ability to learn new skills when managing the patient with cognitive impairments.

Halper et al. (1999) discussed two case studies of TBI patients in which details on the process of swallowing rehabilitation were noted. The first case presented with severe dysphagia and moderately severe cognitive-communicative deficits. The rehabilitative process for this patient involved an oral feeding program with compensatory strategies (modified consistencies, quiet environment, multiple swallows) and simultaneous therapy targeting improving memory, attention, and reasoning. The authors reported concomitant improvements in chewing and swallowing, with improvements in cognitive state. In the second case, the patient presented with a similar pattern of severe dysphagia and moderately severe cognitive-communicative function as that reported for case one. For this case, some improvements in swallowing function were noted following intervention; however, the patient continued to present with moderately severe cognitive deficits. Because of his continued cognitive impairments, he required individual supervision for all oral intake to ensure safe swallowing. The authors concluded that the patient's potential for functional feeding was limited by the cognitive impairments.

Tippet et al. (1987) reported on the management of a single head-injured patient whose cognitive and language impairments complicated dysphagia management. In particular the patient had deficient attention skills, impaired short-term memory, impulsivity, faulty verbal reasoning, and poor abstract thinking, which were contraindicating safe feeding and swallowing. The authors used a combination of processes to address the cognitive factors affecting swallowing function including: behavioral modification techniques such as modeling and verbal cues to reinforce behaviors, including a reduced rate of oral intake, reduced bolus size, and the use of multiple swallows and throat clearing; introducing a structured environment by maintaining staff consistency and reducing distractions in the room and on the food tray; enforcing patient supervision while feeding to encourage monitoring and feedback on behaviors; the use of clear explanations; and family education and involvement to facilitate their understanding and reinforce adherence to dietary recommendations. In the months postinjury, the patient was also encouraged to keep a journal of appropriate dietary consistencies, which could be reviewed by the individual to assist in making safe food choices in environments outside the hospital room, e.g., the hospital cafeteria. This process was introduced to help in the generalization of dietary modifications to other external situations (Tippett et al., 1987).

Avery-Smith and Dellarosa (1994) outlined the various subskills that influence swallowing ability in the TBI population including: alertness and orientation, cognitive behaviors and behavioral dysregulation, positioning and proximal control, self-feeding; oral and pharyngeal sensory disorders, and the physiological impairments (oral and pharyngeal movement disorders). From a range of literature detailing potential strategies employed to improve deficits in any of these areas, the authors identified various techniques that may have application for the brain-injured patient under each of these specific subskills. As yet, however, limited information exists regarding the exact effects of these subskill deficits on swallowing, the prevalence of each with various injury types, how they change in response to intervention, how progress of changes in the subskills affects patient outcome, and the nature of spontaneous recovery in these subskills. Avery-Smith and Dellarosa (1994) stated that such information would lead to the formation of a clinical model for treatment, incorporating the relevant subskills for the dysphagic TBI patient. A significant amount of research has yet to be done to achieve the formulation of such a model.

Summary

It has long been recognized that the literature on the rehabilitation of the dysphagic patient is lacking in efficacy research data (Langmore, 1995; Rosenbek, 1995). This fact remains true for the TBI population. While some efficacy data on the use of specific therapeutic strategies and treatment programs for improving aspects of swallow physiology and oropharyngeal dysphagia have recently been reported, the utility of the application of these techniques and programs with the TBI patient has yet to be determined. Additional research is needed in the area of prognostic indicators and short- and long-term swallowing outcomes for both the adult and pediatric TBI populations. Once again, while some researchers have started to investigate these issues in the adult TBI population, there continues to be a paucity of information on prognostic indicators, intervention programs, and outcomes for the pediatric TBI patient. For both the adult and pediatric TBI patient, dysphagia rehabilitation is a complex issue in which nutritional factors, physiological deficits, cognitive/behavioral impairments and quality-of-life issues must guide each stage of the rehabilitative process to produce the optimal outcome for each individual.

References

Akkersdijk, W.L., van Bergeijk, J.D., & van Egmond, T., Mulder, C.J.J., Henegouwen, G.P.V., Vanderwerken, C., and Vanerpecum, K.J. (1995). Percutaneous endoscopic gastrostomy (PEG): Comparison of push and pull methods and evaluation of antibiotic prophylaxis. *Endoscopy, 27*, 313–316.

Akkersdijk, W.L., Roukema, J.A., & vd Werken, C. (1998). Percutaneous endoscopic gastrostomy for patients with severe cerebral injury. *Injury, 29(1)*, 11–14.

Alexander, R.P. (1987). Oral-motor treatment for infants and young children with cerebral palsy. *Seminars in Speech and Language, 8*, 87–100.

Allison, M.C., Morris, A.J., Park, R.H., & Mills, P.R. (1992). Percutaneous endoscopic gastrostomy tube feeding may improve outcome of late rehabilitation following stroke. *Journal of the Royal Society of Medicine, 85*, 147–149.

Annoni, J.M., Hubert, V., Frischknecht, R., & Uebelhart, D. (1998). Percutaneous endoscopic gastrostomy in neurological rehabilitation: A report of six cases. *Disability and Rehabilitation, 20(8)*, 308–314.

Arvedson, J. (1993). Management of swallowing problems. In J.C. Arvedson & L. Brodsky (Eds.), *Pediatric Swallowing and Feeding: Assessment and Management.* (p. 327–387). San Diego: Singular Publishing.

Arvedson, J. & Lefton-Greif, M. (1998). *Pediatric Videofluoroscopic Swallow Studies: A Professional Manual with Caregiver Guidelines.* San Antonio, Texas: Communication Skill Builders/Psychological Corporation.

Avery-Smith, W. & Dellarosa, D.M. (1994). Approaches to treating dysphagia in patients with brain injury. *The American Journal of Occupational Therapy, 48(3)*, 235–239.

Bisch, E.M., Logemann, J.A., Rademaker, A.W., Kahrilas, P.J., & Lazarus, C.L. (1994). Pharyngeal effects of bolus volume, viscosity, and temperature in patients with dysphagia resulting from neurologic impairment and in normal subjects. *Journal of Speech and Hearing Research, 37(5)*, 1041–1059.

Borzotta, A.P., Pennings, J., Papasadero, B., Paxton, J., Mardesic, S., Borzotta, R., Parrott, A., & Bledsoe, F. (1994). Enteral versus parenteral nutrition after severe closed head injury. *The Journal of Trauma, 37(3)*, 459–468.

Brooke, M.M. & Barbour, P.G. (1986). Assessment of nutritional status during rehabilitation after brain injury. *Archives of Physical Medicine and Rehabilitation, 67(9)*, 634–634.

Burtch, G.D. & Shatney, C.H. (1985). Feeding gastrostomy. Assistant or assassin? *The American Surgeon, 51*, 204–207.

Bussone, M., Lalo, M., Piette, F., Hirsch, J.F., & Senecal, P. (1992). Percutaneous endoscopic gastrostostomy: Its value in assisted alimentation in malnutrition in elderly patients: Apropos of 101 consecutive cases in patients over 70 years of age. *Annales de Chirurgie, 46(1)*, 59–66.

Cherney, L.R. & Halper, A.S. (1989). Recovery of oral nutrition after head injury in adults. *Journal of Head Trauma Rehabilitation, 4*, 42–50.

Cherney, L.R., & Halper, A.S. (1996). Swallowing problems in adults with traumatic brain injury. *Seminars in Neurology, 16(4)*, 349–353.

Ciocon, J.O., Silverstone, F.A., Graver, L.M., & Foley, C.J. (1988). Tube feedings in elderly patients: Indications, benefits and complications. *Archives of Internal Medicine, 148(2)*, 429–433.

Cook, I.J., Dodds, W.J., Dantas, R.O., Massey, B., Kern, M.K., Lang, I.M., Brasseur, J.G., & Hogan, W.J. (1989). Opening mechanism of the human upper esophageal sphincter. *American Journal of Physiology, 257*, G748–G759.

Cope, N. & Hall, K.H. (1982). Head injury rehabilitation: Benefit of early intervention. *Archives of Physical and Medical Rehabilitation, 63*, 433–437.

Crary, M. (1995). A direct intervention program for chronic neurogenic dysphagia secondary to brainstem stroke. *Dysphagia, 10*, 6–18.

Dantas, R.O., Dodds, W.J., Massey, B.T., & Kern, M.K. (1989). The effect of high vs. low density barium preparations on the quantitative features of swallowing. *American Journal of Radiology, 153*, 1191–1195.

Dantas, R.O., Kern, M.K., Massey, B.T., Dodds, W.J., Kahrilas, P.J., Brasseur, J.G., Cook, I.J., & Lang, I.M. (1990). Effect of swallowed bolus variables on oral and pharyngeal phases of swallowing. *American Journal of Physiology, 258 (Gastrointestinal and Liver Physiology)*, G675–G681.

Dikeman, K.J. & Kazandjian, M.S. (1995). *Communication and Swallowing Management of Tracheostomized and Ventilator-Dependent Adults*. San Diego: Singular Publishing.

Dodds, W.J., Man, K.M., Cook, I.J., Kahrilas, P.J., Stewart, E.T., & Kern, M.K. (1988). Influence of bolus volume on swallow-induced hyoid movement in normal subjects. *American Journal of Roentgenology, 150*, 1307–1309.

Ergun, G.A., & Kahrilas, P.J. (1997). Medical and surgical treatment interventions in deglutitive dysfunction. In A.L. Perlman and K. Schulze-Delrieu (Eds.), *Deglutition and Its Disorders, Anatomy, Physiology, Clinical Diagnosis and Management.* (pp. 463–490), San Diego: Singular Publishing.

Fay, D.E., Poplausky, M., Gruber, M., & Lance, P. (1991). Long term enteral feeding: A retrospective comparison of delivery via percutaneous endoscopic gastrostomy and nasoenteric tubes. *American Journal of Gastroenterology, 86(11)*, 1604–1609.

Field, L.H. & Weiss, C.J. (1989). Dysphagia with head injury. *Brain Injury, 3(1)*, 19–26.

Fujiu, M. & Logemann, J.A. (1996). Effect of a tongue holding maneuver on posterior pharyngeal wall movement during deglutition. *American Journal of Speech Language Pathology, 5(1)*, 23–30.

Greenspan, A.I. & Mackenzie, E.J. (1994). Functional outcome after pediatric head injury. *Pediatrics, 94(4)*, 425–432.

Groher, M. (1992). *Dysphagia: Diagnosis and Management*, Third edition. Boston: Butterworth-Heinemann.

Hagen, C. (1981). Language disorders secondary to closed head injury: Diagnosis and management. *Topics in Language Disorders, 1*, 73–87.

Halper, A.S., Cherney, L.R., Cichowski, K., & Zhang, M. (1999). Dysphagia after head trauma: The effect of cognitive-communicative impairments on functional outcomes. *Journal of Head Trauma Rehabilitation, 14(5)*, 486–496.

Har-El, F. & Balwally, A.N. (1995). Transcutaneous cervical minioesophagostomy. *Otolaryngology Head and Neck Surgery, 113*, 387–392.

Hsieh, A.H., Bishop, M.J., Kublis, P.S., Newell, D.W., & Pierson, D.J. (1992). Pneumonia following closed head injury. *American Review of Respiratory Disease, 146*, 20–24.

Huckabee, M.L. & Cannito, M.P. (1999). Outcomes of swallowing rehabilitation in chronic brainstem dysphagia: A retrospective evaluation. *Dysphagia, 14*, 93–109.

Ibuki, T., Ando, N., & Tanaka, Y. (1994). Vocal fold paralysis associated with difficult gastric tube insertion. *Canadian Journal of Anaesthesiology, 41*, 431–434.

Jacob, P., Kahrilas, P.J., Logemann, J.A., Shah, V., & Ha, T. (1989). Upper esophageal sphincter opening and modulation during swallowing. *Gastroenterology, 97*, 1469–1478.

Kahrilas, P.J., Lin, S. Chen, J., & Logemann, J.A. (1996). Oropharyngeal accommodation to swallow volume. *Gastroenterology, 111*, 297–306.

Kahrilas, P.J., Lin, S., Logemann, J.A., Ergun, G.A., & Facchini, F. (1993). Deglutitive tongue action: Volume accommodation and bolus propulsion. *Gastroenterology, 104*, 152–162.

Kahrilas, P.J. & Logemann, J.A. (1993). Volume accommodation during swallowing, *Dysphagia, 8(3)*, 259–265.

Kahrilas, P.J., Logemann, J.A., Krugler, C., & Flanagan, E. (1991). Volitional augmentation of upper esophageal sphincter opening during swallowing. *American Journal of Physiology, 260 (Gastrointestinal and Liver Physiology, 23)*, G450–G456.

Kahrilas, P.J., Logemann, J.A., Lin, S., & Ergun, G.A. (1992). Pharyngeal clearance during swallow: A combined manometric and videofluroscopic study. *Gastroenterology, 103*, 128–136.

Kiel, M.K. (1994). Enteral tube feeding in a patient with traumatic brain injury. *Archives of Physical Medicine and Rehabilitation, 75*, 116–117.

Kirby, D., Clifton, G., Turner, H., Manion, D., Barrett, J., & Gruemer, H.D. (1991). Early enteral nutrition after brain injury by percutaneous endoscopic gastrojejunostomy. *Journal of Parenteral and Enteral Nutrition, 15(3)*, 298–302.

Klonoff, H., Low., M.D., & Clark, C. (1977). Head injuries in children: A prospective five-year follow-up. *Journal of Neurosurgery and Psychiatry, 40*, 1211–1219.

Langmore, S.E. (1995). Efficacy of behavioral treatment for oropharyngeal dysphagia. *Dysphagia, 10*, 259–262.

Larson, D.E., Burton, D.D., Schroeder, K.W., & DiMagno, E.P. (1987). Percutaneous endoscopic gastrostomy: Indications, success, complications and mortality in 314 consecutive patients. *Gastroenterology, 93*, 48–52.

Lazarus, C.L., Logemann, J.A., & Gibbons, P. (1993). Effects of maneuvers on swallowing function in a dysphagic oral cancer patient. *Head and Neck Surgery, 15*, 419–424.

Lazarus, C.L., Logemann, J.A., Rademaker, A.W., Kahrilas, P.J., Pajak, T., Lazar, R., & Halper, A. (1993). Effects of bolus volume, viscosity and repeated swallows in nonstroke subjects and stroke patients. *Archives of Physical Medicine and Rehabilitation, 74*, 1066–1070.

Lazzara, G., Lazarus, C., & Logemann, J. (1986). Impact of thermal stimulation on the triggering of the pharyngeal swallow. *Dysphagia, 1*, 73–77.

Leder, S.B., Cohn, S.M., & Moller, B.A. (1998). Fiberoptic endoscopic documentation of the high incidence of aspiration following extubation in critically ill trauma patients. *Dysphagia, 13*, 208–212.

Linden, P. (1989). Videofluoroscopy in the rehabilitation of swallowing dysfunction. *Dysphagia, 3*, 189–191.

Logemann, J.A. (1983). *Evaluation and Treatment of Swallowing Disorders*. Austin, Texas: Pro-Ed.

Logemann, J.A. (1989). Evaluation and treatment planning for the head-injured patient with oral intake disorders. *Journal Head Trauma Rehabilitation, 4(4)*, 24–33.

Logemann, J.A. (1991). Approaches to management of disordered swallowing. *Bailliere's Clinical Gastroenterology, 5(2)*, 269–280.

Logemann, J.A. (1993). *Manual for the Videoflurographic Study of Swallowing*, Second edition. Austin, TX: Pro-Ed.

Logemann, J.A. (1994). Multidisciplinary management of dysphagia. *Acta-Oto-Rhino-Laryngologica-Belgica, 48(2)*, 235–238.

Logemann, J.A. (1996). Screening, diagnosis and management of neurogenic dysphagia. *Seminars in Neurology, 16(4)*, 319–327.

Logemann, J.A. (1997). Therapy for oropharyngeal swallowing disorders. In A.L. Perlman and K. Schulze-Delrieu (Eds.), *Deglutition and Its Disorders, Anatomy, Physiology, Clinical Diagnosis and Management*. (449–462). San Diego: Singular Publishing.

Logemann, J.A. (1999). Behavioral management for oropharyngeal dysphagia. *Folia-Phoniatrica-et-Logopedica, 51*, 199–212.

Logemann, J.A. (2000). The potential future of dysphagia: Population-specific diagnosis and treatment. *Folia Phoniatrica-et Logopaedica, 52*, 136–141.

Logemann, J.A. & Kahrilas, P.J. (1990). Relearning to swallow post CVA: Application of manoeuvres and indirect biofeedback: A case study. *Neurology, 40*, 1136–1138.

Logemann, J.A., Kahrilas, P., Kobara, M., & Vakil, N. (1989). The benefit of head rotation on pharyngeal dysphagia. *Archives of Physical Medicine and Rehabilitation, 70*, 767–771.

Logemann, J.A., Pauloski, B.R., & Colangelo, L. (1998). Light digital occlusion of the tracheostomy tube: A pilot study of effects on aspiration and biomechanics of the swallow. *Head and Neck, 20(1)*, 52–57.

Logemann, J.A., Pauloski, B.R., Colangelo, L., Lazarus, C., Fujiu, M., & Kahrilas, P.J. (1995). Effects of sour bolus on oropharyngeal swallowing measures in patients with neurogenic dysphagia. *Journal of Speech and Hearing Research, 383*, 556–563.

Logemann, J.A., Pepe, J., & Mackay, L.E. (1994). Disorders of nutrition and swallowing: Intervention strategies in the trauma center. *Journal of Head Trauma Rehabilitation, 9(1)*, 43–56.

Mackay, L.E. (1994). Benefits of a formalized traumatic brain injury program within a trauma center. *Journal of Head Trauma Rehabilitation, 9(1)*, 11–19.

Mackay, L.E., Bernstein, B.A., Chapman, P.E., Morgan, A.S., & Milazzo, L.S. (1992). Early intervention in severe head injury: Long-term benefits of a formalized program. *Archives of Physical Medicine Rehabilitation, 73(July)*, 635–641.

Mackay, L.E., Morgan, A.S., & Bernstein, B.A. (1999a). Factors affecting oral feeding with severe TBI. *Journal of Head Trauma Rehabilitation, 14(5)*, 435–447.

Mackay, L.E., Morgan, A.S., & Bernstein, B.A. (1999b). Swallowing disorders in severe brain injury: Risk factors affecting return to oral intake. *Archives of Physical Medicine Rehabilitation, 80*, 365–371.

Martin, B.J., Corlew, M.M., Wood, H., Olson, D., Golopol, L.A., Wingo, M., & Kirmani, N. (1994). The association of swallowing dysfunction and aspiration pneumonia. *Dysphagia, 9*, 1–6.

Martin, B.J.W., Logemann, J.A., Shaker, R., & Dodds, W.J. (1993). Normal laryngeal valving patterns during three breath hold maneuvers: A pilot investigation. *Dysphagia, 8*, 11–20.

Miller, R.E., Castlemain, B., Lacqua, F.J., & Kotler, D.P. (1989). Percutaneous endoscopic gastrostomy. Results in 316 patients and review of literature. *Surgical Endoscopy, 3(4)*, 186–190.

Morgan, A.S. (1994). The trauma center as a continuum of care for persons with severe brain injury. *Journal of Head Trauma Rehabilitation, 9(1)*, 1–10.

Morris, S.E. & Klein, M.D. (1987). *Pre-Feeding Skills*. Tucson: Therapy Skill Builders.

Norton, J.A., Ott, L.G., McClain, C., Adams, L., Dempsey, R.J., Hauck, D., Tibbs, P.A., & Young, A.B. (1988). Intolerance to enteral feeding in the brain injured patient. *Journal of Neurosurgery, 68*, 62–66.

O'Gara, J.A. (1990). Dietary adjustments and nutritional therapy during treatment for oral-pharyngeal dysphagia. *Dysphagia, 4*, 209–212.

Ohmae, Y., Logemann, J.A., Kaiser, P., Hanson, D.G., & Kahrilas, P.J. (1996). Effects of two breath holding maneuvers on oropharyngeal swallow. *Annals of Otology, Rhinology and Laryngology, 105(2)*, 123–131.

Ott, L., McClain, C., & Young, B. (1989). Nutrition and severe brain injury. *Nutrition, 5*, 75.

Parathyras, A.J. & Kassak, L.A. (1983). Tolerance, nutritional adequacy and cost-effectiveness in continuing drip versus bolus and/or intermittent feeding techniques. *Nutritional Support Surveys, 4*, 556–577.

Park, R.H., Allison, M.C., Lang, J., Spence, E., Morris, A.J., Danesh, B.J., Russell, R.I., & Mills, P.R. (1992). Randomized comparison of percutaneous endoscopic gastrostomy and nasogastric tube feeding in patients with persisting neurological dysphagia. *British Medical Journal, 304(6839)*, 1406–1409.

Pepe, J., Morgan, A.S., & Mackay, L.E. (1997).The metabolic response to acute traumatic brain injury and associated complications. In L.E. Mackay, P.E. Chapman, & A.S. Morgan (Eds.), *Maximizing Brain Injury Recovery: Integrating Critical Care and Early Rehabilitation.* (pp. 396–443), Gaithersburg, MD: Aspen Publishers.

Prosek, R., Montgomery, A., Walden, B., & Schwartz, D. (1978). EMG biofeedback in the treatment of hyperfunctional voice disorders. *Journal of Speech and Hearing Disorders, 43,* 282–294.

Ramig, L.O., Countryman, S., Thompson, L.L., & Horii, Y. (1995). Comparison of two forms of intensive speech treatment for Parkinsons Disease. *Journal of Speech and Hearing Research, 38,* 1232–1251.

Rasley, A., Logemann, J.A., Kahrilas, P.J., Rademaker, A.W., Pauloski, B.R., & Dodds, W.J. (1993). Prevention of barium aspiration during videofluoroscopic swallowing studies: Value of change in posture, *American Journal of Roentgenology, 160(5),* 1005–1009.

Rosenbek, J.C. (1995). Efficacy in dysphagia. *Dysphagia, 10,* 263–267.

Rowe, L.A. (1999). Case studies in dysphagia after pediatric brain injury. *Journal of Head Trauma Rehabilitation, 14,* 5, 497–504.

Rubow, R.T. (1984). Role of feedback, reinforcement, and compliance on training and transfer in biofeedback-based rehabilitation of motor speech disorders. In McNeil, M.R., Rosenbek, J.C., & Aronson, A. (Eds.), *The Dysarthrias: Physiology, acoustics, perception, management* (pp. 207–230). San Diego: College Hill Press.

Sasaki, C.T., Milmoe, Yanagisawa, E., Berry, K., & Kirchner, J.A. (1980). Surgical closure of the larynx for intractable aspiration. *Archives of Otolaryngology, 106,* 7, 422–423.

Schurr, M.J., Ebner, K.A., Maser, A.L., Sperling, K.B., Helgeson, R.B., & Harms, B. (1999). Formal swallowing evaluation and therapy after traumatic brain injury improves dysphagia outcomes. *The Journal of Trauma: Injury, Infection and Critical Care, 46(5),* 817–821.

Schwartz-Cowley, R., Swanson, B., Chapman, P., Kitik, B.A., & Mackay, L.E. (1994). The role of rehabilitation in the intensive care unit. *Journal of Head Trauma Rehabilitation, 9(1),* 32–42.

Scott-Jupp, R., Marlow, N., Seddon, N., & Rosenbloom, L. (1992). Rehabilitation and outcome after severe head injury. *Archives of Disease in Childhood, 67,* 222–226.

Shaker, R., Kern, M., Bardan, E., Arndorfer, R.C., Hofmann, C., & Easterling, C. (1997). Effect of isotonic/isometric head lift exercise on hypopharyngeal intrabolus pressure. Presented at the Fifth Annual Dysphagia Research Society Meeting, 1997 [Abstract]. *Dysphagia, 12,* 107.

Shaker, R., Kern, M., Bardan, E., Taylor, A., Stewart, E., Hoffmann, R., Arndorfer, R., Hofmann, C., & Bonnevier, J. (1997). Augmentation of deglutitive upper-esophageal sphincter opening in the elderly by exercise. *American Journal of Physiology, 272,* G1518–G1522.

Shanahan, T.K., Logemann, J.A., Rademaker, A.W., Pauloski, B.R., & Kahrilas, P.J. (1993). Chin-down posture effect on aspiration in dysphagic patients. *Archives of Physical Medicine and Rehabilitation, 74(7),* 736–739.

Steffes, C., Weaver, D.W., & Bouwman, D.L. (1989). Percutaneous endoscopic gastrostomy. New technique-old complications. *American Surgery, 55,* 273–277.

Stiegman, G.V., Goff, J.S., Silas, D., Pearlman, N., Sun, J., & Norton, L. (1990). Endoscopic versus operative gastrostomy: Final results of a prospective randomized trial. *Gastrointestinal Endoscopy, 36,* 1–5.

Tippett, D.C., Palmer, J., & Linden, P. (1987). Management of dysphagia in a patient with closed head injury. *Dysphagia, 1,* 221–226.

Ward, E.C. & Conroy, A-L. (1999). Validity, reliability and responsivity of the Royal Brisbane Hospital Outcome Measure for Swallowing. *Asia Pacific Journal of Speech, Language and Hearing, 4,* 109–129.

Ward, E.C., Theodoros, D.G., Murdoch, B.E., & Silburn, P. (In press). Changes in maximum capacity tongue pressures in surgical and non-surgical patients with Parkinson Disease following the Lee Silverman Voice Treatment Program. *Journal of Medical Speech Language Pathology.*

Welch, M.W., Logemann, J.A., Rademaker, A.W., & Kahrilas, P.J. (1993). Changes in pharyngeal dimensions effected by chin tuck. *Archives of Physical Medicine and Rehabilitation, 74,* 170–177.

Wicks, C., Gimson, A., Vlavianos, P., Lombard, M., Panos, M., Macmathuna, P., Tudor, M., Andrews, K., & Westaby, D. (1992). Assessment of the percutaneous endoscopic gastrostomy feeding as part of an integrated approach to enteral feedings. *Gut, 33(5)*, 613–616.

Winstein, C.J. (1983). Neurogenic dysphagia: Frequency, progression, and outcome in adults following head injury. *Physical Therapy, 63(12)*, 1992–1997.

Wolf, L.S. & Glass, R.P. (1992). *Feeding and Swallowing Disorders in Infancy: Assessment and Management.* Tucson, AZ: Therapy Skill Builders.

Woratyla, S.P., Morgan, A.S., Mackay, L. Bernstein, B., & Barba, C. (1995). Factors associated with early onset pneumonia in the severely brain-injured patient. *Connecticut Medicine, 59(11)*, 643–647.

Workman, J.R., Pillsbury, H.C., & Hulka, G. (1997). Surgical Intervention in Dysphagia. In M.E. Groher (Ed.), *Dysphagia, Diagnosis and Management*, Third edition. Boston: Butterworth-Heinemann.

Ylvisaker, M. & Logemann, J.A. (1985). Therapy for feeding and swallowing disorders following head injury. In M. Ylvisaker, (Ed.), *Head Injury Rehabilitation: Children and Adolescents* (pp. 195–215), College Hill Press: Boston.

Ylvisaker, M. & Weinstein, M. (1989). Recovery of oral feeding after pediatric head injury. *Journal of Head Trauma Rehabilitation, 4(4)*, 51–63.

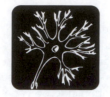

Index